CANCER CHEMOTHERAPY:
Challenges for the Future
Volume 7

International Congress Series No. 1022
ISBN 0 444 89806 9

The series *Cancer Chemotherapy: Challenges for the Future* has been made possible through a grant from Bristol-Myers Squibb K.K.

Publisher: Excerpta Medica

Offices:　P.O. Box 1126　　　　　　3/F, 13 Duddell Street
　　　　　1000-BC Amsterdam　　　Hong Kong

　　　　　P.O. Box 3085　　　　　　15-23, Nishi-Azabu 4-chome
　　　　　Princeton, N.J. 08543　　Minato-ku, Tokyo

　　　　　180 Ocean Street
　　　　　Sydney NSW 2027

Printed in Japan

CANCER CHEMOTHERAPY: Challenges for the Future
Volume 7

Proceedings of the Seventh Nagoya International Symposium on Cancer Treatment, Nagoya, Japan, September 29–30, 1991

Editors:

Kiyoji Kimura
H. Saito
Stephen K. Carter
R. C. Bast, Jr

 1992

Excerpta Medica, Amsterdam–Hong Kong–Princeton–Sydney–Tokyo

Organizing Committee

Chairman
    Kiyoji Kimura   (National Nagoya Hospital)

Vice Chairmen
    Kazuo Ota   (Nagoya Memorial Hospital)
    Kazumasa Yamada   (Nagoya University)

Secretary General
    Hidehiko Saito   (Nagoya University)

Organizing Committee
    Mitsuyuki Abe   (Kyoto University)
    Osahiko Abe   (Keio University)
    Yutaka Ariyoshi   (Aichi Cancer Center)
    Yoshio Aso   (Tokyo University)
    Hiroshi Fujita   (Tsurumi University)
    Hisashi Furue   (Teikyo University)
    Nobu Hattori   (Tokyo Metropolitan Komagome Hospital)
    Masami Hirano   (Fujita-Gakuen Health University)
    Yukio Inuyama   (Hokkaido University)
    Ikuro Kimura   (Okayama University)
    Hisanobu Niitani   (Nippon Medical School)
    Kiichiro Noda   (Kinki University)
    Makoto Ogawa   (Japanese Foundation for Cancer Research)
    Ryuzo Ohno   (Nagoya University)
    Masanori Shimoyama   (National Cancer Center)
    Tetsuo Taguchi   (Osaka University)
    Hiroshi Takagi   (Nagoya University)
    Shigeru Tsukagoshi   (Japanese Foundation for Cancer Research)
    Ryuzo Ueda   (Aichi Cancer Center)
    Akira Wakui   (Tohoku University)
    Kiyokazu Yoshida   (Saitama Cancer Center)

Advisory Board

    J.L. Tyree   (Bristol-Myers Squibb K.K.)
    Genshichiro Fujii   (Shinyamate Hospital)
    Takao Hattori   (Shakaihoken Nakabaru Hospital)
    Susumu Hibino   (National Nagoya Hospital)
    Heizaburo Ichikawa   (National Cancer Center)
    Kiyoshi Inokuchi   (Kyushu University)
    Toshi Kato   (Kurume University)
    Tatsuhei Kondo   (Tokai Central Hospital)
    Yoshiyuki Koyama   (National Medical Center)
    Tadao Niijima   (Tokyo Seamen's Insurance Hospital)
    Tatsuo Saito   (Kyoundo Hospital)
    Yoshio Sakurai   (Kyoritsu College of Pharmacy)
    Ichiro Urushizaki   (Higashi Sapporo Hospital)

Overseas Adviser
    Stephen K. Carter   (Bristol-Myers Squibb Company)

Preface

The Seventh Nagoya International Symposium on Cancer Treatment was held from September 29–30, 1991, and was attended by over 500 oncologists. In the past 6 volumes of the proceedings of this international symposium, many problems of cancer chemotherapy have been reported and discussed from the viewpoint of clinical and basic studies. At this seventh symposium the main topics were new strategies for cancer therapy based on biology and pharmacology. During recent years remarkable achievements have been made in the area of the biology of tumor progression and regression with regard to recessive oncogenes and dose-intensive chemotherapy based on pharmacologic aspects, such as pharmacokinetics and pharmacodynamics in relation to the optimal administration method of anticancer drugs, phase I studies of new anticancer drugs and dose escalation, and the combined modality of anticancer drugs and biological response modifiers.

In addition to the keynote address "New strategies for management of epithelial ovarian and breast cancer based on biology and pharmacology," presentations on the biology of tumor progression and regression covered the molecular basis of cancer suppression by the human tumor suppressor genes, mutation of the p53 gene and accumulation of the p53 protein, tumor suppressor genes involved in the pathogenesis of lung cancer, and lessons learned from studies on tumor suppression by chromosome transfer. On the topic of oncogenes, there were reports on tumor suppressor genes in B cell lymphoma pathogenesis, protein-tyrosine kinases in cellular signal transduction and malignant transformation, suppression of N-cadherin-mediated cell adhesion by v-src transformation with tyrosine phosphorylation of catenins, and biological rationales for modifying radiotherapy and chemotherapy. In other words, many new reports on oncogenes provided the highlights for those chemotherapists present.

For cancer therapy based on pharmacology, papers were presented on drug resistance such as P-glycoprotein (p170) multidrug resistance (MDR) transporter limitations on successful therapy for childhood tumors: possible circumvention of MDR by cyclosporin A, regulation of the MDR gene in response to environmental stimuli, and dose-intensive chemotherapies. Furthermore, in relation to clinical trials based on pharmacokinetics and pharmacodynamics, the investigation of their relevance to medical oncology, pharmacokinetic guided dose escalation in phase I studies, a pharmacokinetic hypothesis for the clinical efficacy of etoposide in small cell lung cancer (SCLC), and the activity of a prolonged schedule of etoposide in patients with SCLC were all documented and evaluated in addition to the combination of cisplatin and carboplatin in vitro and in clinical practice, and the establishment of optimal administration of anticancer agents. The subject of the special lecture was the importance of clinical pharmacokinetics for developing new therapies in the USA.

On the subject of cancer therapies, lung cancer was the focus of attention, and the efficacy of combined modalities, including radiotherapy, was reported and discussed. As chemoradiation therapy, combined chemotherapy and radiotherapy in the treatment of lung cancer, concurrent platinum-etoposide chemotherapy plus thoracic radiotherapy for limited-stage SCLC, and the role of chemotherapy and interferon in lung cancer were reported. New adjuvant chemotherapy for non-small cell lung cancer was also discussed.

I am certain that the Proceedings of the Seventh Nagoya International Symposium on Cancer Treatment will provide new concepts and important information for developing cancer chemotherapy to many oncologists working in both clinical and basic research.

Kiyoji Kimura

CONTENTS

V. CLINICAL TRIALS BASED ON PHARMACOLOGY

Pharmacokinetics and pharmacodynamics

Administration methods of anticancer drugs

SPECIAL LECTURE

Closing remarks

KEYNOTE ADDRESS

New strategies for the management of ovarian and breast cancer based on biology and pharmacology

R.C. Bast, Jr, C.M. Boyer, A. Berchuck, F.J. Xu, S. Wu, Y. Lidor, L.A. Maier, J.R. Crews, M. Rosse, J.J. Vredenburgh, E.J. Shpall, W.P. Peters

Duke University Medical Center, Durham, North Carolina, USA

Introduction

Over the years our group has performed studies aimed to increase our understanding of the biology of ovarian and breast carcinomas. Although this conference, for the most part, concerns lung cancer research, experience with other epithelial neoplasms may ultimately prove relevant to understanding and managing pulmonary neoplasms.

Monitoring of Epithelial Ovarian Cancer

Two thirds of patients with epithelial ovarian carcinoma present with disease that has metastasized throughout the abdominal cavity. Following total abdominal hysterectomy, bilateral salpingo-oophorectomy and cytoreductive surgery, a majority of these patients still have small nodules of tumor that stud the peritoneum. The most careful physical examination or the most sophisticated CT scan is often unable to monitor this disease during chemotherapy.

More than a decade ago my laboratory began to identify serum markers that would permit monitoring of patients with epithelial ovarian carcinoma using the then new monoclonal technology. The 125th promising hybridoma, OC 125, recognized an antigenic determinant designated CA 125 that was associated with a 220 Kd glycoprotein expressed in Mullerian duct and coelomic epithelium during embryonic development (1,2). CA 125 was detected in >80% of ovarian cancers and circulating CA 125 levels were elevated in serum from approximately 80% of ovarian cancer patients (3). If elevated, serum CA 125 levels have

3

correlated with disease course in greater than 80% of instances studied (4). Elevation of CA 125 has preceded clinical disease recurrence by one to eleven months with a median of three months. As in the case of carcinoembryonic antigen for monitoring colon cancer, persistently rising CA 125 values are consistently associated with clinical progression of ovarian cancer.

Elevation of CA 125 at the time of a second look surgical surveillance procedure predicts persistence of disease with great accuracy. An elevated CA 125 has a positive predictive value of 96% in this setting (Jacobs 1989). When CA 125 returns to less than 35 U/ml prior to second look, however, residual disease still has been found at laparotomy in approximately 60% of cases. In addition, failure of CA 125 to normalize within three months of initiation of treatment has been associated with persistence of disease at subsequent surgical surveillance procedures even when CA 125 subsequently returns to less than 35 U/ml. Finally, the apparent half-life of CA 125 has correlated inversely with the survival of ovarian cancer patients. The true half-life of CA 125 is approximately 4.8 days. An apparent half-life of greater than 20 days is associated with a significantly shortened survival (5,6). A 125 can also be used to distinguish malignant from benign pelvic masses (7). In postmenopausal patients with a pelvic mass, a markedly elevated CA 125 (>95 U/ml) predicts malignancy with 96% accuracy (Zurawski, personal communication). Consequently an elevated CA125 should prompt the referral of postmenopausal patients with adnexal masses for exploration at institutions capable of cytoreductive surgery at initial laparotomy.

Early Detection of Epithelial Ovarian Cancer
The clinical problem with ovarian cancer is not simply one of monitoring disease course or of distinguishing malignant from benign pelvic masses. The major difficulty, as in the case of lung cancer, is that the disease is wide-spread at the

time of diagnosis in more than two-thirds of patients. Ovarian cancer may, however, be one of the malignancies that lends itself to early diagnosis using a serum test. Early studies by Suzanne Knauf and Gerald Urbach indicated that a shed tumor product designated OCA could be found in the serum of 70% of patients with early stage disease (8). Elevated levels of the OCA antigen were, however, found in 10% of apparently healthy individuals so that this particular marker could not be used for early detection. These observations did suggest, however, that an ovarian tumor associated antigen could reach the venous circulation at an early stage of tumor growth.

In the case of CA 125, anecdotal reports have suggested that CA 125 values can be elevated ten to twelve months prior to the clinical detection of ovarian cancer (9). In a study using the Janus serum bank from Oslo, Norway, Zurawski, et al, had found elevated CA 125 levels in serum from 50% of the patients destined to develop ovarian cancer within eighteen months (10). Even five years prior to presentation, 24% of individuals had elevated CA 125 levels compared to 7% of an age-matched control population. It is not possible to determine whether ovarian cancer was growing slowly over five years in individuals with an elevated CA125 or whether an elevated serum CA 125 indicated a predisposition to development of the neoplasm.

If CA 125 is to be used for early detection of ovarian cancer the assay must be both sensitive and specific. With regard to sensitivity, CA 125 levels are elevated in 50% of patients with Stage I disease and 90% of patients with Stage II disease at conventional diagnosis (4). Taken together, CA 125 values are elevated in 60% of patients with these early stages of tumor spread. With regard to specificity, in a study of 915 normal healthy nuns from the Philadelphia Archdiocese, CA 125 was elevated in 0.8% (11). If only those women greater than 40 years of age were considered, the false-positive rate was 0.6%. Although this is quite good for a monitoring test, it is not acceptable for screening in that there would be 30 false-positives for each case of ovarian cancer detected.

One approach to improving the specificity of CA 125 would be to monitor serial levels over time. A Phase I study of CA 125 for early detection of epithelial ovarian carcinoma was initiated in 1,082 women who were asked to visit a gynecologic clinic in Stockholm (12). If CA 125 was greater than 35 U/ml, blood tests were repeated. Semi-annual pelvic examinations and trans-abdominal ultrasounds were performed. CA 125 was initially elevated in 34 of the 1,082 women, but on sequential monitoring only one patient had progressively rising values. CA 125 continued to rise over twenty months until a pelvic mass was finally appreciated and a mixed mesodermal tumor diagnosed.

Based on these promising results, a Phase II trial of CA 125 was undertaken in 5,550 women over the age of 40 (13). One hundred seventy-five were found to have an elevated level of CA 125 (>30-35 U/ml). An additional 175 women with normal CA 125 levels were chosen as controls to avoid biasing the clinical observers. Both groups were followed with quarterly serum CA 125 determinations, semi-annual pelvic examinations, and trans-abdominal ultrasounds. In women over 50 years of age, CA 125 was greater than 30 U/ml in only 2%, indicating than an acceptable number of positive values would be obtained to permit additional screening with ultrasound and pelvic examination. Among the group with an elevated CA 125, six patients with ovarian cancer were detected including four with Stage I or II disease . Using the tumor registry in Sweden, it was possible to identify three patients who had normal levels of CA 125 prior to developing ovarian cancer. Although these results are promising, a much larger study of 75-150,000 women will be required to determine whether routine screening with CA 125 can decrease mortality from ovarian cancer.

Early Detection of Lung Cancer
A similar approach might be applied in the case of lung cancer using bronchial secretions or sputum cytologies. The

6

group of Dr. James Mulshine at the National Cancer Institute in Bethesda has identified two antigens associated with dysplastic bronchial epithelial cells that may predict patients who will develop lung cancer up to two years following sputum cytology (14). In our own laboratory, Dr. Margaret Deutsch has developed a monoclonal antibody that binds to apparently normal bronchial epithelium at a distance from lung cancers (15). This antigen is shed into the fluid phase of sputum and might provide a test for patients who are at a high risk for developing a malignancy (16).

Growth Regulation in Normal and Malignant Ovarian Epithelium

Over the last five years we have been particularly interested in the changes that affect cell growth regulation in normal and malignant ovarian epithelium. More than 90% of ovarian cancers arise from a single layer of epithelial cells that cover the normal ovary or that lines cysts immediately beneath the ovarian surface. Using the technique of Kruk, et al (17), we have cultured normal human ovarian epithelial cells. These cells express cytokeratin and retain normal epithelial morphology by electron microscopy. With these cultures it has been possible to study the production of and response to different growth factors.

Epidermal growth factor (EGF) and transforming growth factor alpha (TGFα) stimulate proliferation of normal ovarian epithelium, whereas proliferation of these cells is inhibited by TGFß. In ovarian cancer cell lines an autocrine stimulatory loop may be established by the secretion of TGF-alpha (18) and expression of the epidermal growth factor receptor by ovarian cancers is a poor prognostic sign (19). Although a majority of ovarian cancers retain EGF receptor expression, responsiveness to EGF is often decreased relative to that of normal epithelium (20). Consequently, autocrine stimulation by TGF-alpha may become progressively less important with tumor progression.

Normal ovarian epithelium expresses TGFß1 and TGFß2, but not TGFß3 (21). The normal epithelial cells are also inhibited

(40-70%) by exogenous TGFß. In the one ovarian cancer cell line that retained expression of TGF-ß as well as responsiveness to TGFß, binding of extracellular growth factor with anti-TGFß antibodies stimulated tumor cell proliferation. Consequently, loss of the autocrine inhibitory function of TGFß could be on step in ovarian carcinogenesis.

A number of proto-oncogenes have been described in different human tumor types. The products of these genes are homologous to growth factors, growth factor receptors, transducing proteins and nuclear binding proteins. In studies with Drs. Larry Feig and Geoffrey Cooper we had found an activated Ki-ras oncogene associated with epithelial ovarian carcinoma cells, but not with normal mesothelial cells in ascites from a single patient (22). This was one of the first instances in a human cancer where somatic mutation of a proto-oncogene appeared to be associated with malignant transformation. In subsequent studies, however, ras genes were mutated or amplified in only 12% of the ovarian cancers studied (23-27). Other oncogenes are expressed more frequently in ovarian carcinoma including c-fos, c-myc and Ha-ras (28). Each of these genes can be expressed by rapidly proliferating cells, but ovarian cancers also express fms and erbB-2 which are less widely distributed in normal tissues (28-30).

Expression of fms is of particular interest in that this gene encodes a 150 kd cell surface protein with tyrosine kinase activity. The fms protein binds macrophage colony stimulating factor (M-CSF or CSF-1) and is probably identical to the normal receptor for this factor. In studies with Dr. S. Ramakrishnan we had found that most ovarian cancer cell lines produce M-CSF (31). In addition, substantial amounts of M-CSF are released into the serum of patients with ovarian cancer. Indeed, M-CSF may provide a useful marker to complement CA 125 in those patients whose tumors do not produce or release the antigen (32). The biological significance of M-CSF production may be two-fold. M-CSF may produce autocrine growth stimulation in the 50% of ovarian cancers that express fms (29). In addition,

8

M-CSF is a potent chemo-attractant that may account for the accumulation of macrophages in ascites fluid and within tumors. Our group has found that several macrophage products including tumor necrosis factor (TNF-α), Interleukin-1-α (IL-1) and Interleukin-6 (IL-6) can stimulate ovarian cancer growth (33). Consequently a paracrine growth regulatory loop may exist in ovarian carcinoma.

A tumor suppressor gene that has proven important in lung cancer may also be important in growth regulation of ovarian cancer. Wild type p53 is a nuclear phosphoprotein with a short half-life that is present in small amounts in normal cells. Transfection of wild type p53 suppresses transformation of malignant cells, whereas deletion of both copies of wild type p53 is associated with transformation. Transfection of a mutant p53 that encodes proteins with increased stability causes transformation and mutant p53 can also complex with wild type p53 preventing its effective interaction with DNA.

We have studied the expression of p53 in epithelial ovarian cancers using monoclonal antibodies reactive with the gene product (34). In the case of approximately half of ovarian cancers, little, if any, p53 can be detected. In the other half of ovarian cancers, however, p53 is overexpressed and can be readily detected in the nuclei of tumor cells. We have obtained RNA from tumors that either overexpress p53 or express normal amounts of the protein. The p53 mRNA has been reverse transcribed. Using p53 specific primers for exons 4-9 of p53, cDNA was amplified using the polymerase chain reaction. When the DNA's were sequenced, in each case where p53 was overexpressed, a mutation was detected. Interestingly, p53 expression did not correlate with survival in advanced ovarian cancer. It did, however, correlate with aneuploidy.

Finally, we have studied the expression of c-erbB-2 (HER-2/neu) in epithelial ovarian cancer. When originally described in tumors of rat brain by Dr. Robert Weinberg and his associates, the activated neu oncogene contained a mutation in the intra-membranous domain (35). In human tumors of the breast and ovary, however, it appears that HER-2/<u>neu</u> may be amplified without mutation. There is substantial homology between HER-2/<u>neu</u> and the epidermal growth factor receptor. In epithelial ovarian cancers, HER-2/<u>neu</u> can be amplified and overexpressed (30,28,36). Using the TA1 antibody against the extracellular domain of the p185 gene product, small amounts the HER-2/<u>neu</u> gene produce p185 can be found in normal ovarian epithelium. Some two-thirds of ovarian cancers have comparable amounts of p185. The oncogene product, however, is overexpressed in approximately 30% of ovarian cancers associated with a median survival approximately one-half that of patients whose tumors do not overexpress p185 (36).

In summary, then, there are a number of differences between normal and malignant ovarian epithelium. Malignant ovarian epithelium may be stimulated by TGFα, but tends to lose responsiveness to EGF (TGFα) and TGFß. Maintenance of the former and loss of the latter autocrine inhibitory loops may impact on the proliferation of tumor cells. Both the normal and malignant epithelium express M-CSF. Approximately half of the malignant epithelium expresses c-<u>fms</u> the M-CSF receptor, whereas the normal epithelium does not. Macrophages and malignant epithelium produce IL-1α, IL-6 and TNF. The role of these cytokines in normal epithelial growth remains to be defined. Expression of <u>erb</u>B-2 is increased in approximately 30% of ovarian cancers associated with poor prognosis, whereas p53 is mutated and overexpressed in approximately half of the tumors.

Inhibition of Tumor Cell Growth with Anti-p185 Antibodies.

The frequent expression and overexpression of HER-2/<u>neu</u> may provide a useful target for therapy. Multiple monoclonal antibodies have been prepared by different investigators against the extracellular domain of p185. We have assembled eleven of these reagents and have performed cross-blocking experiments to define epitopes (37). These studies are consistent with a relative epitope map where there are at least two distinct groups of epitopes and where one of the two contains multiple epitopes in a roughly linear array. Several of these antibodies have the ability to inhibit growth of tumor cells in the absence of complement or cellular immune effectors. Overall, seven of the eleven antibodies significantly inhibited tumor growth in soft agar (37). When anchorage dependent growth was studied, only two of the eleven antibodies significantly inhibited growth. In collaborative studies with Dr. Ruth Lupu, these were shown to be the same two antibodies that inhibited binding of the putative ligand that Dr. Lupu has described.

Several mechanisms might account for antibody mediated growth inhibition of tumor cells that overexpress p185. At least in the case of anchorage independent growth, simple blocking of ligand binding is not an adequate explanation. Each of the antibodies might mimic ligand binding or produce allosteric interactions with the extracellular domain that would modulate intracellular kinase activity. In addition, the monoclonals might promote dimerization or aggregate dimers. Against the importance of this mechanism, however, is the observation that univalent Fab fragments are also effective in inhibiting tumor growth. Finally, antibodies might promote internalization and consequently down-regulate these growth factor receptors.

Kinase activity does appear to correlate with growth inhibition in that different patterns of phosphorylation have been observed on 2D gel analysis after treatment with antibodies that inhibit or fail to affect tumor growth. In addition, antibodies that inhibited tumor growth produced a marked inhibition of diacylglycerol levels (38). Thus, other intracellular targets including protein kinase C may be affected. This may have relevance to recent reports that antibodies against p185 can affect multi-drug resistance and cisplatin resistance to the extent that these are regulated by protein kinase C activity.

Inhibition of Tumor Cell Growth with anti-p185 Immunotoxins

The extracellular domain of p185 can also be used as a target for immunotoxins which might have greater potency than unconjugated antibodies. Immunotoxins utilize a plant or bacterial peptide linked to monoclonal reagents. One of the most widely studied group of toxin immunoconjugates utilizes ricin which must be incorporated into endosomes and translocated into the cytoplasm to produce catalytic inhibition of ribosomal protein synthesis. We have studied requirements for internalization and cell killing using ricin immunotoxins that bind to the extracellular domain of p185. In contrast to inhibition of tumor growth with the unconjugated antibody that requires kinase activity, the internalization of immunotoxins does not require the presence of an intracellular kinase (39). Cells that express HER-2/neu constructs which lack the entire intracellular domain or the kinase region, are killed as readily as cells that express the full length wild-type HER-2/neu. Immunotoxins that bind to the extracellular domain are internalized as readily in cells that bear the full length p185 as in those that express the truncated constructs.

Synergistic Cytotoxicity by Immunotoxins in Combination

One potential limitation for serotherapy with immunotoxins is the heterogeneity of antigen expression observed within and between different cancers. Marked heterogeneity has been found from cell to cell within breast and ovarian carcinoma with regard to binding of different monoclonal antibodies. When 16 different monoclonal antibodies were tested against 18 different breast cancers, a different antigeneic phenotype was found in 16 of the 18 tumors (40). Such heterogeneity might be used to advantage if combinations of monoclonal antibodies could be found that bind individually to different groups of normal tissues but that bind coordinately to the same malignant tissue. An improved therapeutic index should be observed if there is additive or synergistic killing by the immunotoxins.

We have used isobolographic analysis to study the interaction of different immunotoxins (41). When the dose response curves for tumor cell killing are linear, isoboles fall on a diagonal line. When these curves are not linear an envelope of additivity must be drawn. Synergistic isoboles fall beneath this curve. We have found that some combinations of immunotoxins produce synergistic cytotoxicity including immunotoxins such as 454A12-rRTA reactive with the transferrin receptor and 260F9-rRTA reactive with a 55 Kd cell surface protein (42). The mechanism in this case may relate to a slowing of the internalization of immunotoxins reactive with the transferrin receptor, permitting a longer interval in the endosome for toxin to translocate.

Synergistic Cytotoxicity by Alkylating Agents and Immunotoxins

Synergistic reactions have also been found against ovarian carcinoma cell lines using different alkylating agents such as cisplatin, thiotepa and 4-hydroperoxycyclophosphamide the activated cyclophosphamide derivative (43). Synergistic interactions have also been found between cisplatin, thiotepa and immunotoxins reactive with a 42 kd cell surface protein (44). For those combinations that are synergistic, an increase in platinum adduct formation has been found. No difference, however, has been detected in the uptake of radiolabelled cisplatin. There has been a significant decrease in glutathione levels and in glutathione S-transferase activity as well as a marked decrease in unscheduled DNA synthesis reflecting inhibition of DNA repair. Consequently, at high concentrations alkylating agents and immunotoxins may interact synergistically, possibly related to the decreased synthesis of enzymes required to generate and transfer glutathione as well as to repair DNA damage.

Treatment of Ovarian Cancer with High Dose Alkylating Therapy with Autologous Bone Marrow Support

To achieve in vitro the concentrations of reagents needed

to observe the cytotoxic effects that can be produced in vitro, bone marrow transplantation is required. The Bone Marrow Transplantation Program at Duke has examined the use of cyclophosphamide, cisplatin and thiotepa to treat patients with ovarian cancer using the intraperitoneal administration of cisplatin and the intravenous instillation of high doses of cyclophosphamide and thiotepa followed by infusion of autologous bone marrow (45). In pilot studies of 16 patients who had been heavily pretreated with 4 or 5 different cytotoxic regimens, there have been 9 objective responses (CR or PR). There have also been 4 toxic deaths, possibly related to the condition of the patients at the time of treatment.

Use of Purged Bone Marrow for Treatment of Breast Cancer

Another application of autologous bone marrow transplantation has been in the management of breast cancer. The Bone Marrow Transplantation Program at Duke has had remarkable success in treating patients with advanced breast cancer and in treating individuals at high risk of recurrence with 10 or more positive nodes (46-48). This form of treatment has generally not been applied to patients who have marrow metastases out of concern that tumor cells would be returned to patients with the autologous marrow. Over the last several years we have developed techniques in the laboratory to remove breast cancer cells selectively from human bone marrow (49). Multiple monoclonal antibodies are used to compensate for heterogeneity in antigen expression. Tumor cells that have bound antibody are recognized using magnetospheres coated with sheep anti-mouse immunoglobulin. Rosettes are formed around the tumor cells but not around the normal marrow precursors. Marrow can be passed over a magnet and 3-4 logs of tumor cells removed. Although this is relatively effective, residual clonogenic tumor cells can still be detected following immunomagnetic purging. Consequently, we have added treatment with 4-hydroperoxycyclophosphamide (4-HC) to the immunomagnetic purging, permitting the elimination of 4-5 logs of malignant

14

cells.

A phase I study has now enrolled more than 60 patients who have received doxorubicin, 5-fluorouracil and methotrexate before undergoing marrow harvest. Bone marrow was purged with immunomagnetic beads, with 4-HC or with both agents. Purged marrow was cryopreserved. An additional course of doxorubicin, adriamycin and methotrexate was given before high dose cyclophosphamide, cisplatin and BCNU was administered. The purged marrow was then thawed and reinfused. In a dose escalation study where marrow was treated with progressively higher doses of 4-HC, engraftment of white cells was significantly delayed after use of 80 μg/ml of 4-HC _ex_ _vivo_ (50). Immunomagnetic purging _per_ _se_ did not significantly affect time to engraftment, but chemoimmunoseparation prolonged time to engraftment (WBC >1,000) from 17 to 36 days. Interestingly, the use of interleukin-3 has substantially accelerated engraftment in these individuals (51). Use of 50 μg/M^2 IL-3 per day was associated with a time to engraftment of 32 days, whereas 500 μg/M^2 IL-3 per day reduced time to engraftment to 22 days. Using purged marrow, approximately 40% of patients have achieved a complete response compared to 68% of patients who had undergone similar treatment without marrow involvement in a previous study.

Conclusion

New technologies are clearly impacting upon the diagnosis, monitoring and treatment of ovarian and breast cancer. In the future the new biology should provide additional insights which will permit both more effective and less toxic therapy.

References

1. Bast RC Jr, Feeney M, Lazarus H, Nadler LM, Colvin RB, Knapp RC. (1981) Reactivity of a monoclonal antibody with human ovarian carcinoma. J Clin Invest 68:1331-1337.

2. Kabawat SE, Bast RC Jr, Bhan AK, Welch WR, Knapp RC, Colvin RB. (1983) Tissue distribution of a coelomic-

epithelium-related antigen recognized by the monoclonal antibody OC 125. Int J Gynecol Pathol 2:275-285.

3.   Bast RC Jr, Klug TL, St. John E, Jenison E, Niloff JM, Lazarus H, Berkowitz RS, Leavitt T, Griffiths CT, Parker L, Zurawski VR, Knapp RC. (1983) A radioimmunoassay using a monoclonal antibody to monitor the course of epithelial ovarian cancer. N Engl J Med 309:883-887.

4.   Jacobs I, Bast RC Jr. (1989) The CA 125 tumour-associated antigen: A review of the literature. Human Reprod 4:1-12.

5.   van der Burg ME, Lammes FB, van Putten WL, Stoter G. (1988) Ovarian cancer: the prognostic value of the serum half-life of CA125 during induction chemotherapy. Gynecol Oncol 30:307-12.

6.   Hunter VJ, Daly L, Helms M, Soper JT, Berchuck A, Clarke-Pearson DL, Bast RC Jr. (1990) The prognostic significance of CA 125 half-life in patients with ovarian cancer who have received primary chemotherapy after surgical cytoreduction. Am J Obstet Gynecol 163:1164-1167.

7.   Malkasian GD Jr, Knapp RC, Lavin PT, Zurawski VR Jr, Podratz KC, Stanhope CR, Mortel R, Berek JS, Bast RC Jr, Ritts RE. (1988) Preoperative evaluation of serum CA 125 levels in premenopausal and postmenopausal patients with pelvic masses: Discrimination of benign from malignant disease. Am J Obstet Gynecol 159:341-346.

8.   Knauf S and Urbach GI. (1980) A study of ovarian cancer patients using a radioimmunoassay for human ovarian tumor-associated antigen OCA. Am J Obstet Gynecol 138:1222-1223.

9.   Bast RC Jr, Siegal F, Runowicz C, Klug TL, Zurawski VR Jr, Schonholz D, Cohen CJ, Knapp RC. (1985) Elevation of serum CA 125 prior to diagnosis of an epithelial ovarian carcinoma. Gynecol Oncol 22:115-120.

10.   Zurawski VR Jr, Orjamaseter H, Andersen A, Jellum, E. (1988) Elevated serum CA 125 levels prior to diagnosis of ovarian neoplasia: relevance for early detection of ovarian cancer. Int J Cancer 42:677.

11.   Zurawski VR Jr, Broderick SF, Pickens P, Knapp RC, Bast RC Jr. (1987) Serum CA 125 levels in a group of nonhospitalized women: Relevance for the early detection of ovarian cancer. Obstet Gynecol 69:606-611.

12.   Zurawski VR Jr, Sjovall K, Schoenfeld DA, Broderick SF, Hall P, Bast RC Jr, Eklund G, Mattsson B, Connor RJ, Prorok PC, Knapp RC, Einhorn N.   (1990) Prospective evaluation of serum CA 125 levels in a normal population. Phase I: the specificities of single and serial determinations in testing for ovarian cancer. Gynecol Oncol 36:299-305.

13.   Einhorn N, Sjovall K, Knapp RC, Schoenfeld DA, Hall P,

Eklund G, Scully RE, Bast RC Jr, Zurawski VR Jr. Specificity of serum CA 125 radioimmunoassay for early detection of ovarian cancer: A prospective study. Submitted for publication.

14. Tockman, MS, Gupta, PK, Myers, JD, Frost, JK, Baylin, SB, Gold, EB, Chase, AM, Wilkinson, PH, Mulshine, JL (1988) Sensitive and specific monoclonal antibody recognition of human lung cancer antigen on preserved sputum cells: A new approach to early lung cancer detection. J Clin Onc 6:1685-1693.

15. Deutsch MA, Pence JC, Kerns BJM, Plate CA, Kinney R, Gooch G, Iglehart JD, Bast RC Jr. Detection of a novel marker in the bronchial secretions of patients with non-small cell lung cancer (NSCLC) using the 4B5 monoclonal antibody. Cancer, In press.

16. Pence JC, Deutsch MA, Kerns BJM, Huper G, Jordan L III, Wolfe WG, Samuelson WM, Fulkerson WJ Jr, Dodge RK, Bast RC Jr, Iglehart JD. Sensitive and specific detection of the 4B5 antigen in bronchial lavage specimens from patients with primary bronchogenic carcinoma. Cancer, In press.

17. Kruk PA, Maines-Bandiera SL, Auersperg N. (1990) A simplified method to culture human ovarian surface epithelium. Lab Invest 63:132-136.

18. Stromberg K, Collins TJ IV, Grodon AW, Jackson CL, Johnson GR. Transforming growth factor-α acts as an autocrine growth factor in ovarian carcinoma cell lines. Cancer Res In Press.

19. Berchuck A, Rodriguez GC, Kamel A, Dodge RK, Soper JT, Clarke-Pearson DL, Bast RC Jr. (1991) Epidermal growth factor receptor expression in normal ovarian epithelium and ovarian cancer. I. Correlation of receptor expression with prognostic factors in patients with ovarian cancer. Am J Obstet Gynecol 164:669-674.

20. Rodriguez GC, Berchuck A, Whitaker RS, Schlossman D, Clarke-Pearson DL, Bast RC Jr. (1991) Epidermal growth factor receptor expression in normal ovarian epithelium and ovarian cancer. II. Relationship between receptor expression and response to epidermal growth factor. Am J Obstet Gynecol 164:745-750.

21. Berchuck A, Rodriguez GC, Olt G, Arrick BA, Clarke-Pearson DL, Bast Jr. Regulation of growth of normal ovarian epithelium and ovarian cancer cell lines by transforming growth factor-ß Am J Obstet Gynecol, In press.

22. Feig LA, Bast RC Jr, Knapp RC, Cooper GM. (1984) Somatic activation of ras^k gene in a human ovarian carcinoma. Science 223:698-701.

23. Zhou DJ, Gonzalez-Cadavid N, Ahuja H, Battifora H, Moore GE, Cline MJ. (1988) A unique pattern of proto-oncogene

abnormalities in ovarian adenocarcinomas. Cancer 62:1573-1576.

24. Fukumoto M, Estensen RD, Sha L, Oakley, GJ, Twiggs, LB, Adcock, LL, Carson, LF, Roninson, IB. (1989) Association of Ki-_ras_ with amplified DNA sequences, detected in human ovarian carcinomas by a modified in-gel renaturation assay. Cancer Res 49:1693-1697.

25. Boltz EM, Kefford RF, Leary JA, Houghton CR, Friedlander ML. (1989) Amplification of c-_ras_-Ki oncogene in human ovarian tumours. Int J Cancer 43:428.

26. van't Veer LJ, Hermens R, van den Berg-Bakker LAM, Cheng, NC, Fleuren, GJ, Bos, JL, Cleton, FJ, Schrier, PI. (1988) _ras_ oncogene activatoin in human ovarian carcinoma. Oncogene 2:157-165.

27. Rodenburg CJ, Koelma IA, Nap M, Fleuren GJ. (1988) Immunohisto-chemical detection of the _ras_ oncogene product p21 in advanced ovarian cancer. Lack of correlation with clinical outcome. Arch Pathol Lab Med 112:151-154.

28. Tyson FL, Boyer CM, Kaufman R, O'Briant K, Cram G, Crews JR, Soper JT, Daly L, Fowler WC Jr, Haskill JS, Bast RC Jr. (1991) Overexpression and amplification of the HER-2/_neu_ (c-_erb_B-2) proto-oncogene in epithelial ovarian tumors and cell lines. Am J Obstet Gynecol 165:640-646.

29. Kacinski BM, Carter D, Mittal K, Yee, LD, Scata, KA, Donofrio, L, Chambers, SK, Wang, KI, Yang-Feng, T, Rohrschneider, LR, Rothwell, VM. (1990) Ovarian adenocarcinomas express _fms_ complementary transcripts and fms antigen, often with coexpression of CSF-1. Am J Pathol 137:135-147.

30. Slamon DJ, Godolphin W, Jones LA, Holt, JA, Wong, SG, Keith, DE, Levin, LJ, Stuart, SG, Udove, J, Ullrich, A, Press, MF. (1989) Studies of HER-2/_neu_ proto-oncogene in human breast and ovarian cancer. Science 244:707-712.

31. Ramakrishnan S, Xu FJ, Brandt SJ, Niedel JE, Bast RC Jr, Brown EL. (1989) Constitutive production of macrophage colony-stimulating factor by human ovarian and breast cancer cell lines. J Clin Invest 83:921-926.

32. Xu FJ, Ramakrishnan S, Daly L, Soper JT, Berchuck A, Clarke-Pearson D, Bast RC Jr. Increased serum levels of macrophage colony-stimulating factor in ovarian cancer. Am J Obstet Gynecol, _In press_.

33. Wu S, Rodabaugh K, Martinez-Maza O, Watson JM, Silberstein DS, Boyer CM, Peters WP, Weinberg JB, Berek JS, Bast RC Jr. Stimulation of ovarian tumor cell proliferation with monocyte products including interleukin-1-alpha, interleukin-6 and tumor necrosis factor-alpha. Am J Obstet Gynecol, _In press_.

34. Marks JR, Davidoff AM, Kerns BJ, Humphrey PA, Pence JC,

Dodge R, Clarke-Pearson DL, Iglehart JD, Bast RC Jr, Berchuck A. (1991) Overexpression and mutation of p53 in epithelial ovarian cancer. Cancer Res 51:2979-2984.

35. Bargmann CI, Hung MC, Weinberg RA. (1986) Multiple independent activations of the neu oncogene by a point mutation altering the transmembrane domain of p185. Cell 45:649-657.

36. Berchuck A, Kamel A, Whitaker R, Kerns B, Olt G, Kinney R, Soper JT, Dodge R, Clarke-Pearson DL, Marks P, McKenzie S, Yin S, Bast RC Jr. (1990) Overexpression of HER-2/neu is associated with poor survival in advanced epithelial ovarian cancer. Cancer Res 50:4087-4091.

37. Xu FJ,. Rodriguez GC, Whitaker R, Boente M, Berchuck A, McKenzie S, Houston L, Boyer CM, Bast RC Jr. (1991) Antibodiesagainst immunochemically distinct epitopes on the extracellular domain of HER-2/neu (c-erbB-2) inhibit growth of breast and ovarian cancer cell lines. Proc Amer Assoc Cancer Res 32:260.

38. Berchuck A, Boente MP, Whitaker RS, Xu FJ, Kalen AE, Bell RM, Bast RC Jr. Anti-erbB-2 (HER-2/neu) antibodies that downregulate growth of SKBr3 human breast cancer cells decrease intracellular levels of diacylglycerol (DAG). Submitted for publication.

39. Maier LA, Xu FJ, Hester S, Boyer CM, McKenzie S, Bruskin AM, Argon Y, Bast RC Jr. (1991) Requirements for the internalization of a murine monoclonal antibody directed against the HER-2/neu (c-erbB-2) gene product. Cancer Res 51:5361-5369.

40. Boyer CM, Borowitz MJ, McCarty KS Jr, Kinney RB, Everitt L, Dawson DV, Ring D, Bast RC Jr. (1989) Heterogeneity of antigen expression in benign and malignant breast and ovarian epithelial cells. Int J Cancer 43:55-60.

41. Yu YH, Crews JR, Cooper C, Ramakrishnan S, Houston LL, Leslie DS, George SL, Lidor Y, Boyer CM, Ring DB, Bast RC Jr. (1990) Use of immunotoxins in combination to inhibit clonogenic growth of human breast carcinoma cells. Cancer Res 1990; 50:3231-3238.

42. Crews JR, Maier LA, Yu YH, Hester S, O'Briant K, Leslie DS, DeSombre K, George SL, Boyer CM, Argon Y, Bast RC Jr. A combination of two immunotoxins exerts synergistic cytotoxic activity against human breast cancer cell lines. Submitted for publication.

43. Lidor YJ, Shpall EJ, Peters WP, Bast RC Jr. (1991) Synergistic cytotoxicity of different alkylating agents for epithelial ovarian cancer. Int J Cancer 49:704-710.

44. Lidor YJ, Hamilton TC, Ozols RF, Bast RC Jr. (1990) Alkylating agents and immunotoxins exert synergistic antitumor activity against ovarian cancer cells lines:

Mechanisms of action. Antibodies Immunoconjugates and Radiopharm 3:74.

45. Shpall EJ, Clarke-Pearson D, Soper JT, Berchuck A, Jones RB, Bast RC Jr, Ross M, Lidor Y, Banacek K, Tyler T, Peters WP. (1990) High-dose alkylating agent chemotherapy with autologous bone marrow support in patients with stage III/IV epithelial ovarian cancer. Gynecol Oncol 38:386-391.

46. Jones RB, Shpall EJ, Shogan J, Affronti ML, Coniglio D, Hart L, Halperin E, Iglehart JD, Moore J, Gockerman J, Bast RC, Peters WP. (1990) The Duke AFM program. Intensive induction chemotherapy for metastatic breast cancer. Cancer 66:431-436.

47. Peters WP. High-dose chemotherapy and autologous bone marrow support for breast cancer. In: Important Advances in Oncology, 1991, eds. DeVita VT, Hellman S, Rosenberg SA. Philadelphia: J.B. Lippincott Co., pp. 135-150, 1991.

48. Peters WP, Ross M, Vredenburgh JJ, Nadel S, Marks L, Kurtzburg J, Jones R, Shpall E, Petros W, Reisner E, Berlangieri SU, Hurd D, Norton L, Gilbert C, Mathias B, Coniglio D, Rosner G. High-dose chemotherapy and autologous bone marrow support as consolidation after standard dose adjuvant therapy for high-risk primary breast cancer. Submitted for publication.

49. Anderson IC, Shpall EJ, Leslie DS, Nustad K, Ugelstad J, Peters WP, Bast RC Jr. (1989) Elimination of malignant clonogenic breast cancer cells from human bone marrow. Cancer Res 49:4659-4664.

50. Shpall EJ, Jones RB, Bast RC Jr, Rosner GL, Vandermark R, Ross M, Affronti ML, Johnston C, Eggleston S, Tepperburg M, Coniglio D, Peters WP. (1991) 4-Hydroperoxycyclophosphamide purging of breast cancer from the mononuclear cell fraction of bone marrow in patients receiving high-dose chemotherapy and autologous marrow support: A phase I trial. J Clin Oncol 9:85-93.

51. Peters WP, Hussein AM, Kurtzberg J, Ross M, Vredenburgh J, Gilbert C, Coniglio D, Dukelow K, Oette D. (1991) Use of recombinant human interleukin-3 (IL-3) in patients (pts) with metastatic breast cancer receiving high-dose chemotherapy (HDC) and chemo-immunologically purged autologous bone marrow transplantation (P-ABMT). Blood 78:162a.

Discussion

Dr Ryuzo Ohno (The Branch Hospital, Nagoya University School of Medicine, Nagoya, Japan): In Japan, M-CSF has recently become commercially available for leukopenia after chemotherapy. If M-CSF is given to patients with ovarian cancer or healthy women with precancerous lesions, do you think it is possible that M-CSF might stimulate tumor growth?

Professor Bast: Dr Barry Kacinski, Yale University, New Haven, Connecticut, USA, has data that suggest that for an ovarian cancer that expresses the *fms* protooncogene, M-CSF increases the aggressiveness and invasiveness of the cancer rather than its proliferative thrust. In the several cell lines that we have studied in our own laboratory, *fms* expression has not been observed, so we have not been able to study the effect of M-CSF on proliferation. I am not aware of extensive studies of M-CSF on the growth of ovarian cancer cells taken directly from ascites fluid or from solid tumors. In the presence and absence of M-CSF. Dr Sidney Salmon's group at the University of Arizona, Tucson has done work with G-CSF and GM-CSF and these do not stimulate tumor growth, but I would be more concerned about altering the aggressiveness or proliferative thrust of avarian tumors with M-CSF. Of course, the tumors themselves are already producing a lot of M-CSF. There is tremendous heterogeneity from patient to patient and how much additional impact we add with pharmacologic administration of M-CSF is not clear.

Dr Toshitada Takahashi (Aichi Cancer Center, Nagoya, Japan): You mentioned bone marrow purging when you do autologous bone marrow transplantation in breast cancer patients. Solid tumors like neuroblastoma often infiltrate into bone marrow and you said also that this also happens in breast cancer, with 50% of patients having metastasis to bone marrow. Do you believe that when you do autologous bone marrow transplantation you should also do bone marrow purging?

Professor Bast: Attempts to purge marrow in leukemia, lymphoma, neuroblastoma, and now in breast cancer have been ongoing for over a decade and you have asked one of the most critical questions. In breast cancer, we may have a patient population for whom one actually can ask whether you needs to purge the bone marrow. One of the problems in designing such a study has been an ethical one. Informed consent has been difficult to obtain when one approaches patients saying, "We are going to randomize you either to have your marrow purged or to give you back tumor cells." In the case of breast cancer patients in an adjuvant setting, however, there is very seldom obvious marrow involvement. Here, you may have a patient population where it would be ethical and feasible to do a randomized study. From the work of about a dozen groups worldwide, including our own, it appears that there is a significant subclinical contamination of bone marrow, at least 28%, even in node-negative patients, if you use monoclonal antibodies to stain latent tumor cells in the marrow. As the studies are maturing, it appears that contamination with antigen-positive cells does have adverse prognostic significance. In 10 node-positive patients who are now undergoing transplantation, the cmarrow ontamination should be even more prevalent. In that setting, where no visible tumor cells are detected by conventional methods, but where you can, by unproven techniques, demonstrate tumor cells using staining with monoclonal antibodies and sorting of the cells, perhaps one can randomize patients to receive either purged or nonpurged marrow, provided you can do it safely. The purpose of our present study was to see whether we could purge all of the tumor cells that we could detect in model systems and still have the marrow reconstitute promptly enough not to jeopardize the well-being of patients in the transplant setting. With the help of IL-3, it seems that this is possible.

I. BIOLOGY OF TUMOR PROGRESSION AND REGRESSION

Recessive oncogenes

Molecular basis of cancer suppression by the human tumor suppressor genes

Wen-Hwa Lee, Phang-Lang Chen, David Goodrich, Yumay Chen, Nan-Ping Wang, Eva Lee

Center for Molecular Medicine/Institute of Biotechnology, University of Texas Health Science Center, San Antonio, Texas, USA

A. Introduction

Tumor suppressor genes are defined as genes for which loss-of-function mutations are oncogenic. Wild-type alleles of such genes may thus function to prevent or suppress oncogenesis (1). Based on the observations of loss of heterozygosity and karyotypic deletion, many such candidate genes have been proposed in the human genome. The retinoblastoma gene (RB) is the prototype of this class (2, 3). A gene located in chromosome band 13q14 has been molecularly cloned that has properties consistent with the RB gene (4). Expression of this gene (as a 4.7 kb mRNA transcript) was found in all normal tissues, but was undetectable or altered in retinoblastoma cells. The gene size is approximately 200 kb and contains total of 27 exons (5). The promoter was similar to a class of promoters that drive so-called "housekeeping" genes which are ubiquitously expressed at a relatively constant level. Evolutionary conservation and ubiquitous expression suggested that this gene may play an important role in basic cellular processes.

B. The RB protein, $pp110^{RB}$

From the predicted protein sequence data, a phosphoprotein of about 110 kD was identified as the RB gene product, $pp110^{RB}$ by using a specific antibody (6). Three biochemical activities of the RB protein have been discovered. First, the carboxy-terminal half of $p110^{RB}$ is capable of binding to DNA, although no sequence specificity for this binding has been demonstrated (7; F. Hong, unpublished observation). Second, the transforming proteins of several DNA tumor viruses, including SV40 T-antigen and adenovirus E1A, can bind $p110^{RB}$ (8, 9). Two regions, also within the carboxy-terminal half of the protein, are required for T-antigen and E1A binding; naturally occurring mutations of RB frequently occur in these regions (10). Mutational analysis of the transforming proteins has demonstrated a correlation between their ability to transform cells and their ability to bind $p110^{RB}$ (8, 11-16), although some transformation related properties are not dependent on binding $p110^{RB}$ (17). Third, several unidentified cellular proteins bind RB protein, apparently within the same binding domain used by T-antigen (18, 19). Although provocative, these biochemical properties have not provided a means to explain the physiological effects of loss of RB function.

Interestingly, p110^{RB} is differentially phosphorylated in concert with the cell cycle (20-24). Underphosphorylated forms of p110^{RB} predominate in the G1 phase where control of cell proliferation often occurs. The RB gene product becomes hyperphosphorylated as cells enter S phase. It undergoes additional phosphorylation as cells enter mitosis, and is converted to an underphosphorylated form, once again, after mitosis. These observations suggest that p110^{RB} may be involved in regulation of the cell cycle.

To test whether RB regulates cell cycle progression, purified RB proteins, either full-length or a truncated form containing the T-antigen binding region, have been injected into cells and the effect on entry into S phase determined. Synchronized cells injected early in G1 with either protein inhibits progression into S phase. This effect is antagonized by co-injection with antibodies directed against RB. Injection of RB protein into cells arrested at the G1/S boundary or 6-10 hours before the end of G1 has no effect on BrdU incorporation suggesting that RB protein does not inhibit DNA synthesis in S phase. These results provide direct evidence that RB may regulate cell proliferation, by restricting cell cycle progression at a specific point in G1.

C. Suppression of the Neoplastic Phenotype by Replacement of the RB gene

Examination of a variety of human tumors and cell lines have suggested a broader role for the RB gene in human oncogenesis than was previously anticipated. Inactivation of the RB gene has been observed in several different types of tumors including osteosarcoma, synovial sarcoma and other soft-tissue sarcomas, small cell lung carcinoma, breast carcinoma, prostate carcinoma, bladder carcinoma and leukemia (25-35). This list of "RB gene-related" tumors may be further extended in future studies.

The existence of inactivating mutations of *RB* in some natural human tumors supports the idea that *RB* normally functions to prevent tumor formation in susceptible precursor cells. However, this does not necessarily imply that replacement of the wild-type gene would revert neoplastic cells to more normal behavior later in their evolution, because multiple additional mutations might occur during oncogenesis that make the process irreversible. Furthermore, *RB* mutation is found in only a subset of cases of most tumor types, and these cancers have no well-defined pattern of inheritance that could be analyzed for linkage to the *RB* locus. Therefore, the biological significance of *RB* mutation in these cancers is not clear. On the other hand, successful suppression of some or all neoplastic properties of tumor cells by replacing wild-type *RB* would validate the identification of this gene, would imply a important role for *RB* inactivation in the genesis of that tumor, and would show that some neoplastic properties were reversible by restoration of a single gene.

We have used infection rather than transfection with recombinant retroviral vectors for expressing exogenous *RB* in cultured cells. The main advantage of the former is that infected, stably transformed cells usually carry only single copies of integrated provirus, allowing for better control of gene dosage. The viral genome of Rb, the test virus, consisted of a long terminal repeat (LTR) of Moloney murine leukemia virus driving *RB* cDNA, followed the Rous sarcoma virus promoter driving *neo*, followed by another LTR. *neo* encodes Tn5 neomycin phosphotransferase that confers resistance to the neomycin analog G418, which was used to select against noninfected cells. The control virus, Lux, was identical except that *RB* was replaced by the gene encoding luciferase, an enzyme that catalyzes luminescence in fireflies as well as in quantitative assays for gene expression. Lux served not only as a control for specific effects of *RB*, but also as a means to examine infection and expression efficiency of the viral constructs in different cell types.

Human tumor cell lines such as retinoblastoma WERI-Rb27, osteosarcoma Saos-2, prostate carcinoma DU145, bladder carcinomas and breast carcinoma carry inactivated RB genes. All these cell lines are referred to as RB⁻ cells had partial deletions of the RB gene and contained no intact RB protein. Another osteosarcoma cell line, U-2OS, expressed normal-sized RB protein and had apparently normal RB alleles. These cell lines were used as recipients for infection by RB and Lux viruses. After infection with RB virus, RB⁻ cell lines expressed normal-sized RB protein when labeled with ^{32}P-orthophosphate; Lux-infected RB⁻ cells expressed no RB protein. RB protein expression in U-2OS cells was not detectably altered after infection with either virus because of the presence of endogenous RB protein. However, neo-resistance of the selected clones indicated that viral infection had occurred.

The biological effects of RB gene replacement in these tumor cells were first examined in culture. Morphologically, there is a significant change in retinoblastoma WERI-Rb27 and Saos-2 cells infected with Rb virus and expressed RB protein. Usually, they are enlarged and flattened and grow slower than the parental cells. However, other tumor cell lines, grown as a monolayer, had a similar appearance and growth rate after infection with either virus.

Neoplastic properties of Rb-infected WERI-Rb27 or Saos-2 cells and clonal sublines have been extensively tested for soft-agar colony formation and tumorigenicity in nude mice in our laboratory and by Klein and his coworkers. Bulk-infected WERI-Rb27 cells or RB⁺ clones are completely nontumorigenic after 2 months, whereas parental cells, Lux-infected cells, and RB⁻ clones are invariably

Table 1: Effects of RB replacement on RB Cell lines

RB cell lines	Biological effects in culture			Tumorigenicity in nude mice
	Morphology	Growth rate	Soft-agar colony	
Retinoblastoma				
Y79	sl. enlarged	reduced	no change	suppressed
WERI-RB-27	sl. enlarged	reduced	no change	suppressed
Osteosarcoma				
Saos-2	v. enlarged	reduced	reduced	suppressed
Breast carcinoma				
MB468	granular/ sl. enlarged	reduced	reduced	suppressed/reduced
BT549	granular	no change	reduced	suppressed/reduced
Prostate carcinoma				
Du145	no change	no change	reduced	suppressed/reduced
Bladder carcinoma				
HT1376	no cahnge	no change	reduced	suppressed/reduced
5637	no change	no change	reduced	suppressed/reduced

tumorigenic within the same period. Several dozen RB$^+$ or RB$^-$ Saos-2 clones have been similarly tested, and again tumorigenicity is strongly and inversely correlated with RB expression. Taken together, these results provide direct evidence for a tumor suppression activity of RB protein, and imply that the tumorigenicity of these reconstituted tumor cells is solely determined by their RB expression status. On the other hand, nonretinoblastoma tumor cells with wild-type endogenous RB expression, such as U2OS osteosarcoma cells, are unaffected by Rb infection. Their genesis and tumorigenic properties must be controlled by a different gene or set of genes.

Because *RB* mutations are apparent in only a minority of breast, prostate and bladder carcinomas, the significance of RB inactivation in the genesis of these common adult cancers is uncertain. To address this question, RB replacement studies using the above methods were performed with prostate carcinoma cell line DU145, which expresses a mutated endogenous RB protein. Infection with Rb virus resulted in mass cultures and numerous subclones that expressed exogenous pp110^{RB}. In contrast to the results with WERI-Rb27 and Saos-2, RB replacement in DU145 cells had no apparent effect on morphology or growth rate in culture. In tumorigenicity studies, equal numbers of pp110^{RB}-expressing or -nonexpressing DU145 cells were injected into the right or left flanks, respectively, of twenty nude mice. After 2 months, most mice had formed tumors on both sides, but right-flank tumors were in every case smaller than those on the left, often by about a 15-fold margin of volume. All tumors had the same histologic appearance (poorly differentiated adenocarcinoma). It was hypothesized that right-flank tumors may have formed from revertant cells that had lost exogenous RB expression. Western blot analysis of some of the right-flank tumors showed that exogenous RB expression was undetectable, whereas endogenous RB protein was easily detectable. We concluded that cells retaining exogenous RB expression were unable to participate in tumor formation, i.e., their tumorigenicity was suppressed by wild-type RB protein. RB replacement studies in human breast and bladder carcinoma cells have generally yielded similar findings (E. Lee et al and D. Goodrich, et al) as listed in table 1, and suggest that *RB* inactivation is a biologically significant alteration when it occurs in adult neoplasms.

D. Replacement with wild type p53 gene suppresses tumorigenicity

p53 was originally identified as a mammalian cellular protein that binds to SV40 T antigen (36), a property that is also shared by RB protein. Deletions or rearrangements of the murine or human gene encoding p53 were found in Friend virus-induced murine erythroleukemias, and in human leukemias and osteosarcomas. On the other hand, many human breast, lung and colon carcinomas expressed high levels of aberrant p53 species with markedly prolonged half-lives due to certain point mutations in the p53 gene. These observations suggested that mutation of p53 could contribute in some way to human oncogenesis. p53 was originally considered to be an oncogene because it could transform primary rat embryo fibroblasts in concert with an activated *ras* gene (37-39). However, the observation of p53 deletions, and point mutations scattered over several exons, also suggested that p53 might be a tumor suppressor gene, i.e., a gene that was *inactivated* by mutation. Indeed, cotransfection of murine wild-type p53 DNA could reduce the transformation efficiency of transfected *ras* and E1A genes in rat embryo fibroblasts, whereas mutated p53 DNA enhanced such transformation (40). The dominant transforming effect was presumed to be due to a "dominant negative" activity of mutated p53 protein that somehow blocked the growth-restricting function of wild-type p53 protein in cells (41). However, that the copy numbers of transfected genes relative to endogenous p53 alleles were not controlled raised the question.

Table 2:   Cancer suppression by the wild-type p53 gene

Cell line / p53 genotype	Biological effects in culture			Tumorigenicity in nude mice
	Morphology	Doubling times	Soft-agar colony	
Osteosarcoma				
Saos-2/ (-/-)	enlarged	increase	diminished	suppressed
	enlarged	increase	diminished	suppressed
Peripheral Neunoepithelioma				
A673/ (-/-)	no change	no change	reduced	suppressed/reduced
Breast cancer				
MB468/ (M/-)	no change	no change	reduced	suppressed/reduced
BT549/ (M/-)	no change	no change	reduced	suppressed/reduced
Hepatocellular carcinoma				
T2/ (-/-)	no change	increase	reduced	suppressed/reduced
HA22T/(-/-)	no change	increase	reduced	suppressed/reduced

We have employed a human osteosarcoma cell line, Saos-2, that lacked endogenous p53 due to complete deletion of the gene as a model system. Single copies of exogenous p53 genes were then introduced by infecting cells with recombinant retroviruses containing either wild type or point-mutated versions of the p53 cDNA sequence. We found that 1) expression of wild-type p53 suppresses the neoplastic phenotype of Saos-2 cells; 2) expression of mutated p53 confers a limited growth advantage to cells in the absence of wild-type p53; and 3) wild-type p53 is phenotypically dominant to mutated p53 in a two-allele configuration. These results strongly suggested that, as with the retinoblastoma gene, mutation of both alleles of the p53 gene is essential for its role in oncogenesis (42).

To generalize this observation, many different kinds of human cancers such as breast carcinoma, peripheral epithelioma and hepatoma cells which have mutated p53 gene were used to test whether reintroduction of wild-type p53 gene would have any effect on these tumor cells. Expression of exogenous wild type p53 was performed by retrovirus mediated gene transfer. The effects of expression of wild-type or mutated p53 on human peripheral neuroepithelioma (PNET) A673, breast carcinoma and hepatoma cells were examined including morphology, growth rate, soft agar colony formation, and tumorigenicity in nude mice. In contrast to osteosarcoma Saos-2 cells, expression of wild-type or mutant p53 protein in A673 cells had no effect on morphology or growth characteristics. However, clones expressing wild-type p53 protein had reduced ability to form colonies in soft agar and tumors in nude mice (43). As listed in table 2, similar results were also obtained from breast carcinoma (E. Lee et al, unpublished) and hepatoma cells (Shew et al unpublished). To substantiate the genotype of wild-type p53 expressing cells, the proviral p53-encoding DNA of one cell clone was amplified by the polymerase chain reaction and sequenced. We concluded that expression of a single allele of the wild-type p53 gene was sufficient to suppress their tumorigenicity.

E. Conclusions

The mutation of tumor suppressor genes in cancer cells, and the suppression effects on their tumorigenicity by replacement with wild type genes, suggest novel approaches for future cancer therapies. The first trials of gene therapy in humans are begining and promise a new era in the treatment of genetic diseases. Although development of a new method to deliver wild-type genes into tumor cells may encounter many difficulties, practical treatments based on tumor suppressor genes may be achieved by delivery to tumor cells of recombinant proteins or infusion of carrier liposomes. Finally, the insights obtained by studies of tumor suppressor genes may be translatable into new drugs designed to mimic their functions.

F. Acknowledgments

The work performed in this laboratory was supported by grants from the National Institute of Health (EY-05758 and CA 51495)

References

1. Sager, R. (1986) Cancer Res. 46: 1573-1580.

2. Cavenee, W. K., T. P. Dryja, R. A. Phillips, W. F. Benedict, R. Godbout, B. L. Gallie, A. L. Murphree, L. C. Strong and R. L. White. (1983) Nature (London). 305: 779-784.

3. Knudson, A. G. (1973) Adv. Cancer Res. 17: 317-352.

4. Lee, W.-H., R. Bookstein, F. Hong, L.-J. Young, J.-Y. Shew and E. Y.-H. P. Lee. (1987) Science. 235: 1394-1399.

5. Bookstein, R., E. Y.-H. P. Lee, H. To, L.-J. Young, T. Sery, R. C. Hayes, T. Friedmann and W.-H. Lee. (1988) Proc. Natl. Acad. Sci. U.S.A. 85: 2210-2214.

6. Lee, W.-H., J.-Y. Shew, F. Hong, T. Sery, L. A. Donoso, L. J. Young, R. Bookstein and E. Y.-H. P. Lee. (1987) Nature. 329: 642-645.

7. Wang, N.-P., P.-L. Chen, S. Huang, L. A. Donoso, W.-H. Lee and E. Y.-H. P. Lee. (1990) Cell Growth Differ. 1: 233-239.

8. DeCaprio, J. A., J. W. Ludlow, J. Figge, J.-Y. Shew, C.-M. Huang, W.-H. Lee, E. Marsillo, E. Paucha and D. M. Livingston. (1988) Cell. 54: 275-283.

9. Dyson, N., R. Bernards, S. H. Friend, L. R. Gooding, J. A. Hassell, E. O. Major,

J. M. Pipas, T. Vandyke and E. Harlow. (1990) J. Virol. 64: 1353-1356.

10. Huang, S., N.-P. Wang, B. Y. Tseng, W.-H. Lee and E. Y.-H. P. Lee. (1990) EMBO J. 9: 1815-1822.

11. Cherington, V., M. Brown, E. Paucha, J. S. Louis, B. M. Spiegelman and T. M. Roberts. (1988) Mol. Cell. Biol. 8: 1380-1384.

12. Lillie, J. W., P. M. Loewenstein, M. R. Green and M. Green. (1987) Cell. 50: 1091-1100.

13. Moran, E., B. Zerler, T. M. Harrison and M. B. Mathews. (1986) Mol. Cell. Biol. 6: 3470-3480.

14. Moran, E. (1988) Nature. 334: 168-170.

15. Smith, D. H. and E. B. Ziff. (1988) Mol. Cell. Biol. 8: 3882-3890.

16. Whyte, P., N. M. Williamson and E. Harlow. (1989) Cell. 56: 67-75.

17. Thompson, D., D. Kalderon, A. Smith and M. Tevethia. (1990) 178: 15-34.

18. Huang, S., W.-H. Lee and E. Y.-H. P. Lee. (1991) Nature. 350: 160-162.

19. Kaelin, W. G. J., D. C. Pallas, J. A. DeCaprio, F. J. Kaye and D. M. Livingston. (1991) Cell. 64: 521-532.

20. Buchkovich, K., L. A. Duffy and E. Harlow. (1989) Cell. 58: 1097-1105.

21. Chen, P.-L., P. Scully, J.-Y. Shew, J. Y.-J. Wang and W.-H. Lee. (1989) Cell. 58: 1193-1198.

22. DeCaprio, J. A., J. W. Ludlow, D. Lynch, Y. Furukawa, J. Griffin, H. Pawnica-Worms, C.-M. Huang and D. M. Livingston. (1989) Cell. 58: 1085-1095.

23. Ludlow, J. W., J. Shon, J. M. Pipas, D. M. Livingston and J. A. DeCaprio. (1990) Cell. 60: 387-396.

24. Mihara, K., X.-R. Cao, A. Yen, S. Chandler, B. Driscoll, A. L. Murphree, A. T'Ang and Y.-K. T. Fung. (1989) Science. 246: 1300-1303.

25. Bookstein, R., J.-Y. Shew, P.-L. Chen, P. Scully and W.-H. Lee. (1990) Science. 247: 712-715.

26. Cheng, J., P. Scully, J.-Y. Shew, W.-H. Lee, V. Vila and M. Haas. (1990) Blood. 75: 730-735.

27. Dryja, T. P., J. M. Rapaport, J. M. Joyce and R. A. Petersen. (1986) Proc Natl.Acad Sci USA. 83: 7391-7394.

28. Friend, S. H., J. M. Horowitz, M. R. Gerber, X.-F. Wang, E. Bogenman, F. P. Li and R. A. Weinberg. (1987) Proc. Natl. Acad. Sci. U.S.A. 84: 9059-9063.

29. Harbour, J. W., S.-H. Lai, J. Whang-Peng, A. F. Gazdar, J. D. Minna and F. J. Kaye. (1988) Science. 241: 353-357.

30. Hensel, C. H., C. L. Hsieh, A. F. Gazdar, B. E. Johnson, A. Y. Sakaguchi, S. L. Naylor, W.-H. Lee and E. Y.-H. P. Lee. (1990) Cancer Res. 50: 3067-3072.

31. Horowitz, J. M., S.-H. Park, E. Bogenmann, J.-C. Cheng, D. W. Yandell, F. J.

Kaye, J. D. Minna, T. P. Dryja and R. A. Weinberg. (1990) Proc. Natl. Acad. Sci. U.S.A. 87: 2775-2779.

32. Lee, E. Y.-H. P., H. To, J.-Y. Shew, R. Bookstein, P. Scully and W.-H. Lee. (1988) Science. 241: 218-221.

33. Shew, J.-Y., N. Ling, X. Yang, O. Fodstad and W.-H. Lee. (1989) Oncogene Res. 1: 205-214.

34. Shew, J.-Y., B. Lin, P.-L. Chen, B. Y. Tseng, T. L. Yang-Feng and W.-H. Lee. (1990) Proc. Natl. Acad. Sci. U.S.A. 87: 6-10.

35. Toguchida, J., K. Ishizaki, M. S. Sasaki, M. Ikenaga, M. Sugimoto, Y. Kotoura and T. Yamamuro. (1988) Cancer Res. 48: 3939-3943.

36. Lane, D. P. and L. V. Crawford. (1979) Nature. 278: 261-263.

37. Eliyahu, D., A. Raz, P. Gruss, D. Givol and M. Oren. (1984) Nature. 312: 646-649.

38. Jenkins, J. R., K. Rudge and G. A. Currie. (1984) Nature. 312: 651-654.

39. Parada, L. F., H. Land, R. A. Weinberg, D. Wolf and V. Rotter. (1984) Nature. 312: 649-651.

40. Finlay, C. A., P. W. Hinds and A. J. Levine. (1989) Cell. 57: 1083-1093.

41. Lane, D. P. and S. Benchimol. (1990) Genes Devel. 4: 1-8.

42. Chen, P.-L., Y. Chen, R. Bookstein and W.-H. Lee. (1990) Science. 251: 1576-1580

43. Chen, Y., P.-L. Chen, N. Arnaiz, D. Goodrich and W.-H. Lee. (1991) Oncogene, in press.

Mutation of the p53 gene and accumulation of the p53 protein: Common steps in human cancer that provide novel targets for chemotherapy

David P. Lane

Cancer Research Campaign Laboratories, Department of Biochemistry, University of Dundee, Dundee, Scotland, UK

INTRODUCTION

The development of human cancer involves multiple genetic changes(9). Until recently most attention has focused on the activation of proto oncogenes such as *ras*. Now new evidence has been obtained for another class of genes that are frequently mutated in human cancer. These are the tumour suppressor genes(34). The normal function of these genes limits cell growth and so their inactivation can allow uncontrolled growth in the tumour. Germ line mutation of these suppressor genes is the basis for some inherited cancer suceptibility syndromes(25)(32)(44). The two best characterised suppressor genes are the p53 gene(26) on chromosome 17p and the retinoblastoma gene on chromosome 13q(29). The p53 genes suppressor activity can be inactivated by a large number of different point mutations(11)(12) or by physical complexing of the p53 protein to viral oncogenes.

The p53 suppressor gene

The p53 protein was discovered because it was found complexed to the SV40 large T antigen the oncogene of this small papova virus(27)(31). Subsequently the gene was cloned and the amino acid sequence deduced. The gene is located on the small arm of chromosome 17 in man and consists of eleven exons encoding a 393 amino acid nuclear phosphoprotein(30). The normal gene product when overexpressed in a range of tumour cells will restore some level of normal growth control(36)(1) Over three hundred mutations in the p53 gene have now been described(21). Most of the mutations are point missense mutations. Many of these mutations seem to activate a growth promoting activity of the p53 protein(23)(20). So unlike any other oncogene so far described p53 seems to have a dual nature. The normal gene acts as a tumour suppressor but many mutant p53's act as tumour promoters or oncogenes. This dual activity of the p53 protein is readily detected in transfection assays. The recent identification of a temperature sensitive mutant in p53 that acts as an oncogene at 37°C but as a suppressor gene at 32°C has given strong support to this idea(37). Both growth suppressing and growth promoting activities are intrinsic to the protein and the the protein may be switched between the two states by a conformational change(13)(16)(15)(35).

Many of the mutations in p53 stabilise the protein. This has an important practical consequence in that mutant protein accumulates to levels capable of ready detection by immunochemical means whereas the normal protein is not readily detected. This has allowed a very rapid analysis of abberant p53 expression using immuohistochemistry in a wide range of human malignancies. This simple method suggests that up to 60% of all human tumours abberantly express p53(5, 6, 7, 17, 22, 38, 41, 46)(4)(18).

MATERIALS AND METHODS

Antibodies

The antibodies to p53 have been recently described(4). CM1 is a rabbit polyclonal antibody to full length human p53(38). PAb421(19),PAb240(13),PAb246,(47) PAb1620 (39)and PAb1801(2)are monoclonal antibodies to different epitopes on p53.

Immunohistochemistry

Proceedures for staining frozen sections methacarn fixed sections (4)and formalin fixed sections of human tissues with anti-p53 antibodies have been recently described(38).

Immunoblotting and Elisa assays

Assays for p53, for p53 complexed to T antigen and assays designed to measure p53 conformation have also been described(13).

RESULTS AND DISCUSSION

Expression of p53 in human tumours.

In order to examine the expression of p53 in human tumours we have developed a panel of monoclonal and polyclonal antibodies to p53. The antibody PAb421 binds to an epitope near the C terminus, the antibody PAb1801 binds near the amino terminus, and the antibody PAb 240 binds to the centre of p53. All of these antibodies work well on frozen sections but are not very satisfactory on conventional sections. Recently we have been able to produce very large quantities of human p53 in bacteria using a T7 polymerase based expression vector system. This has allowed us to produce a new generation of polyclonal and monoclonal anti-p53 antibodies that can be used on conventionally processed histological material. The use of these antibodies has allowed us and our collaboraters to examine p53 expression patterns in nearly all the common neoplasias. The results are remarkable. We find high levels of p53 in about 70% of all malignant lesions examined. These lesions include carcinomas at all sites including breast,lung, colon, stomach,oesophogus,ovary,uterus,cervix,testis, prostate,bladder and oral cavity in addition lymphomas, sarcomas and glioblastomas also show high levels of p53 protein in these simple immunocytochemical tests. These high levels are not found in normal tissue nor in a variety of benign hyperproliferative lesions. High levels of p53 may however be present in early premalignant lesions such as colon adenomas and oesophageal in situ carcinomas. The detection of high levels of p53 is an indicator of poor prognosis in some tumour types for example gastric cancers (Dr I.Fillipe personal communication). High levels of p53 can be detected using this assay in simple cytology samples which may prove to be of diagnostic importance(18). Quantitative measurement of p53 protein level in tumour extracts is possible using two site immunometric ELISA assays(4). In addition to its diagnostic importance this tumour specific accumulation of p53 protein makes it a potential target for attack by novel chemotherapeutic agents.

The molecular basis for the accumulation of high levels of p53 protein.

Molecular analysis of the p53 gene in colon and lung cancer suggested that mutation of the p53 gene and loss of one allele of the p53 gene were frequent events in these neoplasias. When we looked at a sample of 47 primary lung cancers 26 showed accumulation of high levels of p53 as judged by immunohistochemistry. We developed a PCR based sequencing stratergy which did not involve a cloning step. we used this method to amplify and directly sequence p53 cDNA prepared from the tumours we had stained. In a small sample we found a complete correlation betwen high level expression of p53 and the presence of homozygous point mutations in the p53 gene. The mutations altered highly conserved amino acids in the p53 sequence(22). A similar correlation between mutation of the p53 gene and accumultation of the p53 protein has also been seen now in oesophageal cancer(8), breast cancer, colon cancer and ovarian cancer(10, 33). This suggest that a principal mechanism underlying the accumulation of p53 is point mutation in the p53 gene. The result suggests that the mutations found in human tumours may be positively selected for those that stabilise the protein. Other mechanisms could of course be imagined. . It is clear that the viral proteins SV40 large T and Adenovirus E1B can act to stabilise the normal protein. In contrast the E6 protein of Human papilloma virus acts to destabilise p53(42). In addition cellular proteins may also act to stabilise p53 as rare tumour cell lines have been isolated in which the normal p53 protein appears to be stable. The nature of these cellular mechanisms is unclear but will become very important in the future as they represent potential novel tumour suppressor gene products.

<u>The effect of mutations on p53 structure and function.</u>

The mutations in p53 found in human tumours though scattered through the molecule appear to be quite selective(21). While null mutants that result in the complete absence of p53 expression and nonsense mutants that produce truncated p53 proteins do occur that are not nearly as frequent as missense mutations. The missense mutations are quite selective. They nearly always changed a highly conserved amino acid and most are clutered in to the central region of the protein often in one of the four conserved boxes identified by Soussi and his colleagues (43). We have used a panel of human tumour cell lines containing known point mutations in p53 to examine the effect of mutation on p53 function. In all the lines the p53 protein is very stable compared to primary epithelial or fibrobalsts cells. The protein is nuclear in all the lines in contrast to the cytoplasmic location of p53 found in some cells trabsformed by transfection of mutant p53 protein. Using the monoclonal antibodies PAb240 and PAb1620 we have found that most of the point mutations induce a common conformational shift in the tertiary structure of p53. Thus the mutant proteins expose the epitope recognised by the PAb240 antibody and loss the conformationally sensitive epitope recognised by the PAb1620 antibody(6, 13, 41)(4)(13). This conformational shift is also associated with a loss of the ability to bind to T antigen. Since the capacity of p53 to bind T has been highly conserved in evolution it has been suggested that T may be mimicing a cellular p53 binding protein(28). Loss of T binding may therefore reflect loss of an important normal function. It is an attractive model that this allosteric shift acts normally to regulate p53 function and that the PAb1620 form of p53 delivers a growth inhibitory signal while the PAb240 positive form acts as a growth promoter. The point mutations in p53 then work by locking p53 into this growth stimulating form . The mutations thus act both to inactivate the growth inhibitory properties of p53 and also give a positive signal to the cell. This would explain the poor prognosis of those tumours that express high levels of p53 compared to those that do not.

Function of the p53 protein.

The p53 protein is a sequence specific DNA binding protein(3)(24) and can act as a transcriptional transactivator when fused to the gal4 DNA binding element(24)(40). The entry of p53 to the nucleus can be tightly regulated as we found when studying a temperature sensitive mutant of p53. At 37°C this protein is predominantly cytoplasmic while at 32°C it is nuclear. The cytoplasmic retention of p53 requires active protein synthesis(15). In all of these properties p53 resembles known transcription factors such as NFkb. In this model p53 acts to induce the expression of other growth inhibitory genes. The mutations in p53 inactivate this function and so cell growth cannot be so effectivly regulated. Other studies indicate however that p53 may play a more direct role in replication. The p53 protein can certainly act as a direct regulator of SV40 replication by blocking T antigen binding to DNA polymerase a(14). Recently it was found that p53 selectively associates with known host relication proteins in Herpes virus infected cells(45) again suggesting that p53 may interact directly with host replication sites.

The p53 gene in the treatment of cancer.

The identification of a common molecular step in human cancer serves to focus attention on the design of novel therapeutic agents. The accumulation of p53 and the change in its conformation associated with mutation means that the mutant protein may provide a direct chemotherapeutic target. Alternativly the common changes in cellular regulation brought about by p53 mutation may be exploited. We need to know much more about the cellular targets on which p53 acts if p53 specific agents are to be designed. So far p53 has been shown to be involved in the control of viral and cellular DNA synthesis to be a specific DNA binding protein and to carry a transcriptional activation domain. To determine which if any of these properties is essential for its suppressor activity and in mutant form for its growth promoting activituy will require much more detailed work. Nevertheless with the clear goal of developing a novel agent of widespread activity all the work will be 100% worthwhile.

ACKNOWLEDGEMENTS

My work has been supported by the Imperial Cancer Research Fund and the Cancer Research Campaign.

40

REFERENCES

1.   Baker SJ, Markowitz S, Fearon ER, Willson JKV, Vogelstein B.
        Suppression of human colorectal carcinoma cell growth by wild-type p53.
        Science 1990;249:912-915.

2.   Banks L, Matlashewski G, Crawford L. Isolation of human p53 specific
        monoclonal antibodies and their use in the studies of human p53
        expression. Eur J Biochem 1986;159:529-534.

3.   Bargonetti J, Friedman PN, Kern SE, Vogelstein B, Prives C. Wild-Type
        But Not Mutant p53 Proteins Bind to Sequences Adjacent to the SV40
        Origin of Replication. Cell 1991; 65:1083-1091.

4.   Bartek J, Bartkova J, Vojtesek B, et al. Aberrant expression of the p53
        oncoprotein is a common feature of a wide spectrum of human malignancies.
        Oncogene 1991;6:1699-1703.

5.   Bartek J, Bartkova J, Vojtesek B, et al. Patterns of expression of the p53 t
        umour suppressor in human breast tissues and tumours in situ and in vitro.
        Int.J.Cancer 1990;46:839-844.

6.   Bartek J, Iggo R, Gannon J, Lane DP. Genetic and immunochemical analysis
        of mutant p53 in human breast cancer cell lines. Oncogene 1990;5:893-899.

7.   Bennett WP, Hollstein MC, He A, et al. Archival Analysis of p53 Genetic
        and Protein Alterations in Chinese Esophageal Cancer. Oncogene 1991;in
        press

8.   Bennett WP, Hollstein MC, He A, et al. Archival analysis of p53 genetic
        and protein alterations in chinese esophageal cancer. Oncogene 1991;6:in
        press.

9.   Bishop JM. Molecular themes in oncogenesis. Cell 1991;64:235-248.

10.   Davidoff AM, Humphrey PA, Iglehart JD, Marks JR. Genetic basis for p53
        overexprssion in human breast cancer. Proc.Natl. Acad. Sci.U.S.A.
        1991;88:5006-5010.

11. Eliyahu D, Michalovitz D, Eliyahu S, Pinashi-Kimhi O, Oren M. Wild-type p53 can inhibit oncogene-mediated focus formation. Proc. Natl.Acad.Sci.USA. 1989;86:8763-8767.

12. Finlay CA, Hinds PW, Levine AJ. The p53 proto-oncogene can act as a suppressor of transformation. Cell 1989;57:1083-1093.

13. Gannon JV, Greaves R, Iggo R, Lane DP. Activating mutations in p53 produce a common conformational effect. A monoclonal antibody specific for the mutant form. EMBO J. 1990;9:1595-1602.

14. Gannon JV, Lane DP. p53 and DNA polymerase a compete for binding to SV40 T antigen. Nature 1987;329:456-458.

15. Gannon JV, Lane DP. Protein synthesis required to anchor a mutant p53 protein which is temperature-sensitive for nuclear transport. Nature 1991;349:802-806.

16. Ginsberg D, Michael-Michalovitz D, Ginsberg D, Oren M. Induction of growth arrest by a temperature sensitive p53 mutant is correlated with with increased nuclear localisation and decreased stability of the protein. Mol.Cell.Biol. 1991;11:582-585.

17. Gusterson BA, Anbazhagan R, Warren W, et al. Expression of p53 in premalignant and malignant squamous epithelium. Brit J Cancer 1991; in press.

18. Hall PA, Ray A, Lemoine NR, Midgley CA, Krauz T, Lane DP. p53 immunostaining is a marker of malignancy in diagnostic cytopathology. Lancet 1991; 338:513

19. Harlow E, Crawford LV, Pim DC, Williamson NM. Monoclonal antibodies specific for simian virus 40 tumor antigens. J.Virol 1981;39:861-869.

20. Hinds P, Finlay C, Levine AJ. Mutation is required to activate the p53 gene for cooperation with the ras oncogene and transformation. J of Virol 1989;63:739-746.

21. Hollstein M, Sidransky D, Vogelstein B, Harris C. p53 mutations in human cancer. Science 1991;253:49-53.

22. Iggo R, Gatter K, Bartek J, Lane D, Harris AL. Increased expression of mutant forms of p53 oncogene in primary lung cancer. Lancet 1990;335:675-679.

23. Jenkins JR, Rudge K, Chumakov P, Currie GA. The cellular oncogene p53 can be activated by mutagenesis. Nature 1985;317:816-818.

24. Kern S, Kinzler K, Bruskin A, et al. Identification of p53 as a sequence specific DNA binding protein. Science 1991;252:1708-1711.

25. Knudsen AG. Genetics of human cancer. Ann. Rev. Genetics 1987;20:231-252.

26. Lane D, Benchimol S. p53: Oncogene or anti-oncogene. Genes & Development 1990;4:1-8.

27. Lane DP, Crawford LV. T-antigen is bound to host protein in SV40-transformed cells. Nature 1979;278:261-263.

28. Lane DP, Crawford LV. The complex between Simian Virus 40 T antigen and a specific host protein. Proc.Royal.Soc.B. 1980;210:451-463.

29. Levine AJ, Momand J. Tumor suppressor genes: the p53 and retinoblastoma sensitivity genes and gene products. Biochimica et Biophysica Acta 1990;1032:119-136.

30. Levine AJ, Momand J, Finlay CA. The p53 Tumor Suppressor Gene. Nature 1991;351:453-456.

31. Linzer DIH, Levine AJ. Characterization of a 54K dalton cellular SV40 tumor antigen present in SV40 transformed cells and uninfected embryonal carcinoma cells. Cell 1979;17:43-52.

32. Malkin D, Li FP, Strong LC, et al. germline p53 mutations in a familial syndrome of breast cancer,sarcomas and other neoplasias. Science 1990;250:1233-1238.

33. Marks JR, Davidoff AM, Kerns BJ, et al. Overexpression and mutation of p53 in epithelial ovarian cancer. Cancer Research 1991;51:2979-2984.

34. Marshall CJ. Tumor Suppressor genes. Cell 1991;64:313-326.

35. Martinez J, Georgoff I, Martinez J, Levine AJ. Cellular localization and cell cycle regulation by a temperature-sensitive p53 protein. Genes & Development 1991;5:151-159.

36. Mercer WE, Shields MT, Lin D, Appella E, Ullrich SJ. Growth suppression induced by wild-type p53 protein is accompanied by selective down-regulation of proliferating-cell nuclear antigen expression. Proc. Natl. Acad Sci. USA 1991;88:1958-1962.

37. Michalovitz D, Halvey O, Oren M. Conditional Inhibition of Transformation nd of Cell Proliferation by a Temperature-Sensitive mutant of p53. Cell 1990;62:671-680.

38. Midgley CA, Fisher CJ, Bartek J, Vojtesek B, Lane DP, Barnes DM. Analysis of p53 expression in human tumours: an antibody raised against human p53 expresed in *E.coli*. J.Cell.Sci. 1991;In press

39. Milner J, Cook A, Sheldon M. A new anti-p53 monoclonal antibody, previously reported to be directed against the large T antigen of simian virus 40. 1987;1:453-455.

40. Raycroft L, Wu HY, Lozano G. Transcriptional activation by wild type but not transforming mutants of the p53 anti-oncogene. Science 1990;249:1049-1051.

41. Rodrigues NR, Rowan A, Smith MEF, et al. p53 mutations in colorectal cancer. Proc.Natl.Acad.Sci.USA 1990;87:7555-7559.

42.   Scheffner M, Werness BA, Hulbregtse JM, Levine AJ, Howley PM. The E6
       oncoprotein encoded by human papillomavirus types 16 and 18 promotes
       the degradation of p53. Cell 1990;63:1129-1136.

43.   Soussi T, Caron de Fromentel C, May P. Structural aspects of the p53
       protein in relation to gene evolution. Oncogene 1990;5:945-952.

44.   Srivastava S, Zou Z, Pirollo K, Blattner W, Chang EH. Germ-line
       transmission of a mutated p53 gene in a cancer prone family with Li-
       Fraumeni syndrome. Nature 1990;348:747-749.

45.   Wilcock D, Lane DP. Localization of p53, retinoblastoma and host
       replication proteins at sites of viral replication in herpes-infected cells.
       Nature 1991;349:429-431.

46.   Wright C, Mellon K, Johnston P, et al. Expression of Mutant p53, c-erbB-2
       and the Epidermal Growth Factor Receptor in Transitional Cell Carcinoma
       of the Human Urinary Bladder. Br. J. Cancer 1991:63:967-970

47.   Yewdell JW, Gannon JV, Lane DP. Monoclonal antibody analysis of p53
       expression in normal and transformed cells. J.Virol 1986;59:444-452.

Tumor suppressor genes involved in the pathogenesis of lung cancer

Takashi Takahashi

Laboratory of Chemotherapy, Aichi Cancer Center Research Institute, Nagoya, Japan

Introduction

The prevention and treatment of lung cancer should be based on knowledge of the molecular events underlying the pathogenesis of this aggressive disease. Lung cancer patients have had considerable exposure to agents, including those in cigarette smoke, which can damage DNA (1). Recent studies have revealed that the genetic changes which are probably caused by such carcinogenic exposure include activation of dominant oncogenes such as *myc* and *ras* gene families (2) and inactivation of tumor suppressor genes such as *Rb* and p53 (3). Accumulating evidence indicates that changes in both types of genes appear to be necessary for the malignant transformation of normal bronchial epithelial cells. In addition, certain growth factors have been suggested to play an important role as autocrine growth factors in lung cancer (2).

In this paper, I will focus on tumor suppressor genes involved in the pathogenesis of lung cancer and summarize our recent studies regarding inactivation of the p53 gene as well as the results of detailed deletion mapping of 3p.

Inactivation of the p53 gene in lung cancer

Following the discovery of cytogenetic abnormalities and allelic loss by restriction fragment length polymorphism (RFLP) analysis of the short arm of chromosome 17 (4), we initiated to explore the status of the p53 gene, because several reports on murine p53 have suggested the possibility that p53 may act as a tumor suppressor gene (5, 6).

In the initial study of p53 structure and expression in small cell (SCLC) and non-small cell lung cancers (NSCLC), we have found various types of p53 inactivations which include gross DNA alterations such as homozygous deletion and subtle abnormalities such as missense mutation (7). We also found intronic mutations which resulted in abnormal splicing and the production of no or truncated protein (8).

We have recently analysed 17 tumors taken from 15 SCLC patients (9) and 30 NSCLC tumors (30 patients; Suzuki, H. et al., submitted) at the Aichi Cancer Center, and the results are summarized in Tables 1, 2 and Fig. 1 in comparison with those reported by Dr. John Minna's group (7, 8, 10, 11). p53 is frequently mutated both in SCLC tumors (75%) and in NSCLC tumors (47%) and these frequencies of p53 mutations in Japanese lung cancer samples are similar to those in Americans. We note that a strong correlation was seen between the presence of p53 mutations in tumors and the successful establishment of the corresponding cell lines, suggesting that p53 mutations can confer a selective growth advantage *in vitro* (and also probably *in vivo*)(9).

46

The missense mutations found at the Aichi Cancer Center were scattered throughout the low charge region in the central part of p53 (codons 126 to 282, Fig.1), which is consistent with the location of p53 missense mutations in American samples. However, mutation at codon 273 which is the most prominent hot spot in American lung cancer samples was not seen in Japan, suggesting that distinct mutagenic process might be involved in part in these two countries (see below).

TABLE 1

p53 MUTATIONS IN LUNG CANCER

Histologic type	No. cases	Japan[#]	USA[§]
Small cell lung cancer	(15, 20)[¶]	75%	80%
Non-small cell lung cancer	(30, 49)	47	45
Squamous cell carcinoma	(12, 17)	67	65
Adenocarcinoma	(17, 27)	35	33
Large cell carcinoma	(1, 5)	0	40

#, Mutations identified in our laboratory at the Aichi Cancer Center (9)(Suzuki, H. et al., submitted).
§, Mutations identified by Dr. John Minna's group (10, 11).
¶, Numbers in parentheses indicate number of cases studied in Japan and in USA, respectively

TABLE 2

NATURE OF BASE CHANGES IN p53 MUTATIONS IN LUNG CANCER

| | SCLC | | NSCLC | |
Mutation	Japan (12)[§¶]	USA (22)[*]	Japan (12)[¶]	USA (24)[*]
G:C to T:A	50%	36%	50%	54%
G:C to A:T	8	18	25	21
G:C to C:G	8	14	0	17
A:T to T:A	0	9	8	8
A:T to G:C	33	4	8	0
A:T to C:G	0	22	8	0

§　Number in parentheses indicates mutations included in this table.
¶　Base changes identified in our laboratory at the Aichi Cancer Center (9)(Suzuki, H., et al., submitted).
*　Base changes identified in Dr. John Minna's laboratory (7, 8, 10, 11).

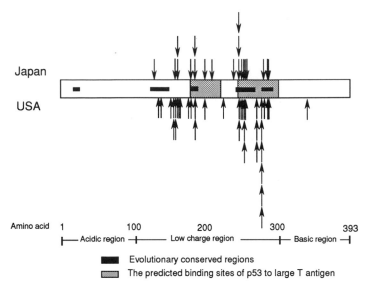

Fig. 1. p53 MISSENSE MUTATIONS IN LUNG CANCER. p53 missense mutations identified at the Aichi Cancer Center in Japan (9)(Suzuki, H., et al., submitted) are shown above the schematic diagram of the p53 protein in comparison with those reported by Dr. John Minna's group in America (7, 8, 10, 11).

In general, the type of mutation reflects the mutagen involved, since specific mutational spectra are associated with individual mutagens. For example, G:C to T:A transversions can be caused by benzoapyrene in some situations (12), while O^4-ethylthymine resulting from alkylating carcinogen exposure can cause A:T to G:C transition through mispairing with guanine (13). G:C to T:A transversions were the most frequent base substitutions both in SCLC and NSCLC in Japan, but interesting difference was observed between these two types of lung cancer, i.e., the second most frequent mutations in SCLC were A:T to G:C transitions, whereas G:C to A:T transitions were the second most frequent in NSCLC (Table 2). Since SCLC and NSCLC are believed to arise from distinct bronchial epithelial stem cells which are committed to differentiate towards neuroendocrine and epithelial cells respectively, it is conceivable that such differentially committed stem cells have differences in sensitivity to certain carcinogens, which result in distinct nucleotide substitution pattern in the corresponding tumor types. We note that clear differences between SCLC and NSCLC can be seen also in American lung cancer samples (Table 2).

Another point of interest is the differences in base changes in SCLC between Japan and America. Although G:C to T:A transversions were the most frequent in both countries, A:T to G:C transitions which are the second most frequent in Japan were seldom found in America. In contrast, G:C to A:T, G:C to C:G and A:T to C:G substitutions frequently found in America were rare in

Japan. Therefore, it is suggested that different mutagenic process may exist in these two countries. To investigate the possibility that these may be due to difference in caricinogen exposures or in sensitivity to certain carcinogens, SCLC samples of Japanese Americans will be analyzed in our laboratory.

We also examined whether introduction of wild-type p53 (wt-p53) into lung cancer cell lines can suppress tumor growth *in vitro* and/or *in vivo* (unpublished data done in collaboration with Dr. John D. Minna, Simmons Cancer Center, TX). Dramatic suppression of *in vitro* tumor growth of a lung cancer cell line with a homozygous deletion was observed by transfecting wt-p53 cDNA. In contrast, mutant p53 cDNAs isolated from lung cancer failed to do so, indicating that subtle mutations in the p53 gene can inactivate its suppressive effects. Furthermore, introduction of wt-p53 into a lung cancer cell line with missense p53 mutation which is the most frequent type of p53 alterations revealed that the clone expressing moderate level of wt-p53 have lost neoplastic phenotype such as tumor growth in soft agar and in SCID mice. Altogether, the p53 gene appears to play significantly important role in the pathogenesis of lung cancer.

An initial step towards positional cloning of tumor suppressor genes on the short arm of chromosome 3

The 3p deletion was first noted by cytogenetic analysis (14) and was later confirmed by several independent studies using RFLP probes (4, 15-17). As an initial step towards positional cloning of the tumor suppressor genes on 3p, we have conducted a collaborative study with Dr. Yusuke Nakamura (Cancer Institute, Tokyo) for a detailed analysis of the minimum deleted regions on 3p using a large number of RFLP probes (13 probes mapped on 3p) and tumor samples (9 SCLC and 39 NSCLC)(Hibi, K., et al., submitted). All SCLC and 79% of NSCLC tumors showed allelic loss at one or more loci mapped on 3p. In addition, three distinct regions were identified as shortest regions of overlap. These include 3p25, 3p21.3 and 3p14-cen. Of note, similar conclusion was drawn recently by Whang-Peng et al. by classic cytogenetic analysis of 61 NSCLC cell lines. These findings strongly suggest that at least three tumor suppressor genes exist on 3p. Further studies aimed at the isolation of the 3p genes are currently under way in our laboratory, which should provide a basis for better understanding of the molecular pathogenesis of lung cancer.

Conclusions

It is now clear that lung cancers frequently suffer inactivation of both copies of several tumor suppressor genes such as p53, in addition to genetic alterations in dominant oncogenes. Future studies addressing when these abnormalities develop and whether their correction reverses the malignant phenotype should help us not only to understand the molecular mechanism of lung cancer but also provide new strategies for prevention, diagnosis and therapy of lung cancer.

Acknowledgements

I would like to thank Drs. Ryuzo Ueda, John D. Minna and Toshitada Takahashi for their supports and encouragements throughout the study. This work was supported in part by a Grant-in-Aid for the Comprehensive Ten-Year Strategy for Cancer Research from the Ministry of Health and Welfare; Grant-in-Aids for Cancer Research for the Ministries of Education, Science, and Culture and of Health and Welfare, Japan; by a grant from the Cancer Research Institute, Inc., New York; and by a grant from the Imanaga Memorial Foundation, Japan.

References

1. Phillips, D., Hewer, A., Martin, C., Garner, R. & King, M. (1988) *Nature (London)* **336,** 790-792.

2. Minna, J. D., Battey, J. F., Brooks, B. J., Cuttitta, F., Gazdar, A. F., Johnson, B. E., Ihde, D. C., Lebacq-Verheyden, A.-M., Mulshine, J., Nau, M. M., Oie, H. K., Sausville, E. A., Seifter, E. & Vinocour, M. (1986) *Cold Spring Harbor Symp. Quant. Biol.* **LI,** 843-853.

3. Minna, J., Kaye, F., Takahashi, T., Harbour, J., Rosenberg, R., Nau, M., Whang-Peng, J., Johnson, B., Birrer, M. & Gazdar, A. (1989) In Cavenee, W., Hastie, N., Stanbridge, E. (eds.) *Recessive oncogenes and tumor suppression. (Current communications in molecular biology.)* Cold Spring Harbor Laboratory Press, New York, pp. 57-65.

4. Yokota, A., Wad, M., Shimosato, Y., Terada, M. & Sugimura, T. (1987) *Proc. Natl. Acad. Sci. USA* **84,** 9252-9256.

5. Mowat, M., Cheng, A., Kimura, N., Bernstein, A. & Benchimol, S. (1985) *Nature (London)* **314,** 633-636.

6. Hinds, P., Finlay, C. & Levine, A. (1989) *J. Virol* **63,** 739-746.

7. Takahashi, T., Nau, M. M., Chiba, I., Birrer, M. J., Rosenberg, R. K., Vinocour, M., Levitt, M., Pass, H., Gazdar, A. F. & Minna, J. D. (1989) *Science* **246,** 491-494.

8. Takahashi, T., D'Amico, D., Chiba, I., Buchhagen, D. L. & Minna, J. D. (1990) *J. Clin. Invest.* **86,** 363-369.

9. Takahashi, T., Takahashi, T., Suzuki, H., Hida, T., Sekido, Y., Ariyoshi, Y. & Ueda, R. *Oncogene* (in press).

10. Chiba, I., Takahashi, T., Nau, M., D'Amico, D., Curiel, D., Mitsudomi, T., Buchhagen, D., Carbone, D., Piantadosi, S., Koga, H., Reissmann, P., Slamon, D., Holmes, E. & Minna, J. (1990) *Oncogene* **5,** 1603-1610.

11. D'Amico, D., Carbone, D., Mitsudomi, T., Nau, M., Fedorko, J., Russell, E., Johnson, B., Buchhagen, D., Bodner, S., Phelps, R., Gazdar, A. & Minna, J. *Oncogene* (in press).

12. Mazur, M. & Glickman, B. (1988) *Somat. Cell. Mol. Genet.* **14,** 393-400.

13. Lawley, P. (1990) In Cooper, C. & Grover, P.(eds.) *Chemical carcinogenesis and mutagenesis I,* Splinger-Verlag, Berlin, pp. 409-469.

14. Whang-Peng, J., Kao-Shan, C., Lee, E., Bunn, P., Jr, Carney, D., Gazdar, A. & Minna, J. (1982) *Science* **215,** 181-182.

15. Naylor, S., Johnson, B., Minna, J. & Sakaguchi, A. (1987) *Nature (London)* **329,** 451-454.

16. Kok, K., Osinga, J., Carritt, B., Davis, M., van der Hout, A., van der Veen, A., Landsvater, R., de Leij, L., Berendsen, H., Postmus, P., Poppema, S. & Buys, C. (1987) *Nature (London)* **330**, 578-581.

17. Brauch, H., Johnson, B., Hovis, J., Yano, T., Gazdar, A., Pettengill, O., Graziano, S., Sorenson, G., Poiesz, B., Minna, J., Linehan, M. & Zbar, B. (1987) *N. Engl. J. Med.* **317**, 1109-1113.

Studies on tumor suppression by microcell-mediated chromosome transfer

Mitsuo Oshimura, Akihiro Kurimasa

Department of Molecular and Cell Genetics, School of Life Science, Tottori University, Yonago, Japan

The suppression of the tumorigenicity of tumor cells by hybridization with normal cells has led to the hypothesis that normal cells contain genes which suppress the neoplastic potential of tumor cells (1). One approach to mapping putative tumor suppressor genes to specific chromosomes was the identification of chromosome which had been lost in the hybrid cells that re-expressed tumorigenicity (2). Another approach for identifying chromosomes which carry putative

Table 1 Summary on suppression type of transformed properties
following chromosome transfer

Type of suppression		Chromosome; Tumor type (cell line)		Ref.
Type I Induction of cellular senescence	# 1	Human,	uterine endometrial carcinoma (HHUA)	(4)*
		Syrian,	hamster immortalized cell (10W)	(5)*
	# 4	Human,	cervical carcinoma (HeLa)	(16)
		Human,	bladder carcinoma (J82)	(16)
		Human,	glioblastoma (J98G)	(16)
	#11	Human,	bladder carcinoma (H-15)	(6)*
Type II Reduction of *in vitro* growth-rate with morphological alteration and suppression of tumorigenicity	# 1	Human,	fibrosarcoma (HT1080)	(7)*
		Mouse,	Kirsten sarcoma virus transformed NIH3T3 (DT)	(8)*
	# 5	Human,	colon cancer (COKFu)	(9)*
	# 6	Human,	malignant melanoma (UACC 903)	(17)
	# 7	Human,	choriocarcinoma (CC1)	(10)*
	#18	Human,	colon cancer (COKFu)	(9)*
Type III Suppression of tumorigenicity	# 1	Human,	neuroblastoma (SK-N-MC)	(11)*
	# 3	Human,	renal cell carcinoma (YCR)	(12)*
		Human,	cervical carcinoma (SiHa)	(13)*
	# 6	Human,	uterine endometrial carcinoma (HHUA)	(4)*
	# 9	Human,	uterine endometrial carcinoma (HHUA)	(4)*
	#11	Human,	uterine endometrial carcinoma (HHUA)	(4)*
		Human,	cervical carcinoma (D98/AH-2)	(18)
		Human,	cervical carcinoma (SiHa)	(14)*
		Human,	Wilms' tumor (G401)	(19)
		Human,	fibrosarcoma (HT1080)	(7)*
		Human,	rhabdomyosarcoma (A204)	(15)*

* Studies done by the present authors and colleagues

tumor suppressor genes is the introduction of specific chromosomes into the tumor cells of interest (3). We examined the ability of human chromosomes derived from normal fibroblasts to suppress or modulate tumorigenicity in nude mice and the _in vitro_ properties in a variety of cell lines (4-16). The following results were obtained (Table 1).

Thus, lessons learned from the above results are as follows. Different members of the family of tumor suppressor genes are present on different chromosomes. More than one normal chromosome suppress the tumorigenicity of a given tumor cell line, which indicates that multiple tumor suppressor genes are involved in cer-

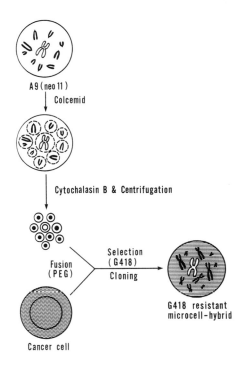

Figure 1   Schematic of Chromosome transfer _via_ microcell-fusion.

Human fibroblasts were first transfected with pSV2neo DNA. G418-resistant fibroblasts were isolated and fused to mouse A9 cells, and hybrid cells were selected in the medium containing 800 µg/ml of G418 plus 10 µM ouabain (Oua). Isolated hybrids were treated with colcemid to induce micronuclei and were enucleated by centrifugation, and the resulting microcells were isolated and karyotyped (3). The A9 microcell clones that had a human chromosome were micronucleated by colcemid; microcells were prepared as above and fused to tumor or transformed cells. G418-resistant microcell hybrids were isolated, and the clones that contained an extra copy of a transferred chromosome were further analyzed.

tain tumors. Three functional classes of suppression were observed, i.e., induction of cellular senescence (Type I), reduction of in vitro growth-rate with morphological alteration and suppression of tumorigenicity (Type II), and suppression of tumori-genicity without alteration of in vitro properties (Type III).

Thus these microcell hybrids of tumor cells suppressed by the introduction of different normal chromosomes are useful in mapping of tumor suppressor genes as well as elucidating their function in cell growth and differentiation.

REFERENCES

1. Klein G, Bregula U, Wiener F, Harris H (1971) J Cell Sci 8:659-672

2. Oshimura M, Koi M, Ozawa N, Sugawara O, Lamb PW, Barret JC (1988) Cancer Res 48:1623-1632

3. Koi M, Shimizu M, Morita H, Yamada H, Oshimura M (1989) Jpa J Cancer Res 80:413-418

4. Yamada H, Wake N, Fujimoto S, Barrett JC, Oshimura M (1990) Oncogene 5:1141-1147

5. Sugawara O, Oshimura M, Koi M, Annab LA, Barrett JC (1991) Science 247:707-710

6. Kugoh M, unpublished data

7. Kugoh MH, Hashiba H, Shimizu M, Oshimura M (1990) Oncogene 5:1637-1644

8. Yamada H, Horikawa I, Hashiba H, Oshimura M (1990) Jpn J Cancer Res 81:1095-1100

9. Tanaka K, Oshimura M, Kikuchi R, Saki M, Hayashi T, Miyaki M (1991) Nature 349:340-342

10. Sasaki M, unpublished data

11. Oshimura M, Kugoh MH, Shimizu M, Yamada H, Hashiba H, Horikawa I, Sasaki M (1990) In: Knudson AG, Stanbridge EJ, Sugimura T, Terada M, Watanabe S (eds) Genetic Basis for Carcinogenesis: Tumor Suppressor Genes and Oncogenes. Jpn Sci Soc Press, Tokyo, Taylor and Francis LTD, London and Bristol, pp249-257

12. Shimizu M, Yokota J, Mori N, Shuin T, Shinoda M, Terada M, Oshimura M (1990) Oncogene 5:185-194

13. Horikawa I, unpublished data

14. Koi M, Morita H, Yamada H, Satoh H, Barrett JC, Oshimura M (1989)· Mol Carcinogen 2:12-21

15. Oshimura M, Morita H, Koi M, Shimizu M, Yamada H, Satoh H, Barrett (1990) J Cell Biochem 42:135-142

16. Ning Y, Weber JL, Killary AM, Ledbetter DH, Smith JR, Pereira-Smith OM, (1991) Proc Natl Acad Sci USA 88:5635-5639

17. Trent JM, Stanbridge EJ, Mcbride HL, Meese EV, Casey G, Araujo DE, Witkowski CM, Nagle R (1990) Science 247:568-571

18. Saxon PJ, Srivatsan ES, Stanbridge EJ (1986) EMBO J 15:3461-3466

19. Weissman BE, Saxon PJ, Pasquale SR, Jones GR, Geiser AG, Stanbridge EJ (1987) Science 236:175-180

Discussion

Dr Takayuki Enomoto (Osaka University, Japan): Dr Lee, in colon tumors it has been established that the activation of the *ras* gene and several antibodies is important for the development of the tumor. In retinoblastoma is inactivation of the RB gene sufficient to cause tumor development?

Dr Lee: This is currently an important concept. Many studies have led to the suggestion that the retinoblastoma gene alone can cause retinoblastoma formation, however I am not sure. The retinoblastoma gene is a key gene predisposed to and important for tumor formation, but I am not sure whether this is the only gene required; I believe there may be more. Maybe other factors are important for the downstream tumor progression.

Dr Akio Matsukage (Aichi Cancer Center, Nagoya, Japan): I am interested in the biological function of the retinoblastoma gene. Am I correct in thinking that the RB gene is involved in cell cycle regulation?

Dr Lee: Yes.

Dr Matsukage: Many tumor cells that have lost the RB gene, however, seem to go through a normal cell cycle. So what point of the cycle is different in cells with and without the RB gene mutation?

Dr Lee: The retinoblastoma protein is involved in the cell cycle, however it is not an essential protein in terms of what makes the cell cycle work or not. These proteins are important in subtle regulation. Recently we were able to demonstrate retinoblastoma in function in early G1. This protein basically controls or regulates a whole group of other factors important for a cell to move from G1 to S phase. The retinoblastoma protein is the key protein at this moment for control, so loss of this protein will leave this reaction unsynchronized and it becomes difficult to coordinate all the necessary steps for entry into the S phase, ie, DNA synthesis. Unsynchronized DNA synthesis will cause a lot of trouble for the cell later on, eg, aneuploidy and damage to DNA. That is the reason why the retinoblastoma gene is important, but may not be the only important gene for cancer formation.

Professor Oshimura: Do you see any dosage effects of transferred retinoblastoma genes on suppression of transformed phenotypes?

Dr Lee: It is possible; however we have not done this experiment purposely. Dr Lane, do you know of any protein that is able to associate completely with the mutated P53 protein or the wild-type P53 protein in terms of degradation?

Dr Lane: Yes. The only model that we have at the moment is the E6 protein of human papillomavirus which seems to be targeting p53 for destruction. It is critical that we identify the cellular proteins with which p53 normally interacts. The sort of protein that I would like to see it interacting with is a protein involved in initiation of replication.

Dr Masao Seto (Aichi Cancer Center, Nagoya, Japan): You showed using the HSV system that p53 is localized at the point where DNA replicates. Is the p53 you showed mutated or is it a normal one?

Dr Lane: In that particular experiment it was a mutant.

Dr Seto: Is there any evidence that normal p53 is localized to the same point?

Dr Lane: We do not know yet in the HSV system. We are not examining viral replication, but cellular replication for colocalization at the moment.

Dr Lee: Regarding RB protein distribution, after you infect with herpes simplex virus, do you see more spotted areas than in the virus-free infection? The original RB seems surrounded in the middle region, but after the infection with herpes simplex virus, more spots are coming out.

Dr Lane: We do not really know why that is yet.

Dr Matsukage: Dr Takahashi, the difference between mutation in lung and colon cancers is striking. What causes this difference: different carcinogens or different mutations of p53? Do they function in both tumors?

Dr Takahashi: I believe that lung cancer and colon cancer arise from a different exposure to carcinogens. In Japanese Americans, the incidence of lung cancer still remains similar to those in Japanese, while for colon cancer, the incidence increases almost comparable to those in white Americans. So tumors have a different mutagenic process and this affects the results.

Dr Lee: You identified one specific probe that is homozygously deleted in small cell lung carcinoma. What is the percentage of tumors with this probe deleted and how did you get the probe?

Dr Takahashi: No, it is not a homozygous deletion, but allelic loss, hence the loss of heterozygosity. I hope we will be able to find a homozygous deletion, because it would be of great use to us in isolating tumor suppressor genes.

Dr Nagahiro Saijo (National Cancer Center, Tokyo, Japan): In your experiment on transfection of wild type p53 gene to tumor cells with mutated p53 gene, does the transfectant contain 2 genes of p53?

Dr Takahashi: That is correct. That clone is expressing wild type and mutant p53. The expression level of wild type is several times lower than that of mutant p53 mRNA. This agrees with the recessive oncogene theory.

Dr Lee: Professor Oshimura, is there any way to produce a large amount of chromosome, such as chromosome 11, 17, or 3P, for this type of experiment?

Professor Oshimura: If chromosomes have a different marker, yes. For example, we have a chromosome 17 marked with the HPRT gene and a chromosome 18 marked with the neogene. Therefore, we can transfer chromosomes 5, 17, and 18 simultaneously.

Dr Shonen Yoshida (Nagoya University, Nagoya, Japan): I believe that if one puts the tumor suppressor gene into the neoplastic state, the transformation characteristics become normal. If you delete the suppressor gene in normal cells, however, does that work for malignant transformation, such as if you put the antisense RB gene, for example, into cells?

Dr Lee: I believe that this type of experiment has been done in vitro, but no results have yet been published. This suggests that the results are not as encouraging as we might have expected. However, in a recent experiment in an animal model, inoculation of the p53 gene, with loss of one allele, produced cancer at a very very late stage. If you make a homozygous deletion in mice they produce cancer in 2–3 months. This applies to many different types of cancer.

Dr Lane: It is important to understand that in the germ line tumors all the cells in the body have only one allele, so there must be a very high frequency of cells arising spontaneously that have lost the other allele. There are clearly enough other genes regulating those cells that they do not mature into full cancer cells. So it is just another example of the multistage nature of human cancer. Loss of one allele produces susceptibility, but it is not sufficient to produce the tumor.

Dr Takahashi: From the clinical point of view, the suppressor oncogene is very useful for diagnosis, as we probably all agree, but we would like to treat tumors with p53 mutation. One possible way might be gene therapy, by infecting tumor cells with the p53 mutation with retrovirus vector or something similar. Do you have any experiments going on in this area?

Dr Lee: Certainly this is the goal that many laboratories—and many pharmaceutical companies—are aiming at. As we learn more about tumor suppressor genes, gene inactivation certainly appears to play an important role in cancer formation, and to put back this gene and return the cell to the normal state would be the ultimate treatment. The problems facing us in doing this, however, are enormous. For example, however we put them back, by retrovirus or by other means, those genes induce cancer cells. Of course, if the cancer is very small in size or has not metastasized, ie, is localized in a certain area, that will be much easier, but for cancer that already has metastasized all over the body, this will be very difficult. The alternative way is the use of proteins or other small chemicals, such as Dr Lane has proposed. I believe that in the near future, maybe in 2–3 years, results from this type of study will appear.

Dr Lane: I think that the gene therapy approach is really very difficult, for the reasons that Dr Lee has pointed out, but also because you will inevitably infect normal cells. I used to wonder whether having an extra couple of copies of the normal p53 gene would make one very resistant to tumor development, but of course it also provides an additional target for mutation; there is a very fine balance between whether that would be helpful or harmful. My own view is that unless we see some radical improvement in the way that we can carry out gene therapy, it is not going to be the right strategy. Events are moving so fast, however, that one cannot make definite statements.

Dr Lee: We hope that in the future a suppressor gene will be discovered that controls signal transductions, particularly at the cell surface, and that this will provide a convenient way to treat cancer, ie, by treating with the tumor suppressor gene product.

Dr Yoshida: Dr Lane, you emphasized that p53 could be a very important target for chemotherapy in the future. Mutated p53 accumulates in the cell, especially in the malignant cell, and if you attack the mutated p53 molecule with a reagent, you may destroy the p53 proteins in the cancer cell. Then what happens? Will the cancer cell die due to some type of cytotoxicity or it could be differentiated to the normal?

Dr Lane: There are various possibilities. One is that if this conformational change is important you might be able to restore some aspect of wild type function. In a few systems it has been shown that inappropriate production of the wild type protein could induce differentiation and apoptosis both in colon and lymphoid systems. Also you might, if this conformational or concentration difference could be exploited, use it to target a cytotoxic chemical. It would have to be a small molecule, readily diffusible, with a short half-life and a high affinity for p53, but it is not unimaginable that such a molecule could be obtained.

Oncogenes

Molecular pathogenesis of non-Hodgkin lymphoma

Gianluca Gaidano, Paola Ballerini, Giorgio Inghirami, Daniel M. Knowles, Riccardo Dalla-Favera

Department of Pathology and Cancer Center, College of Physicians and Surgeons, Columbia University, New York, New York, USA

INTRODUCTION

Non-Hodgkin lymphomas (NHL) include a group of neoplasms which share a common target tissue, B cells, yet are characterized by a high degree of biological and clinical heterogeneity. The most widely used classification system for NHL (1) is based upon the degree of clinical aggressiveness correlated with the stage of differentiation and the pattern of growth (follicular or diffuse) of the tumor (table I). While the etiopathogenesis of these neoplasms remains unclear, one conceivable hypothesis is that their marked heterogeneity may reflect distinct pathogenetic mechanisms whose elucidation is likely to have important biological and clinical implications.

Tumorigenesis in various tissues is associated with two main categories of genetic lesions, activation of dominantly acting oncogenes and deletion/inactivation of tumor suppressor genes. In B cell neoplasms, several oncogenes have been identified which are activated by chromosomal translocations involving antigen receptor genes. More recently, deletions/inactivations of the tumor suppressor genes p53 and Rb1 have also been shown to be associated with specific subtypes of NHL. This chapter will review the distribution and biological significance of these genetic lesions in NHL and discuss their possible use as clinico-prognostic markers.

ACTIVATION OF DOMINANTLY ACTING ONCOGENES

I. Oncogene activation by chromosomal translocations

Non-random chromosomal translocations represent a distinctive feature of lymphoid neoplasia including NHL. These translocations frequently involve antigen receptor genes, immunoglobulin genes (Ig) in B-cells and T-cell receptor genes in T cells (2) and the use of antigen receptor gene probes has been instrumental in cloning the chromosomal breakpoint sequences, thus leading to the identification of the oncogenes involved in the translocations.

Translocations involving the c-myc oncogene. Probably the best characterized group of translocations in human neoplasia are the ones iuxtaposing the c-myc oncogene, on chromosome 8 (3), and the Ig genes on chromosome 2, 14 or 22. In the more frequent t(8;14) translocation, breakpoints located 5' and centromeric to c-myc lead to its translocation into the Ig heavy-chain (IgH) locus on chromosome 14 (4). In the less frequent t(2;8) and t(8;22) translocations, an Ig light-chain locus is translocated 3' and telomeric to the c-myc locus, which remains on chromosome 8 (5,6). Breakpoint sites on chromosome 8 are heterogeneous relative to the c-myc locus, and may occur within the first exon or intron, immediately (<3Kb) 5' to the c-myc promoter region or at an undefined distance (>100 Kb) 5' to the c-myc locus (7). In addition, on chromosome 14, both the J_H and switch region of the IgH locus may be involved in the translocation event (8). Several studies indicate that, in addition to the translocation event, all translocated c-myc alleles contain structural alterations in putative 5' regulatory sequences of the gene, which are either removed or mutated (9,10). The combination of the proximity of Ig transcriptional regulatory elements and the presence of these structural lesions is thought to lead to the deregulated expression of translocated c-myc alleles. Deregulated c-myc expression has been shown to contribute to the transformation of human B cells in vitro and to cause B cell lymphoma in vivo in transgenic animals (11,12). Transfection experiments of lymphoblastoid cell lines have shown that c-myc deregulation also causes phenotypic alterations of cell surface molecules, namely down-regulation of expression of the LFA-1 adhesion receptor (13). Since this molecule is involved in the adhesion of B cells to cytotoxic T cells, NK cells and vascular endothelia (14), its down-regulation by c-myc oncogene may be involved in the ability of tumor cells to escape immunosurveillance and metastatize.

t(14;18) and the bcl-2 oncogene. The bcl-2 gene was identified by molecular cloning of the t(14;18) reciprocal translocation (15, 16), which is the most frequent chromosomal abnormality in B-NHL, being present in virtually all cases of follicular-type as well as in a small fraction of diffuse large cell lymphomas (17,18 and below). Most of the chromosome 18 breakpoints lie within a restricted 2.8 Kb region in the bcl-2 gene known as the "major breakpoint region" (15,16); however, several minor breakpoint clusters have also been described (19,20). The bcl-2 gene does not belong to any known family of proto-oncogenes as it encodes a mitochondrial protein whose function is to increase the cell lifespan by preventing programmed cell death or "apoptosis" (21). Though transfected bcl-2 oncogenes appear to have only subtle effects on B cell growth and transformation in vitro (22), transgenic animals carrying an activated bcl-2 gene develop a pathology similar to that seen in human follicular lymphoma (23).

t(11;14) and the bcl-1 locus. The bcl-1 locus was originally identified as the breakpoint site on chromosome 11 of the t(11;14) (q13;q32) (24), resulting in the juxtaposition of the IgH locus on chromosome 14 to sequences from chromosome 11. Although the search for a transcriptional unit has been performed with probes spanning a region of approximately 60 Kb starting from the major translocation cluster site (25), no

Table I. Lesions associated with NHL.

	bcl-2	c-myc	bcl-1	p53	Rb1
Low Grade					
Small Lymphocytic	-	-	50 % *	-	4 %
Follicular, small cell	90 %	-	-	-	-
Follicular, mixed	90 %	-	-	-	-
Intermediate Grade					
Follicular, large cell	90 %	-	-	-	-
Diffuse, small cell	-	20 %	-	-	30 %
Diffuse, mixed	-	20 %	-	-	30 %
Diffuse, large cell	-	20 %	-	-	20 %
High Grade					
Immunoblastic	-	20 %	-	-	NT
Lymphoblastic	NT	NT	NT	NT	NT
Small non cleaved cell	-	100 %	-	30 %	10 %
"Transformed"**	90 %	10 %	-	-	NT

* This frequency refers only to mantle zone lymphoma (ref. 27)
** NHL which have undergone histological progression from a follicular to a diffuse pattern
NT, not tested

oncogene could be identified. Recently, however, it has been shown that a gene located approximately 200 Kb from the bcl-1 locus is overexpressed in lymphoproliferative disorders showing bcl-1 rearrangements (26). This gene, termed PRAD1, displays homology to cyclins (26), a family of genes involved in the regulation of cell cycle. Among NHL, bcl-1 rearrangements are found at high frequency in tumors derived from the follicular mantle zone (termed as intermediate lymphocytic lymphoma or centrocytic lymphoma) (27); in all the other types of NHL, bcl-1 rearrangements are rare (28) and the sporadic cases reported to be positive may represent diagnostic mismatches. In contrast to previous reports (29), we could not detect any bcl-1 rearrangements in a panel of 100 cases of B-cell chronic lymphocytic leukemia (B-CLL; our unpublished results).

10q24. In 7 % of low-grade NHL and, less frequently, in intermediate and high-grade lymphomas, band 10q24 is involved in a heterogeneous group of aberrations including translocations with the IgH locus (30) . Recently, the molecular cloning of the breakpoint in a B-cell NHL case has led to the identification of a candidate protooncogene for chromosomal abnormalities involving band 10q24 in B cells (31). This gene, which has been named lyt-10, is related to the NF-kB/rel family of transcription factors (32), and, as an effect of the translocation, is deprived of a regulatory region lying at the 3' end of the gene (31). **Curiously, this gene** appears to be distinct from the one reported to be involved in 10q24 aberrations arising in T-cell malignancies (33). The frequency of involvement of the lyt-10 gene in NHL pathogenesis is currently under investigation.

II. Oncogene activation by point mutation.

. Oncogene activation by point mutations is best exemplified in human neoplasia by the case of the ras family of genes , whose mutations at specific codons induce constitutional activation by removing the ability to hydrolize GTP (34). Though the N-, K-, and H-RAS genes are a frequent target in a variety of human tumors (35), including some types of B-cell derived malignancies (36,37), they do not represent a common lesion in NHL, as demonstrated by a large study on more than 100 cases (36). Rather, RAS mutations in NHL appear to be restricted to AIDS-associated lymphomas, which arise in the immunocompromised host and represent very aggressive tumors characterised by an extremely poor prognosis (38). Interestingly enough, when comparing AIDS-associated NHL with lymphomas displaying similar hystologic pattern arising in the non-immunocompromised host, RAS mutations are detected only in the former (38).

LOSS/INACTIVATION OF TUMOR SUPPRESSOR GENES

Inactivation of both alleles, by either chromosomal loss or small mutations, is the feature defining the oncogenic conversion of a tumor suppressor gene (39). Though extensive surveys for loss of molecularly defined chromosomal regions (loss of heterozygosity) have not been performed in NHL, and the evidence of genetic losses is mainly restricted to the level of sensitivity of conventional cytogenetic techniques, the role of at least two tumor suppressor genes in lymphomagenesis is now well established. Recently, we and others have shown that gene loss/inactivation at both the p53 and Rb1 loci is a frequent event in NHL (40-42).

p53. The p53 locus spans around 20 kb and is made up by 11 exons, encoding a 53 kD nuclear phosphoprotein that appears to regulate negatively cell proliferation (reviewed in 43). Several types of human tumors display the monoallelic loss of the short arm of chromosome 17, the site of the p53 locus; in addition, it has been shown that the remaining p53 allele often harbors point mutations which are thought to inactivate the normal protein function (for review, see 43,44). Most mutations are missense mutations which are not randomly scattered along the gene, but rather cluster in four major hotspots within the coding region (exons 5 though 9) corresponding to evolutionarily conserved domains of the protein (43,44).

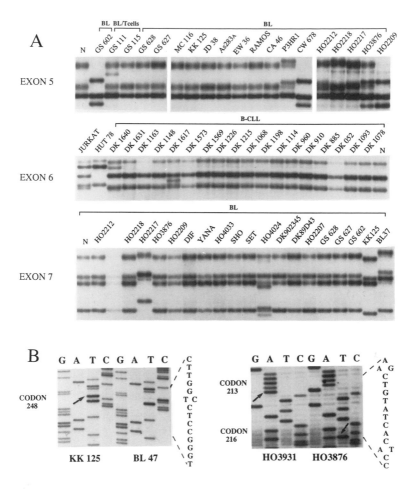

Fig.1.Analysis of p53 mutations in lymphoid malignancies by PCR-SSCP and PCR-direct sequencing. (A) PCR-amplified fragments corresponding to individual exons 5-9 were amplified from genomic DNA and further analyzed by the SSCP method. Representative samples for exons 5-7 are shown. Mutant cases were identified when bands different from the normal control (N) were detectable. (B) Direct sequencing of p53 mutations in NHL. Each mutation is matched to a control DNA. Arrows point to bands corresponding to mutated base pairs; the codon at which the mutation occurs is shown.

p53 mutations can be easily and rapidly detected by polymerase chain reaction (PCR)-single strand conformation polymorphism (SSCP) analysis (45), a technique that can detect single base pair mutant alleles of short stretches of genomic DNA as conformational changes after gel electrophoresis. The sensitivity of this technique is in the order of 1.5 x 10^{-2}, thus allowing the detection of mutations also in tumor samples with a low clonal representation

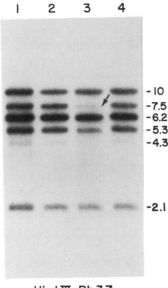

Hind III-Rb 3.7

Fig. 2. Southern Blot representing an example of partial deletion within the Rb1 locus in a case of NHL (lane 3). Genomic DNAs were digested with HindIII and probed with a 3.7 Kb EcoRI/EcoRI fragment from Rb1 cDNA. The size of each band is shown on the right.

(our unpublished observation). By the combination of the PCR-SSCP technique and PCR-direct sequencing (fig. 1), a large number of lymphoid tumors has been screened, showing that mutations in the p53 gene do not represent a general lesion in NHL (table I), but, rather, are specifically associated with Burkitt lymphoma and B-CLL (40).

Rb1. The Rb1 gene encodes a 105 kDa nuclear phosphoprotein which is widely expressed throughout different tissues of the body and is considered to act as a negative regulator of cell growth (reviewed in 46). Though initially associated with retinoblastoma, it is now clear that Rb1 inactivation plays a key role in the pathogenesis of several commonly occurring tumors (46). The molecular mechanisms of Rb1 inactivation are extremely heterogeneous, including complete loss of the locus, partial deletions, rearrangements or small splicing mutations (46). Given the variability in the inactivating lesions and the huge size of the locus (200 Kb; 27 exons), a combination of different technical approaches, including immunohystochemistry, protein fractionation, RFLP studies, Southern blot and PCR-SSCP, has to be used in order to obtain a precise estimate of the lesion. Preliminary results from our group would show that Rb inactivation is a frequent lesion in B-cell lymphomas (42). In particular, when studying high grade lymphomas in the HIV infected individual, 7/20 cases displayed lesions at the Rb1 locus (38).

ASSOCIATION OF DIFFERENT MOLECULAR LESIONS WITH SPECIFIC B-NHL HYSTOTYPES

The identification of the described lesions allows to determine their distribution among and within various NHL subtypes classified according to the Working Formulation (table I).

Low Grade lymphomas

Small lymphocytic lymphoma. Small lymphocytic lymphoma (SLL) represents a tumor of mature B cells which is usually characterized by an indolent clinical course. Though several studies had proposed an association of SLL with bcl-1 rearrangements (reviewed in 47), recent evidence would suggest that translocations involving bcl-1 are found at high frequency (50 %) uniquely in lymphomas arising from the mantle zone (27). Curiously, though SLL and B-CLL are considered to be different manifestations of the same disease, no p53 mutations could be detected in SLL, while present in a small fraction of B-CLL (40). It may be interesting to notice that a higher frequency of p53 alterations are observed in Richter's syndrome, which represents the evolution of B-CLL into a highly aggressive malignancy (40). Studies are in progress to define whether p53 mutations/loss have any prognostic value in the B-CLL tumor progression.

Follicular lymphomas. Follicular lymphomas display a specific hystologic pattern which is characterized by aggregates of neoplastic cells resembling normal germinal centres. Chromosomal translocations involving the bcl-2 oncogene are consistently detected at high frequency (80-90 %) in follicular lymphomas (17,18), independently of the single subtypes (small cleaved cell, mixed cell, large cell), some of which belong to the "intermediate grade" subset. Other oncogenes involved in lymphomagenesis (c-myc, p53, Rb1) do not appear to be altered in this type of NHL.

Intermediate Grade lymphomas

Diffuse lymphomas. Diffuse lymphomas, though further classified in various subtypes by the Working Formulation (table I), can be grouped together as they share common clinical features. Little is known about the molecular pathogenesis of diffuse lymphomas; however, a certain number of these tumors display c-myc translocations (20 %; ref. 48) and Rb1 inactivation (10-30 %; fig. 2; ref. 42). As in follicular lymphomas, p53 is never involved (40). Though previous reports had shown bcl-2 involvement in a small fraction of diffuse lymphomas (17,18), recent evidence would suggest that diffuse NHL carrying a t(14;18) represent the transformation of follicular lymphomas into a more aggressive tumor (49), while bcl-2 rearrangements are never detected in de novo diffuse lymphomas (49).

<u>High Grade lymphomas</u>

    <u>Small non-cleaved cell lymphoma (Burkitt's lymphoma).</u> Burkitt's lymphoma (BL) is a highly aggressive B-cell malignancy of childhood which epidemiologically is distinguished in an endemic and a sporadic type, the former being prevalent in Africa, Papua and New Guinea, the latter occurring at low frequency in North America and Europe. In virtually all cases of BL c-myc deregulation occurs as an effect of chromosomal translocation or point mutations in regulatory regions of the gene (4,9,10). Considering the t(8;14), the endemic type of BL is predominantly associated with breakpoints at an undefined distance (> 100 Kb) 5' to the c-myc locus on chromosome 8 and within or in the proximity of the J_H region on chromosome 14 (7,8); conversely, in the sporadic type, as well as in HIV-associated BL, the translocation involves sequences within or immediately 5' (< 3 Kb) to c-myc on chromosome 8 and sequences within the IgH switch regions on chromosome 14 (7,8,50).

    The role of an activated c-myc in the pathogenesis of BL must also be seen in the context of other lesions which contribute to the development of this malignancy. The Epstein-Barr Virus, present in virtually all cases of endemic type BL and 30 % of cases of sporadic BL, is likely to play an important role (51). More recently, a role is being established for the loss/inactivation of p53 (fig. 1), observed in more than 30 % of cases of BL as well as in its leukemic counterpart known as B-cell L_3-type acute lymphoblastic leukemia (40). Intriguingly, within the spectrum of NHL, p53 lesions appear to be specifically associated with the BL type which also carries an activated c-myc (table I). The possible cooperative role of these two oncogenes in BL pathogenesis is currently under study.

    <u>Immunoblastic lymphomas.</u> The pathogenesis of this highly aggressive lymphoma is still largely unclear. c-myc translocations are found in 20 % of the cases and Rb1 inactivation seems to be a candidate frequent lesion in these tumors when arising in the HIV-infected individual, while p53 loss/inactivation does not appear to be involved (38).

SUMMARY AND PERSPECTIVES

    The complexity of the pathogenesis of lymphoid malignancies is reflected by the accumulation of multiple genetic lesions in the same tumor. Such complexity is best exemplified by the case of AIDS-associated NHL, in which single tumors have been shown to harbour up to four different molecular lesions (38). The total number of genetic lesions detected in NHLs is presently limited by the previous identification of specific oncogenes; it is reasonable to think that additional lesions will become relevant, once the responsible locus has been identified. Ongoing efforts are focusing on identifying the oncogenes or tumor suppressor genes involved in breakpoints involving specific regions of chromosomes 1, 9 and in deletions of the long arm of chromosome 6, which represent well established NHL-associated cytogenetic abnormalities (52,53).

The type and frequency of genetic lesions clearly varies even within the various types of NHL classified according to the Working Formulation (table I), suggesting that tumors which are presently undistinguishable based on phenotype may in fact be distinguishable based on pathogenetic mechanisms. Thus, studies on the identification and distribution of genetic lesions in NHL may provide the framework for a novel classification of these malignancies of potential clinical significance. In breast carcinoma, for example, a precise correlation has emerged between the presence of neu oncogene amplification and the patient's outcome (54). While in NHL comprehensive prognostic studies at the molecular level are still missing, recent cytogenetic evidence (52,53) has clearly demonstrated that breaks on both arms of chromosome 1 as well as at 6q21-q25 are associated with a poor prognosis. The identification of the loci involved in these abnormalities may prove valuable in providing molecular markers to be used at the bedside.

ACKNOLEDGMENTS

Work described in this chapter was supported by National Institutes of Health grants CA-44029 (to R.D.F.), EY06337 and CA40236 (to D.M.K.) . G.G. is partially supported by Gigi Ghirotti Foundation. P.B. is supported by a fellowhip from the Associazione Italiana Ricerca sul Cancro (A.I.R.C.).

REFERENCES

1) National Cancer Institute sponsored study of classifications of non-Hodgkin's lymphomas. Summary and description of a working formulation for clinical usage. (1982) Cancer 49 : 2112-2135

2) Kirsch IR, Morton CC, Nakahara KK, Leder P (1982) Science 216 : 301-303

3) Dalla-Favera R, Martinotti S, Gallo RC, Erikson J, Croce CM (1982) Proc Natl Acad Sci USA 79 : 7824-7827

4) Dalla-Favera R, Bregni M, Erikson J, Patterson D, Gallo RC, Croce CM (1983) Science 219 : 963-967

5) Hollis GF, Mitchell KF, Battey J, Potter H, Taub R, Lenoir GM, Leder P (1984) Nature 307 : 752-755

6) Davis M, Malcom S, Rabbits TH (1984) Nature 308 : 286-288

7) Pelicci PG, Knowles DM, Magrath I, Dalla-Favera R (1986) Proc Natl Acad Sci USA 83 : 2984-2988

8) Neri A, Barriga F, Knowles DM, Magrath I, Dalla-Favera R (1988) Proc Natl Acad Sci USA 85 : 2748-2752

9) Cesarman E, Dalla-Favera R, Bentley D, Groudine M (1987) Science 238 : 1272-1275

10) Murphy JP, Neri A, Richter H, Dalla-Favera R, in preparation

11) Lombardi L, Newcomb EW, Dalla-Favera R (1987) Cell 49 : 161-170

12) Adams JM, Harris AW, Pinkert CA, Corcoran LM, Alexander WS, Cory S, Palmiter RD, Brinster RL (1985) Nature 318 : 533-538

13) Inghirami G, Grignani F, Sternas L, Lombardi L, Knowles DM, Dalla-Favera R (1990) Science 250 : 682-686

14) Springer TA, Dustin HL, Kishimoto TK, Marlin SD (1987) Annu Rev Immunol 5 : 223-252

15) Bakshi A, Jensen JP, Goldman P, Wright JJ, McBride WO, Epstein AL, Korsmeyer SJ (1985) Cell 41 : 899-906

16) Tsujimoto Y, Finger LR, Yunis J, Nowell PC, Croce CM (1984) Science 226: 1097-1099

17) Lipford E, Wright JJ, Urba W, Whang-Peng J, Kirsch IR, Raffold M, Cossman J, Longo DL, Bakshi A, Korsmeyer SJ (1987) Blood 70 : 1816-1823

18) Lee M-S, Blick MB, Pathak S, Trujillo JM, Butler JJ, Katz RL, McLaughlin P, Hagemeister FB, Velasquez WS, Goodacre A, Cork A, Gutterman JU, Cabanillas F (1987) Blood 70 : 90-95

19) Cleary ML, Galili N, Sklar J (1986) J Exp Med 164 : 315-320

20) Tsujimoto Y, Cossman J, Jaffe E, Croce CM (1985) Science 228 : 1440-1443

21) Hockenberry D, Nunez G, Milliman C, Schreiber RD, Korsmeyer S (1990) Nature 348 : 334-336

22) Nunez G, Seto M, Seremetis S, Ferrero D, Grignani F, Korsmeyer SJ, Dalla-Favera R (1989) Proc Natl Acad Sci USA 86 : 4589-4593

23) McDonnell TJ, Deane N, Platt FM, Nunez G, Jaeger U, McKearn JP, Korsmeyer SJ (1989) Cell 57 : 79-88

24) Tsujimoto Y, Yunis J, Onorato-Showe L, Erikson J, Nowell PC, Croce CM (1984) Science 224 : 1403-1406

25) Meeker TC, Grimaldi JC, O'Rourke R, Louie E, Juliusson G, Einhorn S (1989) Blood 74 : 1801-1806

26) Motokura T, Bloom T, Goo Kim H, Juppner H, Ruderman J, Kronenberg HM, Arnold A (1991) Nature 350 : 512-515

27) Williams ME, Meeker TC, Swerdlow SH (1991) Blood 78 : 493-498

28) Athan E, Foitl DR, Knowles DM (1991) Am J Pathol 138 : 591-599

29) Tsujimoto Y, Jaffe E, Cossman J, Gorham J, Nowell PC, Croce CM (1985) Nature 315 : 340-343

30) Offit K, Wong G, Filippa DA, Tao Y, Chaganti RSK (1991) Blood 77 : 1508-1515

31) Neri A, Chang CC, Lombardi L, Salina M, Corradini P, Maiolo AT, Chaganti RSK, Dalla-Favera R, submitted

32) Lenardo MJ and Baltimore D (1989) Cell 58 : 227-229

33) Hatano M, Roberts CWM, Minden M, Crist WM, Korsmeyer SJ (1991) Science 253 : 79-82

34) Barbacid M (1987) Annu Rev Biochem 56 : 779-827

35) Bos JL (1989) Cancer Research 49 : 4682-4689

36) Neri A, Knowles DM, Greco A, McCormick F, Dalla-Favera R (1988) Proc Natl Acad Sci USA 85 : 9268-9272

37) Neri A, Murphy JP, Cro L,Ferrero D, Tarella C, Baldini L, Dalla-Favera R (1989) J Exp Med 170 : 1715-1725

38) Ballerini P, Gaidano G, Inghirami G, Gong JZ, Saglio G, Knowles DM, Dalla-Favera R, manuscript in preparation

39) Stainbridge EJ (1990) Annu Rev Genet 24 : 615-617

40) Gaidano G, Ballerini P, Gong JZ, Inghirami G, Neri A, Newcomb EW, Magrath IT, Knowles DM, Dalla-Favera R (1991) Proc Natl Acad Sci USA 88 : 5413-5417

41) Ginsberg AM, Raffeld M, Cossman J (1991) Blood 77 : 833-840

42) Inghirami G, Corradini P, Gu W, Knowles DM, Dalla-Favera R, manuscript in preparation

43) Levine AJ, Momand J, Finlay CA (1991) Nature 351 : 453-456

44) Hollstein M, Sidransky D, Vogelstein B, Harris CC (1991) Science 253 : 49-53

45) Orita M, Suzuki, Y, Sekiya T, Hayashi K (1989) Genomics 5 : 874-879

46) Goodrich DW and Lee WH (1990) Cancer Surveys 9 : 529-554

47) Raffeld M and Jaffe E (1991) Blood 78 : 259-263

48) Ladanyi M, Offitt K, Jhanwar SC, Filippa DA, Chaganti RSK (1991) Blood 77 : 1057-1063

49) Athan E, Dalla-Favera R, Tarella C, manuscript in preparation

50) Subar M, Neri A, Inghirami G, Knowles DM, Dalla-Favera R (1988) Blood 72 : 667-671

51) Neri A, Barriga F, Inghirami G, Knowles DM, Neequaye J, Magrath IT, Dalla-Favera R (1991) Blood 77 : 1092-1095

52) Offit K, Jhanwar SC, Ladanyi M, Filippa DA, Chaganti RSK (1991) Genes, Chromosomes and Cancer 3 : 189-201

53) Offit K, Wong G, Filippa DA, Tao Y, Chaganti RSK (1991) Blood 77 : 1508-1515

54) Slamon DJ, Clark GM, Wong SG, Levin WJ, Ullrich A, McGuire WL (1987) Science 235 : 177-182

Role of *Src*-like protooncogenes in lymphocyte signaling

Tadashi Yamamoto

Institute of Medical Science, University of Tokyo, Tokyo, Japan

INTRODUCTION

Protein-tyrosine kinases can be divided into receptor-type kinases and nonreceptor-type kinases (or Src-like kinases). The Src-like kinases are generally associated with the internal portion of the plasma membrane, and may act as signal transducers in association with surface receptors that lack an intracellular catalytic domain (1,2). This concept was originally established by the observation that the Src-like kinase Lck is physically and functionally associated with T cell surface antigens CD4 and CD8, receptors for major histocompatibility complex molecules (3-5). Successively associations of the B cell antigen receptor and T cell antigen receptor with the Src-like kinases Lyn and Fyn, respectively, were also reported (6-8). However, the physiological substrates or targets of these Src-like kinases in receptor-mediated signalling have yet to be identified. Here we show that Fyn and Lyn are functionally involved in lymphocytes activation.

RESULTS

Activation of Lyn on mIgM cross-linking

WEHI-231 and Daudi cells are murine and human B-lymphoblastoid cells, respectively, and carry membrane-bound immunoglobulin M (mIgM) on their surface (9-12). Both lines behave as normal B cells in terms of initial biochemical events such as PI turnover, Ca^{2+} mobilization and tyrosine phosphorylation of proteins after mIgM cross-linking (9,10,13,14,15). The physical association of Lyn with mIgM (13) suggests that Lyn plays a role in mIgM-mediated signalling. This possibility was tested by incubating WEHI-231 cells with goat antibody to IgM (μ chain) for 1 min and measuring kinase activity of Lyn by immune-complex kinase assay using monoclonal antibody Lyn-8, which reacts with both murine and human Lyn. The cross-linking of mIgM resulted in about 2- to 3-fold increase in activity as measured by *in vitro* autophosphorylation (Fig. 1, A). The amount of Lyn protein immuno-precipitated with Lyn-8 did not increase during the incubation period (data not shown). Similar activation of the Lyn kinase was observed when splenic B cells of a Balb/c mouse were incubated with antibody to IgM (unpublished observation). Goat antibody to human IgG (γ chain) had no effect on the kinase activity of Lyn of WEHI-231 cells (Fig. 1, A). Curiously, however, the level of phosphorylation of enolase, which was added to the reaction mixture as an exogenous substrate, was not increased following antibody-mediated stimulation (unpublished observation). To test whether this discrepancy depended on the nature of the monoclonal antibody used, we examined the effect of mIgM cross-linking on Lyn kinase using the human B cell line Daudi and the monoclonal antibody Lyn-9, which is specific for human Lyn. One minute of mIgM cross-linking resulted in 4- to 5-fold increase of Lyn kinase activity, as measured by both *in vitro* autophosphorylation and phosphorylation of the exogenous substrate enolase (Fig. 1, B), with no change in the amount of Lyn (data not shown). Antibody to murine IgG (γ chain) had no effect on Lyn kinase activity (Fig. 1, B). Again, the level of phosphorylation of enolase was not affected in the assay using Lyn-8 immunoprecipitates (data not shown). Thus Lyn-8 seems to inhibit mIgM-mediated activation of Lyn kinase to phosphorylate enolase *in vitro* by some unknown mechanism. From the above findings, we conclude that the cross-linking of mIgM activates Lyn kinase.

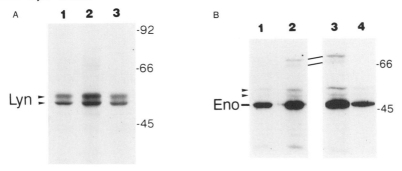

Figure 1, Activation of Lyn kinase after mIgM crosslinking. (A) Murine WEHI-231 B cells (3×10^6) were incubated in the absence (lane 1) or presence of antibody to murine IgM (lane 2) or human IgG (lane 3) and lysed with TNE buffer. The lysates were subjected to immunoprecipitation with monoclonal antibody Lyn-8 and immune-complex kinase assay without enolase. (B) Human Daudi B cells (3×10^6) were incubated in the absence (lane 1) or presence of antibody to human IgM (lanes 2 and 3) or murine IgG (lane 4) and lysed with TNE buffer [1% (vol/vol) Nonidet P-40/50 mM Tris-HCl, pH 8.0/20 mM EDTA/0.2 mM sodium orthovanadate with aprotinin at 10μg/ml]. The lysates were subjected to immunoprecipitation with monoclonal antibody Lyn-9 and immune-complex kinase assay with enolase. Positions of Lyn (arrowheads), enolase (Eno), and protein standard markers ($M_r\times10^{-3}$) are indicated.

In parallel with the mIgM-mediated activation of Lyn kinase, about 70 kDa phosphoproteins were detected after mIgM cross-linking of both WEHI-231 cells (Fig. 1, A, lane 2) and Daudi cells (Fig. 1, B, lanes 2 and 3, and Fig. 2). This suggests that the stimulation induces association of Lyn with these 70 kDa proteins in B cells. Since faint bands of about 70 and 75 kDa proteins were also detected before the treatment (Fig. 2, lane 5), very small amount of these molecules may be associated before the stimulation.

Tyrosine phosphorylation of cellular proteins reaches a peak within 2 to 15 min after cross-linking of the B cell antigen receptor (13,14,16). Moreover, the level of tyrosine phosphorylation of PLC-γ of Daudi cells is increased 2-fold within 90 seconds and 4-fold (the peak activity) within 30 min after mIgM cross-linking (10). We analyzed the time course of the activation of Lyn kinase after mIgM cross-linking (Fig. 2). The *in vitro* kinase activity of Lyn was increased 2- to 3-fold within 15 seconds, and 4- to 5-fold (the peak activity) within 1 min of the cross-linking. This rate of activation is rapid enough to explain up-regulation of cellular tyrosine phosphorylation, which suggests that Lyn transduces at least part of the mIgM-mediated signals to intracellular targets. Veillette *et al.* showed that only Lck co-immunoprecipitated with CD4 is activated after CD4 cross-linking, while non-CD4 associated Lck is not activated (3). We have previously shown that Lyn is co-immunoprecipitated with mIgM from 1% digitonin lysates of B cells (13). However, the level of Lyn co-immunoprecipitated with mIgM after mIgM cross-linking is very low, because mIgM changed rapidly (more than 90% within 1 min) to a digitonin-insoluble form after the stimulation (unpublished observation). Thus, it was difficult to evaluate the kinase activity of Lyn co-immunoprecipitated with mIgM after the cross-linking.

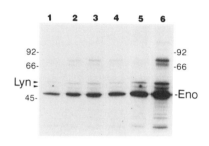

Figure 2, Rapid activation of Lyn kinase by mIgM crosslinking. Daudi cells (3×10^6) were incubated with antibody to IgM for various times and then the kinase activity of Lyn was examined as described for Fig. 1B. Lane 1, untreated control; lane 2, 15-sec incubation; lane 3, 1-min incubation; lane 4, 5-min incubation; lanes 5 and 6, longer exposure of lanes 1 and 3, respectively. Positions of Lyn, enolase (Eno), and protein markers ($M_r \times 10^{-3}$) are indicated.

Above data together with our prliminary data that PI3-kinase is tyrosine phosphorylated and activated by Lyn support the notion that Lyn is an intracytoplasmic signal transducing molecule of B cell antigen receptor. Another line of study has suggested that CD45, membrane-bound tyrosine phosphatase, regulates mIgM-mediated signalling (17). It is important to examine possible functional or physical interactions between Lyn and CD45, G-proteins, GAP, PLC-γ or another regulators/substrates.

Possible involvement of Fyn in T cell activation

T lymphocytes recognize antigens that are physically associated with self major histocompatibility complex (MHC) molecules on the surface of the antigen presenting cells. The antigen-MHC receptor on T cells (TCR) is a heterodimer of covalently linked two polypeptides chains designated α and β. The function of αβ heterodimer requires its association with the CD3 complex that consists of at least five distinct integral membrane proteins, γ, δ, ε, ζ, and η chains. The response of T cells to the antigen-major MHC complex consists of a series of cellular events collectively called T cell activation, which includes activation of protein-tyrosine kinase and induction of a number of genes whose products are essential for the function of T cells. Among these the *fos* and *IL-2* genes are of particular interest because of their pivotal roles in regulation of T cell growth. We and others have previously shown that Fyn is associated with T-cell antigen receptor (18 and our unpublished data). Then we analyzed if Fyn is involved in T cell antigen receptor-mediated transactivation of the *fos* and *IL2* genes.

Transactivation of the c-fos promoter through SRE by active T-Fyn kinase

To examine the effect of the Fyn kinase on c-*fos* expression in T cells, we first cloned the cDNA of active T-*fyn* that encoded the thymus-type Fyn protein (19) with Phe-528 instead of Tyr-528 (T-fynF) into the expression plasmid (pβAM) containing chicken β-actin promoter. A reporter plasmid (c-*fos*CAT) containing the bacterial *CAT* gene for the chloramphenicol acetyl transferase downstream to the 445-bp 5'-flanking sequence of the c-*fos* gene (20) was used as a monitor for its transcriptional activity. These plasmids were cotransfected into Jurkat T cells. As shown in Figure 3, transfection of T-fynF enhanced the c-*fos* promoter activity by 5.5-fold as compared with that of the control plasmid.

Since the c-*fos* promoter contains SRE, TRE and CRE, we examined which element was responsible for the T-fynF-mediated stimulation of the c-*fos* promoter. The result clearly showed that T-fynF greatly stimulated SRE while less stimulation of TRE and CRE was observed by the expression of T-fynF (Fig. 3, and data not shown). The degrees of stimulation of SRE, TRE, and CRE by T-fynF were about 18-, 4-, and 3-folds as compared with control experiments. These data showed that the c-*fos* promoter was activated by T-fynF primarily through SRE.

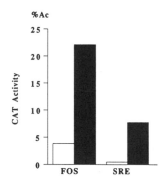

Figure 3, Activation of c-*fos*CAT and SRECAT by cotransfection with active T-*fyn* cDNA to Jurkat cells. c-*fos*CAT or SRECAT plasmid was cotransfected with pβAM vector plasmid or pβT*fyn*F plasmid into Jurkat cells. Then the CAT activity of the cell lysates were measured, the activity being shown as the percentage of conversion of chloramphenicol into acetylated form. Open and solid bars represent CAT activity with pβAM and pβT*fyn*F, respectively.

Transactivation of IL-2 promoter by active T-Fyn

Within an hour of binding of the ligands to the TCR/CD3 complex, T cell begins transcribing the *IL-2* gene. In order to examine whether the Fyn kinase is involved in the TCR-mediated transactivation of the *IL-2* gene, a reporter plasmid (*IL-2*CAT) in which the promoter region of the *IL-2* gene was ligated upstream to the CAT gene was prepared. Cotransfection of T-fynF construct in which *fyn* cDNA coding for T-fynF was ligated under the chimeric promoter of SV40 and HTLV-1 promoters (SRα) into Jurkat cells showed only a slight activation of CAT activity of *IL-2*CAT as compared with that from cells cotransfected with the vector plasmid (unpublished data). This result indicates that elevated tyrosine kinase activity alone is not sufficient for the induction of the *IL-2* gene.

Then T cells cotransfected with *IL-2*CAT and the T-fynF construct were stimulated by TPA and/or mitogens such as ConA or phytohemaglutinin (PHA). The effect of the elevated kinase activity of T-fynF on *IL-2* promoter was remarkable when the transfectants were treated with a combination of TPA and ConA (data not shown). The *IL-2* promoter activity with T-fynF was about eight times greater than that without TfynF. Next, we cross-linked the CD3 molecule by anti-CD3ε antibodies on the surface of the Jurkat T cells that had been transfected with the *IL-2*CAT and T-fynF constructs. When TPA treatment was accompanied with the CD3 cross-linking, significant transactivation of the *IL-2* promoter was observed. Treatment with TPA and anti-CD3 without exogenous T-fynF had little effect (data not shown). These data showed that active Fyn kinase could transactivate the *IL2* promoter in combination with extracellular mitogenic stimulants of the T cells.

DISCUSSION

Recently, Burkhardt *et al.* reported that Blk and Fyn were activated after either mIgM or mIgD cross-linking by using rabbit polyclonal antibodies to these Src-like kinases (21). Thus, Lyn, Blk and Fyn may share pathway(s) in B cell antigen receptor-mediated signalling, and comparison of their role(s) in the signalling should be performed. They also reported that mIgM cross-linking did not result in reproducible changes in activity of Lyn. The apparent discrepancy between this and our observations may reflect differences of antibodies and/or cells used in the experiments.

Our data also provide evidence that Fyn plays an important role in transactivation of c-*fos* and *IL-2* promoter when the cells received mitogenic stimulation that mimiced TCR-mediated activation. This suggests a critical importance of Fyn in transducing membrane signals into more distal cellular events. This is consistent with the observation that overexpression of Fyn in thymocytes of transgenic mice results in a augmented TCR response (22).

The CD3 ζ chain has been implicated in T-cell signalling via TCR. We have evidence that Fyn interacts with the CD3 ζ chain (unpublished data). This interaction would be a prerequisite for tyrosine phosphorylation of ζ by the Fyn kinase. The ζ chain thus phosphorylated might in turn recruit SH2-containing signalling molecules such as PLC-γ , GAP, and PI3-kinase as insulin receptor-associated p185, which becomes tyrosine phosphorylated by the insulin receptor upon insulin stimulation, interacts with PI3-kinase (23). Recently a molecule termed Zap was shown to interact with the ζ chain (24). This interaction might be important to specify T-cell specific response to antigenic activation. It would be important to examine if Zap can be a target of Fyn kinase, although data in ref. 41 do not support this in particular condition. It is also required to identify a target protein of Lyn and/or Blk in B lymphocytes which would specify B cell response to antigenic activation.

References
1. Cooper JA (1990) In; Kemp BE, Alewood PF (eds) Peptides and Protein Phosphorylation. CRC. Boca Raton, Florida, pp85-113

2. Semba K, Toyoshima K (1990)In: Sikora K and Carney D (eds) Genes and Cancer. John Wiley & Sons, Chichester, pp73-83

3. Veillette A, Bookman MA, Horak EM, Samelson LE, Bolen J B (1989) Nature 338: 257-259

4. Barber EK, Dasgupta JD, Schlossman SF, Trevillyan JM, Rudd CE (1989) Proc Natl Acad Sci USA 86: 3277-3281

5. Abraham N, Miceli MC, Parnes JR, Veillette A (1991) Nature 350: 62-66

6. Hatakeyama M, Kono T. Kobayashi N, Kawahara A, Levin SD, Perlmutter RM, Taniguchi T (1991) Science 252: 1523-1528

7. Samelson LE, Phillips AF, Luong ET, Klausner RD (1990) Proc Natl Acad Sci USA 87: 4358-4362

8. Cooke MP, Abraham KM, Forbush KA, Purlmutter RM (1991) Cell 65: 281-291

9. Mizuguchi J, Tsang W, Morrison SL, Beave MA, Paul WE (1986) J Immun137: 2162-2167

10. Carter RH, Park DJ, Rhee SG, Fearon DT. (1991) Proc Natl Acad Sci USA 88: 2745-2749

11. Boyd AW, Schrader JW (1981) J Immun 126: 2466-2469

12. Adams VE, Lieberman R, Sandlund J, Kiwanuka J, Novikovs L, Kirsch I, Hollis G, Magrath IT (1989) Cancer Res 49: 3235-3241

13. Yamanashi Y, Kakiuchi T, Mizuguchi J, Yamamoto T, Toyoshima K (1991) Science 251: 192-194

14. Gold MR, Law DA, DeFranco AL (1990) Nature 345: 810-813

15. Skolnik EY, Margolis B, Mohammadi M, Lowenstein E, Fischer R, Drepps A, Ullrich A, Schlessinger J (1991) Cell 65: 83-90

16. Campbell M, Sefton BM (1990) EMBO J 9: 2125-2131

17. Justement LB, Campbell KS, Chien NC, and Cambier JC Science 252: 1839-1842

18. Samelson LE, Philips AF, Luong ET, Klausner RD (1990) Proc.Natl Acad Sci USA 87: 4358-4362

19. Cooke MP, and Perlmutter RM (1989) New Biologist 1: 66-74

20. Deschamps J, Meijlink F, Verma IM (1985) Science 230: 1174-1177

21. Burkhardt AL, Brunswick M, Bolen JB, and Mond JJ (1991) Proc Natl Acad Sci USA 88: 7410-7414

22. Cooke MP, Abraham KM, Forbush KA, Perlmutter RM (1991) Cell 65: 281-291

23. Shoelson SE, Chattrrjee S, Chaudhuri M, White MF (1992) Proc Natl Acad Sci USA 89: 2027-2031

24. Chan AC, Irving BA, Fraser JD, Weiss A (1991) Proc Natl Acad Sci USA 88: 9166-9170

Suppression of cell-cell adhesion by v-*src* transformation: A molecular base of tumor invasion and metastasis

Michinari Hamaguchi

Research Institute for Disease Mechanism and Control, Nagoya University School of Medicine, Nagoya, Japan

STRUCTURAL FEATURES OF V-SRC GENE PRODUCT

The structure and functions of p60^{v-src}, the oncogene product of Rous sarcoma virus (RSV), has been extensively studied (1). p60^{v-src} is a tyrosine-specific kinase located primarily at the cytoplasmic face of the plasma membrane of transformed cells. p60^{v-src} has three domains functionally distinguished (1). Kinase activity is localized in the carboxy terminal half and this region is called catalitic domain. Area closed to the catalitic domain are called moduratory domain, which contains a sequence called SH2 that directly bind to phosphotyrosine residues of target proteins and appears to regulate the recognition of substrates. Fourteen amino acids of amino terminal end are called membrane binding domain which is necessary for stable association of p60^{src} with plasma membrane. After the translation p60^{src}, myristic acid attaches covalently to its amino terminus. Nonmyristylated forms of p60^{v-src}, which have deletion or mutation in the membrane binding domain, are active protein kinase but defective in myristylation and membrane association (2). Studies with these nonmyristylation mutants clearly demonstrated that membrane association of p60^{v-src} is required for cell transformation (2,3). In other words, critical substrates for cell transformation are phosphorylated in the vicinity of the plasma membrane. Several well characterized proteins such as p36, vinculin, ezrin, glycolitic enzymes and enolase are known as substrates of p60^{v-src}. However, these proteins are phosphorylated in nonmyristylation mutants-infected cells, suggesting that their phosphorylation is not critical for cell transformation (3). Thus, critical substrates are yet to be identified.

IDENTIFICATION OF POTENTIAL SUBSTRATES OF p60^{v-src} BY USE OF ANTIPHOSPHOTYROSINE ANTIBODY

To identify phosphotyrosine-containing proteins in RSV-transformed cells systematically, we examined the utility of antiphosphotyrosine antibody (4). We found that more than 90% of phosphotyrosine-containing proteins in RSV-transformed cells were recognized by our antibody, and more than 30 protein bands were detected by immunoblotting with this antibody. To analyzed subcellular localization of major phosphotyrosine-containing proteins, RSV-transformed cells were fractionated by hypotonic disruption followed by differential centrifugation, and phosphotyrosine-containing proteins in each fraction were analyzed by immunoblotting. We found that most of phosphotyrosine-containing proteins were found to be localized in membrane-matrix fraction, a structure associated with plasma membrane and resistant to extraction with nonionic detergents (5). Subcellular localization of phosphotyrosine-containing proteins in RSV-transformed cells was further studied by immunoelectron microscopic technique. We found most of phosphotyrosine-containing proteins in RSV-transformed cells were associated with cytoskeletal structure localized in submembranous region. These results suggest that membrane-matrix functions as

a place where ealy events of transformation take place, and
proteins localized in this structure could be the critical
substrates.

CADHERIN-MEDIATED CELL ADHESION AND TRANSFORMATION

Given these findings, we focused on cadherin (6). Cadherins
are a group of glycoprotein that mediates Ca^{2+}-dependent
homophilic adhesion among cells (Fig. 1). We think that studies
on cell-cell interaction in oncogenesis are important to clarify
the molecular mechanism of tumor invasion and metastasis.
Cadherins are expressed in tissue specific manner and primarily
mediate stable cell-cell association. Thus, suppression of
cadherin-fuction could be crucial for tumor cell invasion.

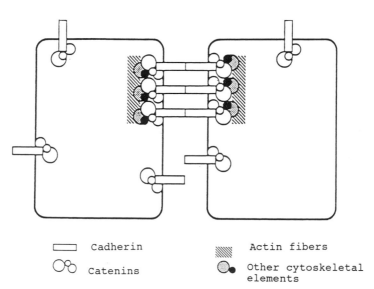

☐ Cadherin   ▨ Actin fibers

◐◐ Catenins   ◑● Other cytoskeletal
                       elements

Association of cadherin-catenin complex
with cytoskeleton in zonula adherens

Cadherin-dependent cell aggregation activity in normal and transformed chicken embryonic fibroblasts which express N-cadherin were examined. We found Ca^{2+}-dependent cell adhesion was strongly suppressed in RSV-transformed cells, but was well maintained in nonmyristylation mutant-infected cells. In cells infected with temperature sensitive mutant of RSV, tsNY68, suppression of cell adhesion was observed in temperature-dependent manner. Although the suppression of cell adhesion was observed in RSV-transformed cells, expression and intracellular transport of cadherin were not inhibited by transformation. Then, we examined catenins, which associate with cadherin and appear to regulated cadherin-function (Fig. 1). In transformed cells association of cadherin with catenins was not disturbed. We found, however, cadherin-catenin complex was phosphorylated at their tyrosine residues in RSV-transformed cells. Moreover, in tsNY68-infected cells, tyrosine phosphorylation of cadherin and catenins were temperature-dependent.

PHOSPHORYLATION OF CADHERIN-CATENINS COMPLEX IN HUMAN CANCER CELLS

We have been screening the phosphotyrosine-level in various human cancer cells. We found certain types of cells derived from human gastric cancer had aberrantly elevated levels of phosphotyrosine (7), and one of these cells showed phosphorylation of E-cadherin and catenins. Thus, tyrosine phosphorylation of cadherin-catenin complex indeed takes place in human cancer cells and may play a role in tumor invasion and metastasis of human cancer (8). Further characterization of cadherin-function and tumor invasion and metastasis of human cancer cells is currently underwent.

ACKNOWLEDGEMENTS

Some part of these studies were underwent in collaboration with Dr. Masatoshi Takeichi. I am greatly indebted to Dr. Hidesaburo Hanafusa and Dr. Yoshiyuki Nagai for their continuous encouragement and support. I am grateful to Dr. Jean Wang for the gift of bacteria that express v-abl-encoded protein.
I thank Miss Yukano Ohnishi and Miss Fumiko Yamauchi for their excellent assistance. This work was supported by a Gant-in-Aid for Cancer Research from the Ministry of Education, Science and Culture, Japan.

REFERENCES

1. Jove R, Hanafusa H (1987) Ann. Rev. Cell Biol. 3:31-56

2. Cross FR, Garber EA, Pellman D, Hanafusa H (1984) Mol. Cell. Biol. 4:1834-1842

3. Kamps MP, Buss JE, Sefton BM (1986) Cell 45:105-112

4. Hamaguchi M, Grandori C, Hanafusa H (1988) Mol. Cell. Biol. 8:3035-3042

5. Hamaguchi M, Hanafusa H (1989) Oncogene Res. 4:29-37

6. Hamaguchi M, Matsuyoshi N, Ohnishi Y, Goto B, Takeichi M, Nagai Y submitted

7. Takeshima E, Hamaguchi M, Watanabe T, Akiyama S, Kataoka M, Ohnishi Y, Xiao H, Nagai Y, Takagi H Jpn. J. Cancer Res. in press

8. Ohnishi Y, Hamaguchi M in preparation

Discussion

Dr Masami Hirano (Fujita Health University, Aichi, Japan): Do you have any evidence to suggest that *fyn* and *lyn* are oncogenes?

Dr Yamamoto: Not in the human tumor. One experiment in our laboratory, however, showed that *fyn* can be oncogenic by mutation. We made a retrovirus containing normal *fyn* cDNA. When this *fyn* virus was injected into chickens, there was no tumor initially, but after a few months, tumors appeared. We recovered the virus from those tumors and sequenced the *fyn* gene, in which we found deletion of *fyn* in the SH2 domain. So by mutation, *fyn* can be activated as an oncogene.

Dr Masahide Takahashi (Nagoya University, Nagoya, Japan): Do you have any evidence that c-*erb*B-2 overexpression in tumor cells is associated with an increase in tyrosine kinase activity? Also, what kind of substrate for the c-*erb*B-2 gene have you identified?

Dr Yamamoto: In answer to your first question, we have not looked for this in human tissue. If you overexpress the normal *erb*B-2 protein in the NIH3T3 cell line, there is high tyrosine kinase activity. That can be done by Western blotting with antiphosphotyrosine antibody. Thus overexpression of *erb*B-2 seems to be active, but this is probably because we are doing it in cell culture, due to the stimulatory factor present in calf serum. The possible target we have identified is PI3-kinase. Association of PI3-kinase is not so important here, but tyrosine phosphorylation of PI3-kinase can occur if the *erb*B-2 kinase is active. We do not know about GAP or PLCγ. We have no direct evidence, but believe that PILγ and GAP also become tyrosine phosphorylated. The reason is in *erb*β-2 transformed cells, the GTP-bound form of *ras* accumulates, suggesting that GAP may be activated. Also in *erb*β-2-transformed cells, the TRE enhancer is up-regulated, which is inhibited by protein kinase C inhibitor, suggesting that C kinase is involved. This suggests also that PLCγ is involved in the signaling pathway.

Dr Toshitada Takahashi (Aichi Cancer Center, Nagoya, Japan): Dr Hamaguchi, when you stain cadherin with antibody, do you find any difference between transformed and untransformed cells?

Dr Hamaguchi: Some data have already been published by Dr Benjamin Geiger's group, Department of Chemical Immunology, the Weizmann Institute of Science, Rehovot, Israel. In normal cells, cadherin forms clusters, resulting in a tight junction known as the zona adherens. However, in RSV-transformed cells, the zona adherens are absent. Cadherin is distributed diffusely on the cell surface, so one can see the difference in pattern between these 2 cell types.

Dr Wen-Hwa Lee (University of Texas Health Science Center, San Antonio, Texas,

USA): You showed in 3 different transformed cells that this protein was phosphorylated. Which tyrosine kinase is the kinase that normally regulates these cadherins, in terms of phosphorylation? Your data seem to suggest that different types of phosphotyrosine kinases can phosphorylate cadherins in the cell.

Dr Hamaguchi: This may be possible but we did not examine it.

Dr Masao Seto (Aichi Cancer Center, Nagoya, Japan): Both Dr Della-Favera and Dr Hamaguchi showed that oncogene introduced into cells down-regulates the function of the adhesion molecule. Are there any data on how these molecules are down-regulated?

Dr Dalla-Favera: The theme of transformation down-regulating adhesion is an evolving theme. I believe that there are several studies showing that different transforming genes regulate different adhesion molecules. More directly, there are also genes that are deleted which appear to be related to adhesion, typically in colon cancer. More specifically related to c-*myc*, in lymphoid cells, *myc* family members, ie, c-*myc* and N-*myc* both seem to down-regulate the LFA-1 adhesion receptors. Other transforming genes in the same cells, *ras*, *BCL2,* and c-*myb* do not do that. The mechanism is quite obscure; *myc* is supposed to be a transcriptional regulator. I believe the target sequences have now been identified also. However, 2 of the 3 genes that have been identified as regulated by c-*myc*, namely LFA-1 and the plasminogen activator inhibitor 1 (PAI-1) are regulated by c-*myc* posttranscriptionally. Obviously, one possibility is that *myc* regulates another gene transcriptionally which in turn regulates LFA-1 and PAI-1 or that *myc* can work at different levels than we think, ie, transcriptionally and posttranscriptionally.

Dr Hamaguchi: Dr Masatoshi Takeichi's group, at the Department of Biophysics, Faculty of Science, Kyoto University, Kyoto, has reported that in certain types of human gastric cancer, expression of E-cadherin is clearly suppressed. It gives the cell more invasive and metastatic ability. It is also interesting how, for example, *ras* or *myc* nontyrosine kinase type oncogenes affect cadherin function. We are currently studying this.

Dr Lee: There are 3 *src* oncogenes that readily produce cancer in chickens, but I have not heard anything about any human cancer caused by *src*. Can you explain this? It also occurs in reverse; retinoblastoma occurs in humans, but there is no known chicken retinoblastoma caused by retinoblastoma gene inactivation.

Dr Yamamoto: We looked for many human tumors to determine whether the *src* gene is amplified or overexpressed, but we could not find any. There is a report that in colon cancer, tyrosine kinase activity of the *src* protein is activated, not due to overexpression. That may be functioning for tumor progression. I do not have any data about the amplification or overexpression of *src* family members, although receptor type kinases are often overexpressed in human tumors. Possibly involvement of *src* kinase is just a change in the specific activity.

Dr Hamaguchi: We are studying many human cancer cell lines and human cancer tissues in the hope of identifying activated *src* using antiphosphotyrosine antibody. We detected this in some types of human gastric cancer cell lines and also in certain types of esophageal cancer tissue, we detected elevated levels of phosphotyrosine. Unfortunately we did not obtain conclusive data that *src* is actually activated in these cells or tissues. In the case of gastric cancer cell lines, however, we found 2 different mechanisms. We examined the effect of the serum or growth factor on these cell lines with elevated levels of phosphotyrosine, and one type of cell line showed no dependency on the serum stimulation. On the other hand, another type shows clear dependency. We believe tyrosine kinase is involved in human cancer immortalization or transformation, and that sometimes it could be of the growth factor receptor type and another type could be of the nonreceptor type. We are trying to identify which tyrosine kinase is involved in these cell lines.

Dr David P. Lane (University of Dundee, Dundee, Scotland, UK): The absence of mutations in the T cell lymphomas is a surprising observation given the frequent occurrence in so many other tumors. Do you have any feeling as to why that particular tumor type might not use that gene?

Dr Dalla-Favera: I do not have any particular explanation, but I want to stress again that even in B cell lymphoma it is quite rare. It is just Burkitt lymphoma p53 that has mutated. The most frequent non-Hodgkin lymphoma is follicular lymphoma and that never displays inactivation of p53.

Dr Hirano: Dr Dalla-Favera, you showed that the c-*myc* oncogene is related not only to oncogenesis, but also to the biological or possibly clinical behavior of the tumor cells. Among the many patients you have studied, were there any genetic lesions that may be related to the morphologic changes in non-Hodgkin lymphoma?

Dr Dalla-Favera: I do not know, but certainly the pattern is developing that there are essentially 2 growth types of non-Hodgkin lymphoma if you look at it from a molecular lesion point of view. There is a low-grade lymphoma, including all the follicular lymphoma, to the intermediate grade, according to the working formulation, that seems to be associated with *BCL2* activation and never has p53 or RB mutation or loss. In the middle of the intermediate grade category, there are diffuse lymphoma, high grade, Burkitt, and non-Burkitt, those are variable levels of *myc* activation, RB inactivation, and p53 activation only in Burkitt. So those seem to be the major categories biologically. One may speculate that those are completely different pathways of transformation and that has less to do with the final phenotype of the tumor.

Dr Lee: Why does v-*src* cause tumors in chickens so readily? In many humans with very early cancer we find the c-*src* gene expressed, but there is no activation of the c-*src* gene that causes cancer.

Dr Yamamoto: I think that in the chicken system, activation of *src* can induce some target genes that may activate *myc* immediately after *src* activation. That pathway may not be present in the mammalian cells.

Dr Dalla-Favera: Are we sure that *src* is never involved in human tumors? The mechanism may be subtle. We did not know anything about the involvement of p53 mutations in many types of human cancer until the gene was sequenced completely by Dr Bert Vogelstein's group at the Oncology Center, Johns Hopkins University, Baltimore, Maryland. Many researchers had looked at the rearrangements and never suspected anything. I would suggest that there could be mutation of *src* in some tumors. Second, I think an oncogene may be active biologically under certain experimental conditions, but still may not be accessible to accidents in vivo. So it may not just be the biological function that determines oncogenicity, but a number of complex factors, of which how an oncogene can be hit may be one. For example, all the family of *myc* genes are expressed in lymphoid cells. Under experimental conditions, they all act the same way, ie, they can transform B cells. Nevertheless, only c-*myc* is involved in rearrangements with the immunoglobulin genes, possibly due to its chromosomal location—or the overall configuration of the locus which makes it more prone to translocation.

II. CANCER THERAPY BASED ON PHARMACOLOGY

Drug resistance

The P-glycoprotein multidrug resistance transporter limits successful therapy of childhood tumors: Possible circumvention by chemosensitizers

Helen S.L. Chan, Paul S. Thorner, George Haddad, Gerrit Deboer, Victor Ling

Department of Pediatrics, Divisions of Hematology/Oncology and Immunology and Cancer, Department of Pathology, The Hospital for Sick Children, Division of Clinical Trials and Epidemiology, Toronto-Bayview Regional Cancer Center, Division of Molecular and Structural Biology, Department of Medical Biophysics, The Ontario Cancer Institute, The University of Toronto, Toronto, Ontario, Canada

INTRODUCTION

Failure of cancer chemotherapy is a significant problem which could be due to pharmacokinetic factors, host factors, sanctuary sites, tumor biology, and drug resistance.[1] The best characterized mechanism of drug resistance is classical multidrug resistance (MDR) mediated by P-glycoprotein (P170).[2] This protein causes cross-resistance to structurally unrelated anticancer drugs by functioning as an ATP-dependent plasma membrane transporter, removing vinca alkaloids, podophyllotoxins, cytotoxic antibiotics and anthracyclines from cancer cells.[3] Human tumors generally express increased amounts of P170 without *mdr*1 gene amplification, probably due to alterations of regulation of expression at transcriptional, translational or post-translational levels.[4] Although high levels of P170 have been described in many human tumors, the evidence that these levels affect the outcome of chemotherapy often remains inconclusive.[5-13] In this study, we tested sequentially biopsied tumor samples in three childhood malignancies that were extensively treated with chemotherapy. We found strong correlations between any detected P170 and poor outcome, and conversely between absence of P170 and long-term survival in patients. We conclude that the expression of P170 appears to be an important factor in limiting the success of chemotherapy. Thus, it appears that these tumors may be good candidates for anticancer drug therapy combined with a chemosensitizing agent capable of reversing P170-related MDR.

MATERIAL AND METHODS

Study Population

The study population included 30 cases of childhood soft tissue sarcoma (rhabdomyosarcoma and undifferentiated sarcoma) treated at a single institution from 1980-1988, 67 cases of neuroblastoma, treated from 1964-1989, and 62 cases of osteogenic sarcoma, treated from 1980-1989. Sequential tumor samples obtained at diagnosis and at different timepoints as clinically indicated during the course of treatment were available for study, and the medical records were reviewed.

Soft Tissue Sarcoma

The soft tissue sarcomas were staged, and prognostic factors and responses to therapy evaluated according to Intergroup Rhabdomyosarcoma Study (IRS) criteria.[14] They included 8 Group I, 3 Group II, 14 Group III, and 5 Group IV tumors. The conventional prognostic factors evaluated included age, gender, tumor size, stage, and histology.[15] Ages under 1 and over 7 years, females, pretreatment lymphocyte counts less than $2x10^9/L$, tumor sizes 5 cm or greater, Groups III and IV, parameningeal head and neck, extremity, torso, intrathoracic sites, and alveolar histology were associated with an unfavorable prognosis; ages between 1 and 7 years, males, lymphocyte counts $2x10^9/L$ or greater, tumor sizes less than 5 cm, Groups I and II, orbital, nonparameningeal head and neck, pelvic, paratesticular sites, and embryonal and undifferentiated histology, a more favorable prognosis.[15] Treatment consisted of chemotherapy with vincristine, dactinomycin, cyclophosphamide, ifosfamide, and/or etoposide,[14-16] surgical resection and radiation according to IRS guidelines.[14]

Neuroblastoma

The neuroblastomas were staged, and prognostic factors and responses to therapy evaluated according to the International Criteria.[17] There were 2 Stage I, 21 Stage II, 17 Stage III, 19 Stage IV, and 8 Stage IVS tumors. The conventional prognostic factors evaluated included age, stage, urinary vanillylmandelic acid (VMA):homovanillic acid (HVA) ratio, serum ferritin, Shimada classification of histology, and N-*myc* oncogene copy numbers.[18,19] Neuron-specific enolase, tumor karyotype, and DNA ploidy were not available for study.[20-22] Ages 2 years or older, Stages III and IV, VMA:HVA ratio less than 1, ferritin greater than 150µg/L, unfavorable Shimada histology, and N-*myc* gene copies of three or greater were associated with an unfavorable prognosis; ages less than 2 years, Stages I and II, VMA:HVA ratio of 1 or greater, ferritin 150 µg/L or less, favorable Shimada tumor histology, and N-*myc* gene copies less than three, a more favorable prognosis. Stage IVS tumors can have prognoses ranging from moderately favorable to unfavorable.[18, 23] Treatment consisted of primary surgical resection for localized Stages I and II tumors. Treatment consisted of chemotherapy with vincristine, cyclophosphamide, doxorubicin, dacarbazine, cisplatinum and/or teniposide, surgical resection and radiation for nonlocalized Stages III and IV tumors, and allogeneic or autologous bone marow transplantation for Stage IV tumors.[25-27] Despite these intensive therapies, the survival rate of Stage IV neuroblastoma is currently still below 15%.[27] Nonlocalized Stage IVS tumors in infants were generally treated with less intensive therapy.[23, 28]

<u>Osteogenic Sarcoma</u>

The osteogenic sarcomas were staged, and prognostic factors and responses to therapy evaluated according to American Joint Committee on Cancer criteria and published guidelines.[29-31] They included 2 Stage I, 56 Stage II, no Stage III, and 4 Stage IV tumors. The conventional prognostic factors evaluated included tumor size, grade and metastatic status. DNA ploidy was not available for study.[32] Tumor sizes 10 cm or greater, poor or lack of differentiation, and metastases were associated with an unfavorable prognosis; tumor sizes less than 10 cm, moderate or good differentiation, and absence of metastases, a more favorable prognosis. More favorable sites (jaw) and types (surface variants), and unfavorable sites (head, torso, pelvis) and types of tumors (multicentric, postradiation and Paget's disease-related) were absent in this study.[31] Treatment consisted of chemotherapy with methotrexate, vincristine, bleomycin, cyclophosphamide, actinomycin D, cisplatinum, doxorubicin, ifosfamide, and/or etoposide, surgical resection (amputation or limb-salvage procedure), and radiation if surgery was not feasible.[33]

<u>P-Glycoprotein Determination and Interpretation of Results</u>

A previously described multilayer immunoperoxidase method was used for determinations of P-glycoprotein in 62, 194, and 313 formalin-fixed tissue sections and bone marrow biopsies of soft tissue sarcoma, neuroblastoma and osteogenic sarcoma, respectively.[34,35] Two murine monoclonal antibodies, C219 (*mdr1* gene and *mdr2/mdr3* genes-specific) and C494 (*mdr1* gene-specific) were used, and normal mouse ascites IgG, as controls.[36,37] C494 is specific for the only isoform of P170 (*mdr1*) that confers MDR in human tumors in gene transfection experiments.[37] P170-negative SKOV3 parental cells, and 5 MDR human ovarian carcinoma cell lines with 8-, 16-, 64-, 510- and 1000-fold enhanced resistance to vincristine relative to drug-sensitive SKOV3, were used as controls to allow semiquantitative grading of 5 levels of increased P170 from 1+ to 5+.[34,38] This method has been determined to be as sensitive as northern blot analysis, more sensitive than conventional western blot analysis, and allows measurements of P170 within single cells to provide an assessment of tumor heterogeneity.[34,35]

<u>Statistical Analysis of Results</u>

The patients with all 3 types of tumors were divided into P170-positive and negative groups, according to whether the protein was detectable in tumor biopsies. P170 status at diagnosis was used for analysis of outcome in neuroblastoma and osteogenic sarcoma, but overall expression of the protein was used in the case of soft tissue sarcoma because the patient numbers were small. Response rates in the 2 groups were compared by Fisher's exact test, and relapse-free and survival durations were estimated by Kaplan-Meier life-tables.[39] Logrank analysis was used to determine whether P170 expression directly, and with adjustment for conventional prognostic factors, had a significant impact on relapse and death.[40] Two-sided statistical tests were used throughout for analysis of results.

RESULTS

Overall, immunohistochemical staining with C219 and C494 reproducibly detected P170-positive and negative samples in replicate experiments, and mouse ascites IgG controls were negative. Three observers concurred in their interpretation of positive and negative samples, without knowing the response to treatment. Negative samples contained no P170-positive cells, and positive samples contained at least 20%. Several important observations were made.[35] Therapeutic failures which were originally P170-negative became positive at relapse, in contrast to successfully treated tumors which remained consistently negative. All initially P170-positive tumors remained positive at relapse. Each relapse saw an increase in the number of positive cells, and an increase in their P170 levels, as did metastatic compared to primary tumors. Although it is beyond the scope of this report to correlate P170 levels with intensity of chemotherapy, and with degree of tumor differentiation, we did observe higher levels of the protein in more heavily treated later relapses compared to earlier biopsies, and in tumor cells that appeared to be more primitive compared to those that were differentiated. Considerable heterogeneity of P170 expression was observed in every positive tumor, both with respect to P170 levels in different cells, and the numbers of positive cells in different tumors. Yet, an equally unfavorable outcome was apparent in cases with small numbers of cells expressing high levels of P170, as in cases with larger numbers of cells expressing lower levels of the protein.

Overall, 13% (4/30) of soft tissue sarcomas were initially P170-positive in Groups II, III and IV, but not in Group I tumors.[35] The incidence of P170-positivity increased to 31% at posttreatment. About 19% (13/67) of neuroblastomas were initially P170-positive, with a striking 63% (12/19) in Stage IV, 6% (1/17) in Stage III, and none in Stages I, II and IVS tumors. The incidence of P170-positivity increased to 43% post-chemotherapy in nonlocalized tumors. About 44% (27/62) of osteogenic sarcomas were initially P170-positive, with 100% (4/4) in metastatic, and 40% (23/58) in non-metastatic tumors. The incidence of P170 positivity increased to 47% at posttreatment.

In all 3 types of tumors, there was a strong association between a less favorable response to chemotherapy and increased P170 expression. In soft tissue sarcoma, a complete response rate of 80% in the P170-negative group was superior to 55% in the positive group. In nonlocalized neuroblastoma, a complete response rate of 84% in the initially P170-negative group was superior to 46% in the positive group (P=0.023, Fisher's exact test). Similarly, in osteogenic sarcoma, a favorable response rate ($\geq$90% tumor necrosis) of 48% in the initially P170-negative group was superior to 17% in the positive group (P=0.030, Fisher's exact test). Even more striking were the consistently strong correlations between

94

detected P170 and poor outcome, and conversely between absence of P170 and long-term survival in patients with all 3 types of tumors. For instance, in soft tissue sarcoma, the actuarial relapse-free rate of 95% in the P170-negative group was superior to 0% in the positive group (P=0.0018, logrank analysis with stratification by stage and site). In nonlocalized neuroblastoma, the actuarial relapse-free rate of 78% in the P170-negative group was superior to 0% in the positive group (P=0.0011, logrank analysis with stratification by stage and age). Similarly, in osteogenic sarcoma, the actuarial relapse-free rate of 94% in the P170-negative group was superior to 4% in the positive group (P<0.00005, logrank analysis with stratification by tumor size, grade and metastatic status). Kaplan-Meier curves were used to compare the probability of remaining relapse-free and surviving in the P170-negative and positive groups. The actuarial survival rates in the P170-negative groups were statistically significantly superior to the P170-positive groups with soft tissue sarcoma, nonlocalized neuroblastoma and osteogenic sarcoma. These findings are summarized in Figure 1. The details of logrank analysis and the prognostic factors stratified for are beyond the scope of this report[35] (Chan et al, unpublished data). The outcomes are likely to remain durable because of the prolonged followup (median of 5.5, 5.5 and 5.7 years, respectively, for living patients with soft tissue sarcoma, neuroblastoma and osteogenic sarcoma).

Fig. 1A

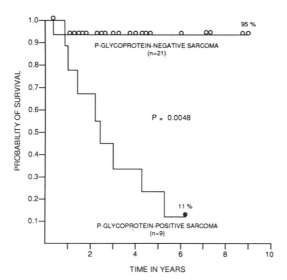

Fig. 1B

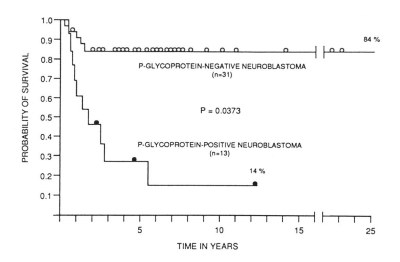

Fig. 1C

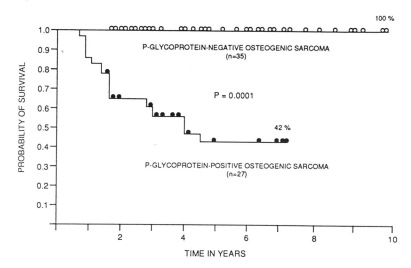

Fig. 1 Kaplan-Meier curves of the probability of surviving in P-glycoprotein-positive versus negative: (A) soft tissue sarcoma, (B) nonlocalized neuroblastoma, and (C) osteogenic sarcoma. The P values are from logrank analysis with stratification for the previous prognostic factors described.

96

DISCUSSION AND CONCLUSIONS

In these studies, significant proportions of soft tissue sarcoma, neuroblastoma and osteogenic sarcoma were P170-positive at diagnosis, as were those tumors that failed treatment.[35] Increased P170 expression was predominantly observed in advanced rather than localized tumors. A strong correlation was observed between any detected P170 and poor outcome, and conversely between absence of increased P170 and long-term survival in patients. Thus, expression of P170 appears to be an important factor in limiting the success of chemotherapy in these 3 childhood malignancies.

The multilayer immunohistochemistry employed in this study allowed retrospective analysis of sequential archival tumor samples from each patient during the course of disease. The information on evolution of P170 expression was crucial for correlation with the long-term outcome of therapy. These longitudinal studies were more valuable than horizontal studies performed at a single timepoint, which were often inconclusive as to whether the levels of P170 detected were prognostic of the durability of response to chemotherapy.[5-12] We were able to address some of the key issues raised in an editorial on the clinical relevance of MDR.[13] First, P170 expression predicted the response to chemotherapy and the outcome of patients. Second, any detected P170 proved clinically relevant to the ability of tumor cells to survive chemotherapy. However, two other issues needed to be emphasized. Studies of different types of tumors have still to be performed, since the prognostic impact of P170 expression identified for soft tissue sarcoma of childhood, neuroblastoma, and osteogenic sarcoma might not be broadly applicable to all chemotherapy-treated malignancies. Additionally, although P170 expression at diagnosis had considerable prognostic significance, the amount of protein could change during the course of treatment. These changes have such profound implications on the subsequent outcome of therapy that continuous surveillance of all followup tumor biopsies is crucial. What is currently at stake is the potential for early detection of nonresponsive disease. This may have important therapeutic significance, since it is now recognized that a group of compounds known as "chemosensitizers" are able to reverse the MDR phenotype *in vitro*.[10,41] Thus, it would appear that the tumors in which it has been shown that the P170 transporter limits successful treatment might be the ideal candidates for the use of chemosensitizers to reverse MDR to anticancer chemotherapy.

ACKNOWLEDGMENTS

Supported by grants from National Cancer Institute of Canada (H. Chan, V. Ling) and Public Health Service Grant CA37130 from National Institutes of Health (V. Ling). H. Chan is a Research Scientist of the National Cancer Institute of Canada.
We thank Dr. H. Yeger for N-myc studies, and Drs. M.L. Greenberg, S.S. Weitzman and

H. Solh for allowing us to study their patients.

REFERENCES

1. Chan HSL, Erlichman C (1991) In: MacLeod SM, Radde IC (eds) Textbook of Pediatric Clinical Pharmacology. 2nd edition. Mosby-Year Book, Inc, St. Louis, Chapter 31 (in press)

2. Gerlach JH, Kartner N, Bell DR, *et al* (1986) Cancer Surv 5:25

3. Gerlach JH, Endicott JA, Juranka PF, *et al* (1986) Nature (London) 324:485

4. Chabner BA, Fojo A (1989) J Natl Cancer Inst 81:910

5. Bell DR, Gerlach JH, Kartner N, *et al* (1985) J Clin Oncol 3:311

6. Gerlach JH, Bell DR, Karakousis C, *et al* (1987) J Clin Oncol 5:1452

7. Ma, DDF, Davey RA, Harman DH, *et al* (1987) Lancet 1:135

8. Goldstein LJ, Galski H, Fojo A, *et al* (1989) J Natl Cancer Inst 81:116

9. Bourhis J, Bénard J, Hartmann O, *et al* (1989) J Natl Cancer Inst 81:1401

10. Dalton WS, Grogan TM, Meltzer PS, *et al* (1989) J Clin Oncol 7:415

11. Goldstein LJ, Fojo AT, Ueda K, *et al* (1990) J Clin Oncol 8:128

12. Noonan KE, Beck C, Holzmayer TA, *et al* (1990) Proc Natl Acad Sci USA 87:7160

13. Ling V (1989) J Natl Cancer Inst 81:84

14. Maurer HM, Beltangady M, Gehan EA, *et al* (1988) Cancer 61:209

15. Gehan EA, Glover FN, Maurer HM, *et al* (1981) Natl Cancer Inst Monogr 56:83

16. Miser JS, Kinsella TJ, Triche TJ, *et al* (1988) J Clin Oncol 5:1191

17. Brodeur GM, Seeger RC, Barrett A, *et al* (1988) J Clin Oncol 6:1874

18. Evans AE, D'Angio GJ, Propert K, *et al* (1987) Cancer 59:1853

19. Seeger RC, Brodeur GM, Sather H, *et al* (1985) N Engl J Med 313:1111

20. Zeltzer PM, Marangos PJ, Parma AA, *et al* (1983) Lancet 2:361

21. Christiansen H, Lampert F (1988) Br J Cancer 57:121

22. Look AT, Hayes FA, Nitschke R, *et al* (1984) N Engl J Med 311:213

23. Mancini AF, Rosito P, Vitelli A, *et al* (1984) Med Pediatr Oncol 12:155

24. O'Neill JA, Littman P, Blitzer P, *et al* (1985) J Pediatr Surg 20:708

25. Hayes FA, Green AA, Casper J, *et al* (1981) Cancer 48:1715

26. Green AA, Hayes FA, Hustu HO (1981) Cancer 48:2310

27. Philip T, Zuker JM, Bernard JL, *et al* (1991) J Clin Oncol 9:1037

28. D'Angio GJ, Evans AE, Koop CE (1971) Lancet 1:1046

29. Beahrs OH, Henson DE, Hutter RVP, Myers MH (eds) (1988) In: Manual for staging of cancer. 3rd edition. J.B. Lippincott, Philadelphia, pp 123

30. Taylor WF, Ivins JC, Unni K, *et al* (1989) J Natl Cancer Inst 81:21

31. Raymond AK, Chawla SP, Carrasco H, *et al* (1987) Semin Diag Pathol 4:212

32. Look AT, Douglass EC, Meyer WH (1988) N Engl J Med 318:1567

33. Rosen G, Caparros B, Huvos AG, *et al* (1982) Cancer 49:1221

34. Chan HSL, Bradley G, Thorner P, *et al* (1988) Lab Invest 59:870

35. Chan HSL, Thorner PS, Haddad G, *et al* (1990) J Clin Oncol 8:689

36. Kartner N, Everden-Porelle D, Bradley G, *et al* (1985) Nature (London) 316:820

37. Georges E, Bradley G, Gariepy J, *et al* (1990) Proc Natl Acad Sci USA 87:152

38. Bradley G, Naik M, Ling V (1989) Cancer Res 49:2790

39. Kaplan EL, Meier P (1958) J Am Stat Assoc 53:457

40. Peto R, Pike MC, Armitage P, *et al* (1977) Br J Cancer 35:1

41. Slater LM, Sweet P, Stupecky M, *et al* (1986) J Clin Invest 77:1405

Circumvention of multidrug resistance (MDR) and regulation of the MDR gene in response to environmental stimuli

Michihiko Kuwano, Kimitoshi Kohno

Department of Biochemistry, Oita Medical School, Oita, Japan

INTRODUCTION

Drug resistance, both intrinsic and acquired, remains a major clinical obstacle in chemotherapy of tumors in human. Acquisition of resistance to multiple anticancer agents such as vinca alkaloids, anthracyclines and epipodophyllotoxins is often correlated with enhanced expression of P-glycoprotein, a membranous glycoprotein with molecular weight of 170,000 coded by the MDR1 gene: P-glycoprotein catalyzes the outward efflux of drugs, resulting in reduced cellular accumulation of chemotherapeutic agents (1-3). P-glycoprotein or its structural MDR1 gene has been detected in tumor cells from patients with ovarian cancer, soft tissue sarcoma, acute leukemia, multiple myeloma, non-Hodgkin's lymphoma, and several other human tumors (4-5). Goldstein et al. (4) investigated the MDR1 mRNA levels in many types of human cancers, and proposed that the expression of MDR1 was associated with several intrinsically resistant cancers. They also observed the increased level of the MDR1 gene expression in certain cancers after chemotherapy, suggesting a correlation of the expression of the MDR1 gene with acquired drug resistance. In this study, we present our study on two projects – development of multidrug resistance (MDR) – reversal agents and regulation of MDR1 gene expression in response to environmental stresses.

CIRCUMVENTION OF DRUG RESISTANCE

To find a way to overcome MDR, a combination chemotherapy of anticancer agents and other agents which may block the drug efflux in MDR cells has been tested on drug-resistant tumor cells. Most of the second agents that can reverse MDR inhibit the photoaffinity labeling of gp170 by azidopine or a vindesine analog (6, 7). By targeting P-glycoprotein, Tsuruo et al. (8) have developed verapamil, a calcium channel blocker, which is a potent MDR-reversal agent. In our laboratory, we have also demonstrated that cepharanthine (a biscoclaurine alkaloid), retinyl palmitate, dipyridamole (persantin) and thioridazine among clinically used compounds could show drug-resistance reversing activities in vitro and/or in vivo (9-15).   We have also looked for MDR-reversing agents among about 100 newly synthetic compounds.   So far tested, a synthetic isoprenoid and two synthetic dihydropyridines are found to overcome drug-resistance.

Figure 1 shows structures of isoprenoid, solanesyl-dimetyl benzylethylenediamine (SDB-ethylenediamine) and verapamil.   SDB-ethylenediamine contains nine isoprene units and shows some similarity in the structure to verapamil, but this isoprenoid has no calcium channel blocking activity.   This isoprenoid has some unique properties.   It can dramatically potentiate bleomycin and other anticancer agents in vitro as well as in vivo against drug-sensitive and drug-resistant tumor cells (16-19).   It is lysosomotropic with cationic and amphipathic property which is specific in MDR-reversing agents including verapamil and cepharanthine (20-24).   Another interesting property of this isoprenoid is its MDR-reversing activity.   SDB-ethylenediamine can almost completely reverse drug-resistance to vincristine, vinblastine, Adriamycin, actinomycin D and daunomycin in MDR cell lines which express P-glycoproteins.   It enhances intracellular accumulation of combined anticancer agents, and binds specifically to the P-glycoprotein (25).

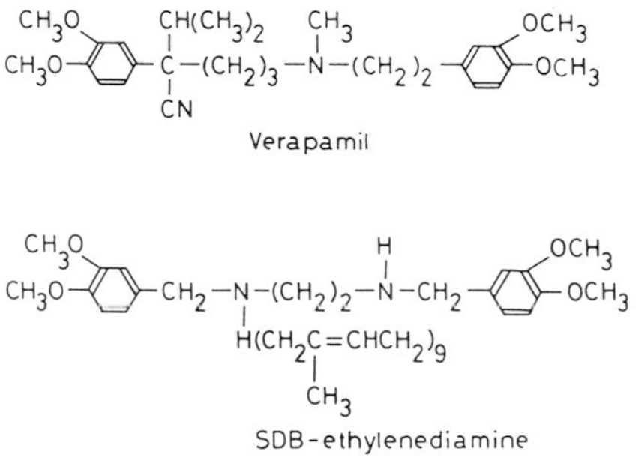

Fig. 1. Chemical structures of verapamil and SDB-ethylenediamine

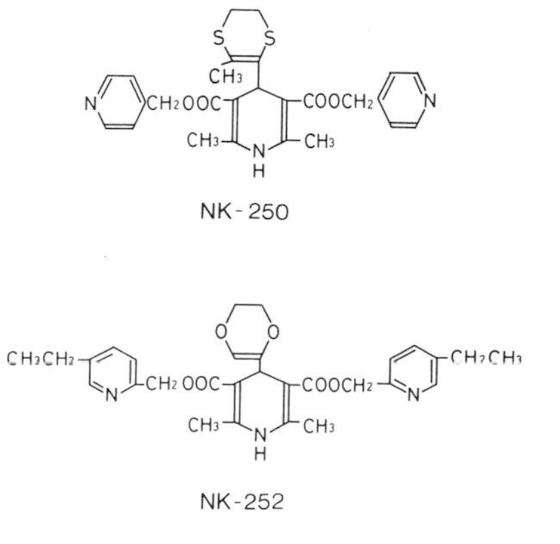

Fig. 2. Chemical structures of two dihydropyridine derivatives, NK-250 and NK-252.

Animal therapeutic experiments with mice carrying vincristine-resistant leukemia show a potent drug-resistance reversal activity by the isoprenoid. In comparison with vincristine alone, much better therapeutic effect is observed when combined with SDB-ethylenediamine.   Similar therapeutic effect of SDB-ethylenediamine are also observed by Suzuki and his colleagues (26, 27). This compound is expected to improve the clinical therapeutic effects.

We further anticipate that potent MDR-reversing agents with few side effects and low calcium channel blocking activity may be useful second agents in practical cancer chemotherapy. From this standpoint, dihydropyridine derivatives with few side effects have been screened to see if they could overcome MDR. In our laboratory, among the many dihydrophyridines tested, lipophilic 1,4-dihydrophyridines were found to effectively overcome MDR in vitro as well as in vivo (28-32). Representative 1,4-dihydrophyridine derivatives, NK-250 and NK-252 (Figure 2), which have low calcium channel blocking activity and very high affinity for gp170, could potentiate the antitumor activity of vincristine in mice inoculated i. p. with drug-resistant tumor cells (29). The p. o. administration of NK-250 and NK-252 is shown to potentiate the antitumor activity of MDR-related anticancer drugs in mice with drug-sensitive and drug-resistant tumor cells (30). These NK-250 and NK-252 can also potentiate the cytocidal action of another antitumor agent, etoposide, a semi-synthetic derivative of epipodophyllotoxin (31) and the anticancer activity of etoposide when the tumor cells and antitumor drugs were administered by various routes (30).

EXPRESSION OF MDR GENE

The physiological function of P-glycoprotein is still unknown, but the P-glycoprotein is supposed to function as an active efflux pump of drugs, hormones and other small molecules. In many MDR cell lines established in vitro, the MDR1 gene is either amplified (Figure 3A) or regulated through transcriptional activation (Figure 3B) (33). In normal tissues and cancer cells, expression of MDR1 gene is regulated at transcriptional levels as seen as in Figure 3B, but no amplification appears. Introduction of a 700-base genomic DNA from a site located at 10 kb upstream of the initiation site increases the transcription of the MDR1 promoter-CAT gene in adrenal or kidney cell lines. The 700-base sequences thus carry a tissue specific transcriptional enhancer (34).

On the other hand, MDR1 mRNA levels are increased in many types of human cancers and the enhanced expression of the MDR1 gene appears to be associated with several intrinsically drug resistant cancers (4). In several types of tumors, expression of MDR1 gene is further increased after cancer chemotherapy (4). Concerning MDR1 expression and drug sensitivity in human tumors, MDR-negative tumors are sensitive to cancer chemotherapy and MDR-positive tumors are refractory to cancer chemotherapy. However, MDR-negative tumors are changed into MDR-positive during chemotherapy and tumors are then refractory to the therapy. In this third case, we can expect that P-glycoprotein-positive cells

102

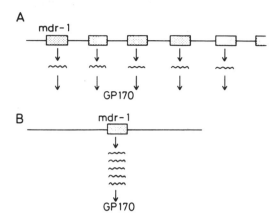

Fig. 3. Two types of multidrug resistance-1 (mdr-1) gene expression. Amplification type (A) and enhanced activation type of one copy of mdr-1 gene (B).

might be enriched during chemotherapy, maybe through selection mechanism as described before.   One possibility is that cancer cells may induce a self-defense mechanism to protect from anticancer agents, plausibly by MDR1 gene activation, and by pumping-out of drugs.   Consistent with this idea, administration of carcinogens and partial hepatectomy increase the expression of the MDR1 gene in the liver in animals.   Marino et al (35) have further demonstrated that increased levels of MDR1 mRNA in regenerating rat liver may result from a posttranscriptional event in response to the liver injury.   Heat shock or arsenite increases the expression of MDR1 gene in a human kidney cancer cell line (36) and some of the cytotoxic chemotherapeutic agetns increase MDR1 mRNA levels in rodent cells, but not in human cells (37).   Differentiating agents such as retinoic acid, sodium butylate and dimethyl sulfoxide can also enhance the MDR1 gene expression in a neuroblastoma cell line and human colon cancer cell lines. Various environmental stresses appear to regulate the expression of this drug-resistance gene.

We have previously demonstrated that the human MDR1 gene expression increases in response to anticancer agents when monkey kidney cell lines transfected with MDR1 promoter fused CAT gene are assayed in transient expression system (38).   Vincristine, daunomycin and adriamycin can activate MDR1 gene expression, and this drug-induced activation does not require the

103

presence of the MDR1 gene enhancer element.   We further construct human cancer cell lines which can show stable expression of CAT gene driven by the MDR1 gene promoter, and examine how the promoter is regulated in response to anticancer agents and other environmental stimuli.   Following exposure to a wide variety of cytotoxic agents including ethylmethane sulfonate, 4-nitroquioline-N-oxide, 5-azacytidine, cisplatinum, etoposide, aphidicolin and ultraviolet irradiation, the expression of CAT gene could be efficiently activated about 3-30-fold higher. Figure 4 demonstrates an example for MDR1 gene promoter activation: treatment of Kst-6 cells, carrying pMRDCAT1 with cisplatinum shows enhanced CAT activity (Kohno, K., Uchiumi, T., Sato, S., Miyazaki, M., Tanimura, H., Kuwano, M., paper submitted).   We also find that inhibitors of DNA topoisomerase I and II such as etoposide, teniposide and camptothecin could activate the MDR1 gene promoter (Sato, S., Uchiumi, T., Tanimura, H., Miyazaki, M., Kohno, K., Kuwano, M., paper submitted).   The promoter of MDR1 gene is found to be activated by other growth inhibitory signals including serum starvation and heat shock (manuscripts in preparation).   These data may propose that MDR1 gene activation by environmental stimuli is mediated through a SOS signal (Fig. 5).   One may expect that some tumor cells respond to anticancer agents, resulting in induction of P-glycoprotein and acquirement of a self-defense mechanism.   However, this model is highly speculative until further understanding of the underlying mechanism(s).

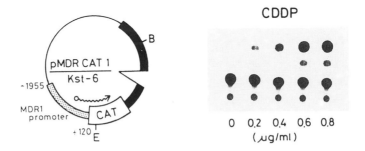

Fig. 4. Induction of CAT by cisplatinum in Kst-6 cells.   Kst-6 cell line is established after introduction of a construct of pMDRCAT1 containing 2kb MDR1 promoter and CAT gene.   Kst-6 cell are incubated for 48 hr with cisplatinum (CDDP) and the CAT assays are performd.

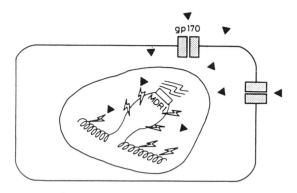

Fig. 5. A model of P-glycoprotein (gp170) induction by environmental stresses. environmental stresses (Δ)

ACKNOWLEDGEMENTS

We thank our colleagues, S. Sato, H. Takano, M. Miyazaki, T. Uchiumi, H. Tanimura, S. Sato, A. Kiue, K. Matsuo, M. Ono (Oita Medical School) and S. Akiyama (Kagoshima University School of Medicine) for collaboration of our present study. This study is supported by cancer research funds from Ministry of Education, Science and Culture of Japan, Ministry of Health and Welfare of Japan, Japanese Foundation for Multidisciplinary Treatment of Cancer, Osaka Cancer Research Fund and Pricess Takamatsu Cancer Research Fund.

REFERENCES

1. Gottesman, M. M., and Pastan, I. 1988.   J. Biol. Chem., 263: 12163- 12166.

2. Beck, W. T. 1987.   Biochem. Pharmacol., 36: 2879-2887.

3. Bradley, G., Juranka, P. F., and Ling, V. 1988.   Biochim. Biophy. Acta, 948: 87-128.

4. Goldstein , L J., Galski, H., Fojo, A., Willingham, M., Lai, S-L., Gazdar, A., Dirker, R., Green, A., Crist, W., Brodeur, M. G., Lieber, M., Cossman, J., Gottesman, M. M. and Pastan, I. 1989.   J. Natl. Cancer, Inst., 81: 116-124.

5. Nakagawara, A., Kadomatsu, K., Sato, S., Kohno, K., Takano, H., Akazawa, K., Nose, Y. and Kuwano, M. 1990.   Cancer Res., 50: 3043-3047.

6. Akiyama, S., Cornwell, M. M., Kuwano, M., Pastan, I. and Gottesman, M. M. 1988.   Molecul. Pharmacol., 33: 144-147.

7. Akiyama, S., Kuwano, M., Cornwell, M. M., Pastan, I. and Gottesman, M. M. 1988. In Cancer Chemotherapy: Challenges for the Future ed. by K. Kimura Excerpta Medica (Tokyo) 3: 26-29.

8. Tsuruo, T., Iida, H., Tsukagoshi, S. and Sakurai, Y. 1981. Cancer Res. 41: 1967-1973.

9. Nogae, I., Kikuchi, J., Yamaguchi, T., Nakagawa, M., Shiraishi, N. and Kuwano, M. 1987. Brit. J. Cancer 56: 267-272.

10. Shiraishi, N., Akiyama, S., Nakagawa, M., Kobayashi, M. and Kuwano, M. 1987. Cancer Res., 47, 2413-2418.

11. Komiyama, S., Matsui, K., Kudoh, S., Nogae, I., Kuratomi, Y., Saburi, Y., Asoh, K., Kohno, K. and Kuwano, M. 1989. Cancer, 63, 675-681.

12. Asoh, K., Saburi, Y., Sato, S., Nogae, I., Kohno, K. and Kuwano, M. 1989. Jpn. J. Cancer Res., 80: 475-481.

13. Kuwano, M., Nakagawa, M., Shiraishi, N., Yamaguchi, T., Kikuchi, J. and Akiyama, S. 1986. In Cancer Drug Resistance ed. by T. C. Hall. A. R. Liss, Inc., New York, 163-171.

14. Akiyama, S., Shiraishi, N., Kuratomi, Y., Nakagawa, M. and Kuwano, M. 1986. J. Nat. Cancer Inst. 76: 839-844.

15. Kuwano, M., Yamaguchi, T., Shiraishi, N., Nakagawa, M. and Akiyama, S. 1986. In Cancer Chemotherapy: Challenges for the Future ed. by K. Kimura. Excerpta Medica (Tokyo) 37-44.

16. Ikezaki, K., Yamaguchi, T., Miyazaki, C., Ueda, H., Kishie, T., Tahara, Y., Koyama, H., Takahashi, T. Fukawa, H., Komiyama, S. and Kuwano, M. 1984. J. Nat. Cancer Inst. 73: 895-901.

17. Yamaguchi, T., Ikezaki, K., Kishie, T. Tahara, Y., Koyama, H., Takahashi, T., Fukawa, H., Komiyama S., Akiyama, S. and Kuwano, M. 1984. J. Nat. Cancer Inst. 73: 903-907.

18. Nakagawa, M., Akiyama, S., Yamaguchi, T., Shiraishi, N., Ogata, J. and Kuwano, M. 1986. Cancer Res., 46: 4453-4457.

19. Yamaguchi, T., Nakagawa, M., Shiraishi, N., Yoshida, T., Kiyosue, T., Arita, M., Akiyama, S. and Kuwano, M. 1986. J. Natl. Cancer Inst., 76: 947-953.

20. Shiraishi, N., Akiyama, S., Kobayashi, M. and Kuwano, M. 1986. Cancer Lett. 30: 251-259.

21. Kuratomi, Y., Akiyama, S., Ono, M., Shiraishi, N., Shimada, T., Okumura, S. and Kuwano, M. 1986. Expt. Cell Res., 162: 436-448.

22. Akiyama, S., Shiraishi, N., Yoshimura, A., Nakagawa, M., Yamaguchi, T., Shimada, T. and Kuwano, M. 1987. Biochem. Pharmacol. 36: 861-868.

23. Shiraishi, N., Shimada, T., Hagino, Y., Kohno, K., Kobayashi, M., Kuwano, M. and Akiyama, S. 1988. Cancer Res. 48: 1307-1311.

24. Akiyama, S., Tomita, K. and Kuwano, M. 1875. Expt. Cell Res. 158: 192-204.

25. Akiyama, S., Yoshimura, A., Kikuchi, H., Sumizawa, T., Kuwano, M. and Tahara, Y. 1989. Molecul. Pharmacol., 36, 730-735.

26. Suzuki, H., Tomida, A. and Nishimura, T. 1990.   Jpn. J. Cancer Res. 81: 298-303.

27. Tomida, A. and Suzuki, H. 1990.   Jpn. J. Cancer Res., 81: 1184-1190.

28. Nogae, I., Kohno, K., Kikuchi, J., Kuwano, M., Akiyama, S., Kiue, A., Suzuki, K., Yoshida, Y., Cornwell, M. M., Pastan, I. and Gottesman, M. M. 1989. Biochem. Pharmacol., 38: 519-527.

29. Kiue, A., Sano, T., Suzuki, K. Inada, H., Okumura, M., Kikuchi, J., Sato, S., Kohno, K. and Kuwano, M. 1990.   Cancer. Res., 50: 310-317.

30. Kiue, A., Sano, T., Naito, A., Inada, H., Suzuki, K., Okamura, M., Sato, S., Takano, H., Kohno, K. and Kuwano, M. 1990.   Jpn. J. Cancer Res., 81: 1057-1064.

31. Kiue, A., Sano, T., Naito, A., Okamura, M., Kohno, K. and Kuwano, M. 1991. Brit. J. Cancer, 63: in press.

32. Watanabe, Y., Takano, H., Kiue, A., Kohno, K., and Kuwano, M. 1991. Anti-cancer Drug Design, 6: 47-57.

33. Kohno, K., Kikuchi, J., Sato, S., Takano, H., Saburi, Y., Asoh, K., and Kuwano, M. 1988.   Jpn. J. Cancer Res. 79: 1238-1246.

34. Kohno, K., Sato, S., Uchiumi, T., Takano, H., Kato, S., and Kuwano, M. 1990. J. Biol. Chem., 265: 19690-19696.

35. Mario, P., Gottesman, M. M., and Pastan, I. 1990.   Cell Growth & Differ., 1: 57-62.

36. Chin , K.- V., Tanaka, S., Darlington, G., Pastan, I., and Gottesman, M. M. 1990.   J. Biol. Chem., 265: 221-226.

37. Chin, K.- V., Chauhan, S. S., Pastan, I., and Gottesman, M. M. 1990. Cell Growth & Differ., 1: 361-365.

38. Kohno, K., Sato, S., Takano, H., Matsuo, K., and Kuwano, M., 1989.   Biochem Biophy. Res. Commun. 165: 1415-1421.

Discussion

Dr Takeo Fujimoto (Aichi Medical University, Aichi, Japan): Dr Chan, there is an age factor in the outcome of the neuroblastoma, which, under the age of 1 year is treatable, with a good prognosis. Have you found P-glycoprotein associated with infant neuroblastoma?

Dr Chan: Yes, we have found P-glycoprotein in the tumors of 4 infants under the age of 1 year at diagnosis and in 2 other infants at relapse; 4 have died, one has had several relapses, and one is still in remission at 2.3 years. In stage 4, 63% of the tumors are positive at diagnosis and all tumors that relapsed had acquired P-glycoprotein, as did the relapses in stages 3 and 4S. All cases positive for P-glycoprotein have relapsed except for one and 16 of 19 have died.

Dr Fujimoto: So under 1 year of age of the neuroblastoma, is P-glycoprotein still found?

Dr Chan: Yes. We have shown that despite stratification for age and stage, P-glycoprotein is observed and its prognostic value still holds true. There are still highly significant differences between the outcomes of therapy for the negative and positive groups for P-glycoprotein.

Dr Ryuzo Ueda (Aichi Cancer Center Research Institute, Nagoya, Japan): Recently, many laboratories have detected P-glycoprotein by the PCR method. Have you ever checked or have you compared data obtained by your staining method with those obtained by PCR detection?

Dr Chan: No. Ours is a retrospective study. However, Dr Igor B. Roninson, Department of Genetics, University of Illinois, Chicago, has commented that both our studies have arrived at the same point—his by using the PCR and mine by using a very sensitive immunohistochemical method. We may be looking at relatively small amounts of P-glycoprotein present on the tumor cells and whatever can be detected seemed to be relevant to the response to chemotherapy. The sensitivity of our immunohistochemical method has been confirmed in tumor cell lines with very low levels of P-glycoprotein.

Dr Atsuya Karato (National Cancer Center Hospital, Tokyo, Japan): Did you modify the dose of cyclosporin according to its concentration?

Dr Chan: No. Ours is a phase I/II trial where we escalated the dose of cyclosporin A for every 3 patients who tolerated it. We did not modify the dose of chemotherapy.

Dr Karato: Did you check the concentration of cyclosporin?

Dr Chan: Yes. All the profiles of cyclosporin A and its major metabolites are checked and we will ultimately be able to develop the concentration versus time peripheral compartment data for every treatment cycle for correlation with the response and toxicity.

Dr Ryuzo Ohno (Nagoya University, Nagoya, Japan): In Japan we can use antibody for P-glycoprotein, mainly MRK16, developed by Dr Takashi Tsuruo, University of Tokyo. Do you think that we could repeat your data using MRK16?

Dr Chan: I am sure it would be possible to use MRK16 for frozen sections of tumors in prospective studies, but I have no personal experience with it. Our method can be used in formalin-fixed tumors and we can do both retrospective and prospective studies. MRK16 does not work in formalin-fixed material. It is easier to establish that P-glycoprotein is relevant to the outcome of therapy in retrospective studies; then we can use this marker to predict prognosis. Prospective studies are now ongoing at our institution and other centers.

Dr Kuwano, have any of the agents that you proposed that might be useful been started in clinical trials in Japan?

Dr Kuwano: No. Isoprenoid is now in phase I studies in Japan. I do not know of any information from the clinical field.

Dr Nagahiro Saijo (National Cancer Center, Tokyo, Japan): Is the mechanism of sensitization of bleomycin affected by isoprenoids? Does it have some suppressing effect on bleomycin hydrolase, etc?

Dr Kuwano: Isoprenoid can potentiate bleomycin as remarkably in vitro as in vivo. Dr Hideo Suzuki, Institute of Applied Microbiology, University of Tokyo, has reported that isoprenoid could not inhibit bleomycin hydroxylase. Concerning the possibility of enhanced permeability of bleomycin by isoprenoid, we do not have a suitable assay system to determine the cellular permeability of bleomycin. The underlying mechanism for isoprenoid-induced potentiation of bleomycin appears to be different from that of P-glycoprotein, however.

Dr Saijo: Under very stressful conditions, such as anticancer drug treatment or heat shock, glutathione transferase or methylcyanate levels are also increased. Do you have any data similar to the *mdr* gene promotor as to these genes?

Dr Kuwano: Experiments to determine the stress-responsive sequence specificity of the *mdr*1 promoter are now in progress. We have recently found that heat shock stress activated the *mdr*1 promoter deleting the typical heat shock element. We do not know whether a common sequence between the *mdr*1 promoter and the glutathione-thiol transferase promoter exists or not.

Dr Ohno: Maybe in future, when we use drugs that overcome the resistance clinically, what will concern us is it that these agents may increase the toxicity of anticancer drugs to normal tissues. In your in vivo experiment, did the 2 compounds you used show any such adverse toxicity in animals?

Dr Kuwano: Yes. On one hand we know that the P-glycoprotein is expressed in normal tissues, on the other we are talking about the P-glycoprotein targeting agent in cancer cells, so these are 2 very paradoxical points. So far as our drug is concerned, within the tested doses we have not observed any loss of body weight or any severe toxicity in animal experiments.

Dr Ohno: May I ask the same question concerning your clinical experience with cyclosporin A?

Dr Chan: We used a different method for administering cyclosporin A compared to our colleagues, for example, the groups of Dr William S. Dalton, at the Cancer Pharmacology Program, Arizona Cancer Center, Tucson, Arizona, and of Dr Branimir I. Sikic, at the Oncology Division, Department of Medicine, Stanford University School of Medicine, Stanford, California. There they have used continuous infusions for several days and have shown that there is an increase in both direct and indirect bilirubin and other side effects of chemotherapy. We use a similar total dose given as much shorter infusions over 3–6 h. Thus, we reached very high levels during our time of infusion but did not see accentuation of chemotherapy toxicity. So far, all of our patients seem to be able to receive chemotherapy on time. We saw no increased bilirubin or liver or renal toxicity.

Dr Ohno: The study of *mdr*1 and P-glycoprotein has been ongoing for several years, but it has not yet proved convincing clinically that P-glycoprotein is clinically relevant in cancer patients. I think Dr Chan showed us very convincing data that *mdr*1 and P-glycoprotein really do something clinically for drug resistance. Dr Kuwano showed us that maybe we can reverse this resistance with new agents.

Dose intensity

Dose intensity: Retrospective reviews and prospective trials

William M. Hryniuk*

OCF Hamilton Regional Cancer Centre and McMaster University, Hamilton, Ontario, Canada
Current address: Cancer Center, University of California at San Diego, San Diego, California, USA

INTRODUCTION

In animal model systems, outcome of chemotherapy depends upon drug dose, tumour sensitivity, and tumour burden. Animal models do not provide for reduced dosage or delay due to toxicity, and optimum treatment can be determined by treating beyond lethal toxicity. This is not possible in humans. Instead, attempts to define optimum treatment in the clinic have resulted in a plethora of schemes, combinations, and a variety of schedules to reduce doses and delay treatments. However, these schemes and schedules have obscured dose-response relationships. We suggest that important dose-response relationships can be rediscovered and studied by reducing all to how much drug is given per unit time, as $mg/m^2/wk$. This we refer to as dose intensity (1). Dose intensity may be calculated from intended drug doses ("projected dose intensity") or from doses received after reductions and delays for toxicity ("received dose intensity"). To calculate received dose intensity, treatment delays are assumed to be equivalent to dose reductions and therefore are accorded equal weight arithmetically (2).

In addition to dose intensity, two other variables may determine outcome: cumulative dose given over the course of treatment (total dose); and the rate of administration of drug into the circulation when each dose is administered (dose rate). Dose rate can be arbitrarily designated as $mg/m^2/min$.

For regimens containing only one drug, dose intensity can be calculated simply by recalculating the drug dosage specified in the protocol into the standard form of $mg/m^2/wk$, regardless of the schedule used. There are limits to this assumption, imposed by the dose rate. For calculating dose intensity and plotting response vs dose intensity, schedules of differing dose rate can be intermingled to the extent that metabolism and excretion of the drug does not alter the area under the curve. The range of differences in dose rate which it is permissible to ignore while calculating dose intensity is not well characterized for any drug.

Dose intensity can also be calculated not only for single drugs but also for regimens containing more than one drug. To do this it is necessary to assume: (1) scheduling does not directly determine antitumour effect; (2) different administration routes produce equivalent effects; (3) drugs in a combination are equivalent in activity; and (4) no significant interactions occur between drugs given simultaneously. These assumptions required validation, but are probably acceptable within limits (2). Consider as an example the treatment of advanced breast cancer using the combinations that contain the three drugs cyclophosphamide (C), methotrexate (M) and 5-fluorouracil (F). For a series of such regimens, any member of the series can be arbitrarily designated as the "standard". Then, for each of the other regimens in the series, the dose intensities for C, M, and F can be calculated and expressed as decimal fractions of the dose intensities of C, M, and F in the "standard". These decimal fractions can then be averaged to give the "average relative dose intensity" for each combination (Table 1). As an extension of this approach, regimens missing one or two of the drugs in the "standard" regimen can still be incorporated into the series by assigning a dose intensity of zero to the missing drug(s) (3). A similar approach allows analysis of other drug combinations, besides CMF.

TABLE 1

Sample Calculation			
	Step 1	Step 2	Step 3
Test Regimen	Convert to standard form mg/m²/wk	Express as fractions of corresponding dose intensities in standard regimen*	Calculate fractions and average them
Cyclophosphamide 100 mg/m²/d d 1-14 Q28d	350	350/560	.62
Methotrexate 40 mg/m²/d d 1 & 8 Q28d	20	20/28	.71
Fluorouracil 600 mg/m²/d d 1 & 8 Q28d	300	300/480	.62
			$\bar{x}$ = .65

*   assume "standard" regimen to be CMF content of CMFVP regimen of Cooper et al. (4)

Retrospective reviews of the clinical literature indicate that dose intensity of *single agent* therapy correlates well with outcome in carcinoma of the breast, lung, colon, and ovary. Also from retrospective reviews, it is clear that dose intensity of *combination chemotherapy* correlates with outcome in carcinoma of breast, ovary, endometrium and lung, in lymphoma, and in neuroblastoma. Within combinations, the dose intensity of some of the drugs correlates with outcome better than for other drugs (5). These retrospective reviews are summarized in Table 2. It should be noted that by and large the positive outcome was seen as improved response rate (CR + PR). Survival may also have been improved in some instances.

114

TABLE 2

RETROSPECTIVE REVIEWS OF DOSE INTENSITY			
Disease	Drugs(s)*	Result**	Reference
Breast	CMF combination	+	3
"	CMF "	+	6
"	CMF "	+	7
Ovary	CHAP combination	+	5
Endometrium	C,A,P	+	8
Colon	5-fluorouracil	+	9
Lung-SCLC	various	-	10
"	various	+	11
" -NSCLC	Cisplatin	+	12
Lymphoma	various	+	13
Osteosarcoma	Adriamycin	+	14
Neuroblastoma	VM-26, C,A,P	+	15

*   Abbreviations are: A=adriamycin; C=cyclophosphamide; E=epirubicin; F=5-fluorouracil; H=hexamethylmelamine; M=methotrexate; P=cisplatin.

**   [+] = Correlation observed between dose intensity and response rate; [-] = no correlation

The reviews summarized in Table 2 were all retrospective and with one or two exceptions (9, 10) did not contain any randomized trials specifically testing dosage questions. Thus, the results suggest but do not prove a causal relationship between dose intensity and outcome because some other factor may be causing the observed correlations with outcome. For example, the total dose may actually be the causative factor, with dose intensity related to total dose. Alternatively, tumours most sensitive to chemotherapy may occur for some reason in patients able to tolerate high dose intensity chemotherapy. Perhaps investigators using high dose intensity chemotherapy intuitively select predominantly patients with drug sensitive disease.

Prospective randomized trials are required to determine whether dose (dose intensity) is an independent determinant of outcome and if so, in which situations is this clinically important. Results of such trials are summarized in Table 3.

In the trials in which single agent adriamycin and cisplatin were tested in advanced breast cancer and ovarian cancer respectively (36, 46, 47), the dose intensity was shown to be the operative factor because the studies were designed to ensure that the two arms in each study were of equivalent total dose. The other prospective tests of dose shown in Table 3, reported as positive, did not control total dose and

TABLE 3

PROSPECTIVE TESTS OF DOSE (INCLUDING DOSE INTENSITY)			
Disease	Drug(s)*	Result**	Reference
ALL***	6 MP-M	+, -	16, 17
Cervix	Cisplatin	+	18
H & N	Methotrexate	-	19
	Cisplatin	-	20
TESTICULAR	Cisplatin	+, +, -	21, 22, 23
LUNG-SCLC+	Cyclophosphamide	+	24
	VP-16	+	25
	Cisplatin	-	26
	Methotrexate	-	27
	Various	+, +, -, -	28, 29, 30, 31
Lung-NSCLC	Cisplatin	-, -, -, -	32, 33, 34, 35
BREAST	Adriamycin	+, +	36, 37
"	Epirubicin	+, +, -, -	38, 39, 40, 41
"	CMF	+, +	42, 43
"	FAC	-	44
" Stage II	FAC	+	45
OVARY	Cisplatin	+, +, +	46, 47, 48
LYMPHOMA	Adriamycin	-	49
	Antifolates	+	50

*   Drug abbreviations as for Table 2
**   [+] = Correlation observed between dose intensity and response rate; [-] = no correlation.
***   Acute Lymphoblastic Leukemia
+   Previously Untreated

dose intensity as independent variables, therefore we are unsure if either or both were responsible for the positive outcome. Nevertheless, these studies suggest improvements could follow further increases in total dose or dose intensity. This is particularly true for breast cancer and SCLC.

Table 3 also shows that some prospective tests of dose have been reported as negative. Some of these negative trials suffer from methodologic flaws: the trials did not have a sufficient number of cases (19, 27, 30); or inadequate differences in dose intensity were tested or dose intensity and total dose were not controlled as separate variables (17, 26, 30, 31, 41, 44, 49). Nevertheless the results from some trials particularly in ovarian cancer and testicular cancer suggest we may be approaching a plateau with respect to dose intensity of cisplatin as a determinant of outcome (21, 23, 46, 47). In the case of NSCLC cisplatin is simply not active enough (32, 33, 34, 35).

Of the prospective tests of dose intensity shown in Table 3, the results of the study of Tannock et al (42) are particularly instructive: they validate the retrospectively derived dose-response line for CMF in advanced breast cancer by firmly anchoring its lower end. These results are shown in Figure 1.

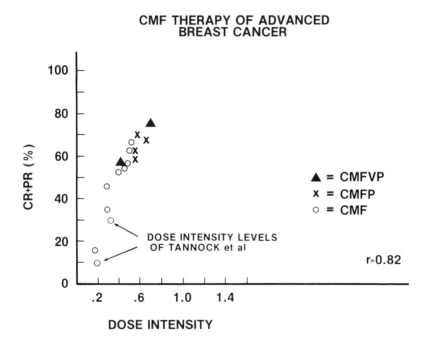

Fig. 1   Response rate v average relative dose intensity of CMF-containing chemotherapy in advanced breast cancer. Calculations are from doses delivered after reductions for toxicity. Dose intensities are relative to the Cooper regimen [4]. Tannock et al [42] study results are superimposed on results from a retrospective analysis[7].

The negative study by Hortobagyi et al (table 3, ref 44) also deserves comment. These authors treated patients with advanced breast cancer using two FAC chemotherapy regimens of differing dose intensity. They found no difference in outcome. However, upon subsequent review of their data, it was found that delays caused by toxicity resulted in an identical received dose intensity in the two arms of the study. This may explains why the outcome was identical in the two arms (52).

FUTURE DIRECTIONS

It will be important to explore dose intensification using methods to increase host tolerance for chemotherapy to see if increases in dose intensity translate into improvements in outcome. Such explorations are underway testing various schedules (53), including fitting the schedule to circadian rhythms (54), use of chemical protectors (55), stem cell rescue (56), and cytokine stimulation (57). We await with great interest the results emerging from such trials, but we also hope that such studies will be properly designed so that the results can be accepted with confidence (58).

It would be logical to increase the dose intensity of the treatment to overcome the *relatively* resistant cells. However, even if complete remission were induced with chemotherapy using the optimal combination of dose intensity and total dose, a small residual tumour burden may persist and cause fatal recurrence. Some of these tumour cells surviving remission induction may be *mutants* and therefore resistant by an order of magnitude to the initial inducing drug or drugs. In order to overcome such *mutant* clones it would be necessary to add non cross-resistant drugs as described by Goldie and Coldman (59). To simultaneously cover both the *relatively* resistant and the *mutant*-resistant tumour cells, it might be desirable to consolidate intensively with several drugs used together as with the mega-dose-then-marrow-rescue treatment. However, one should also consider the combination at dose levels just below those requiring marrow rescue but repeating the treatment two or three times. This would give a smaller increase in dose intensity compared to mega-dose-then-marrow-rescue but would deliver a larger *total* dose. Animal model experiments suggest that in some situations such repeated treatments are superior to the one-shot approach (60).

Another "clean-up" strategy would be augmentation of *immune attack* upon a minimal residual tumour burden. This could be by general stimulation with agents such as interferon or levamisole, or specific passive boosting of immunity with infusion of monoclonal antibodies or stimulated autologous lymphocytes, or by specific active boosting with vaccines.

Finally, it seems possible to permanently suppress residual cells by adjuvant Tamoxifen.

REFERENCES

1.   Green JA, Dawson AA, Fell LF (1980) Measurement of drug dosage intensity in MVPP in Hodgkin's disease. Br J Clin Pharmacol 9:511-514

2.   Hryniuk WM (1988a) The importance of dose intensity in outcome of chemotherapy. In: Hellman S, Devita V, Rosenberg S, (eds) Important advances in oncology. JB Lippincott, Philadelphia 121-141

3.   Hryniuk WM, Levine MN (1986) Analysis of dose intensity for adjuvant chemotherapy trials in stage II breast cancer. J Clin Oncol 4:1162-1170

118

4.   Cooper RG, Holland JF, Glidewell O (1979) Adjuvant chemotherapy of breast cancer. Cancer 44:793-798

5.   Levin L, Hryniuk WM (1987) Dose intensity analysis of chemotherapy regimens in ovarian carcinoma. J Clin Oncol 5:756-767

6.   Bonadonna G, Valagussa P (1981) Dose-response effect of adjuvant chemotherapy in breast cancer. N Engl J Med 304:10-15

7.   Hryniuk W, Bush H (1984) The importance of dose intensity in chemotherapy of metastatic breast cancer. J Clin Oncol 2:1281-1288

8.   Levin L, Hryniuk W (1987) The application of dose intensity to problems in chemotherapy of ovarian and endometrial cancer. Semin Oncol 14(4)(Suppl 4):12-19

9.   Hryniuk W, Figueredo A, Goodyear M (1987) Applications of dose intensity to problems in chemotherapy of breast and colorectal cancer. Semin Oncol 14(4)(Suppl 4):3-11

10. Klasa RJ, Murray N, Coldman AJ (1991) Dose-intensity meta-analysis of chemotherapy regimens in small cell carcinoma of the lung. J Clin Oncol 9(3):499-508

11. Hryniuk W, (1990) Dose intensity in lung cancer chemotherapy. 26th OCTRF Clinical Conference, Sudbury, Ontario, Canada

12. Gandara DR, Wold H, Perez EA (1989) Cisplatin dose intensity in non-small cell lung cancer: Phase II results of a day 1 and day 8 high-dose regimen. J Natl Cancer Inst 81(10):790-794

13. Meyer R, Hryniuk WM, Goodyear M (1991) The role of dose intensity in determining outcome in intermediate grade non-Hodgkin's lymphoma. J Clin Oncol 9:(2)339-347

14. Smith, MA, Ungerleider, RS, Horowitz ME, et al (1991) Doxorubicin dose intensity influences response and outcome for patients with osteogenic sarcoma and Ewing's sarcoma. Manuscript in preparation

15. Cheung NKV, Heller G (1991) Chemotherapy dose intensity correlates strongly with response, median survival, and median progression-free survival in metastatic neuroblastoma. J Clin Oncol 9:1050-1058

16. Pinkel D, Hernandez K, Borella L, et al (1971) Drug dosage and remission duration in childhood lymphocytic leukemia. Cancer 27:247

17. van Eys J, Berry D, Crist W, et al (1989) Treatment intensity and outcome for children with acute lymphocytic leukemia of standard risk. A Pediatric Oncology Group study. Cancer 4:1466-1471

18. Bonomi P, Blessing JA, Stehman FB, et al (1985) Randomized trial of three cisplatin dose schedules in squamous-cell carcinoma of the cervix: A Gynecologic Oncology Group Study. J Clin Oncol Vol 3, No 8:1079-1085

19. Woods RL, Fox RM, Tattersall MHN (1981) Methotrexate treatment of squamous-cell head and neck cancers: Dose-response evaluation. British Medical Journal 282:600-602

20. Tumolo S, Veronesi A, Tirelli U, et al (1983) High-dose (HD) vs low-dose (LD) cis-platinum (DDP) in advanced head and neck squamous carcinoma (HNSC). Proc Am Soc Clin Onc C-635:163

21. Samson JK, Rivkin SE, Jones SE, et al (1984) Dose-response and dose-survival advantage for high versus low-dose cisplatin combined with vinblastine and bleomycin in disseminated testicular cancer. A Southwest Oncology Group (SWOG) project. Cancer 53:1029-1035.

22. Ozols, RF, Ihde DC, Linehan WM, et al (1988) A randomized trial of standard chemotherapy vs a high-dose chemotherapy regimen in the treatment of poor prognosis nonseminomatous germ-cell tumours. J Clin Oncol 6(6):1031-1040

23. Nichols CR, Williams SD, Loehrer PJ, et al (1991) Randomized study of Cisplatin dose intensity in poor-risk germ cell tumors: A Southeastern Cancer Study Group and Southwest Oncology Group Protocol. J Clin Oncol 9(7):1163-1172

24. Mehta C, Vogl SE (1982) High-dose cyclophosphamide (C) in the induction (IND) chemotherapy (CT) of small cell lung cancer (SCLC) - minor improvements in rate of remission and survival. Proc Am Assn Can Res 612:155

25. Cavalli F, Sonntag RW, Jungi F, et al (1978) VP-16 213 monotherapy for remission induction of small cell lung cancer: A randomized trial using three dosage schedules. Cancer Treat Rep 62:473-475

26. Ihde DC, Mulshine JL, Kramer BS, et al (1991) Randomized trial of high vs standard dose etoposide (VP16) and cisplatin in extensive stage small cell lung cancer (SCLC). Proc Am Soc Clin Onc 819:240

27. Hande KR, Oldham RK, Fer MF, et al (1981) A randomized trial of high-dose (HD) vs low dose (LD) methotrexate (MTX) in the treatment of extensive stage small cell lung cancer. Proc Am Soc Clin Onc C-675:505

28. O'Donnell MR, Ruckdeschel JC, Baxter D, et al (1985) Intensive induction chemotherapy for small cell anaplastic carcinoma of the lung. Cancer Treat Rep 69(6):571-575

29. Cohen MH, Creaven PJ, Fossieck BE, et al (1977) Intensive chemotherapy of small cell bronchogenic carcinoma. Cancer Treat Rep 61(3):349-354

30. Figueredo AT, Hryniuk WM, Strautmanis I, et al (1985) Co-trimoxazole prophylaxis during high-dose chemotherapy of small-cell lung cancer. J Clin Oncol 3(1):54-64

31. Johnson, DH, Einhorn LH, Birch R (1987) A randomized comparison of high-dose vs conventional-dose cyclophosphamide, doxorubicin, and vincristine for extnesive-stage small-cell lung cancer: A phase III trial of the Southeastern Cancer Study Group. J Clin Oncol 5(11):1731-1738

32. Klastersky J, Sculier JP, Ravez P, et al (1986) A randomized study comparing a high and a standard dose of cisplatin in combination with etoposide in the treatment of advanced non-small-cell lung carcinoma. J Clin Oncol (4)12:1780-1786

33. Gandara DR (1991) Sixth International Symposium on Platinum and Other Metal Coordination Complexes. San Diego, California

34. Citron M, Brereton H, Huberman M, et al (1986) Randomized phase II study of dichloromethotrexate (DCM) alone, DCM+low-dose cisplatin (CP), and DCM+high-dose CP in non-small cell lung cancer (NSCLC). Proc Am Soc Clin Onc 5(726):185

35. Gralla RJ, Casper ES, Kelsen DP, et al (1981) Cisplatin and vindesine combination chemotherapy for advanced carcinoma of the lung: A randomized trial investigating two dosage schedules. Ann Intern Med 95:414-420

36. Carmo-Pereira J, Costa FO, Henriques E, et al (1987) A comparison of two doses of Adriamycin in the primary chemotherapy of disseminated breast carcinoma. Br J Cancer 56:471-473

37. Creech, RH, Catalano RB, Hopson RC (1980) A comparison of standard dose adriamycin (SDA) and low dose adriamycin (LDA) as primary chemotherapy for metastatic breast cancer. Proc Am Assn Can Res 568:142

38. Habeshaw T, Paul J, Jones R, et al (1991) Epirubicin at two dose levels with Prednisolone as treatment for advanced breast cancer: the results of a randomized trial. J Clin Oncol 9(2):295-304

39. Focan C, Closon MT, Andrien JM (1991) Dose-response relationship with epirubicin (e) as neoadjuvant chemotherapy for advanced breast cancer (BC). End results of a prospective randomized trial. Third International Congress on Neo-Adjuvant Chemotherapy. Paris, France B29:17

40. Ebbs SR, Saunders JA, Graham H, et al (1989) Advanced Breast Cancer: A randomized trial of epidoxorubicin at two different dosages and two administration systems. Acta Oncologica 28:887-892

41. The French Epirubicin Study Group (1991) A prospective randomized trial comparing Epirubicin monochemotherapy to two Fluorouracil, Cyclophosphamide, and Epirubicin regimens differing in Epirubicin dose in advanced breast cancer patients. J Clin Oncol (9) 2:305-312

42. Tannock IF, Boyd NF, DeBoer G, et al (1988) A randomized trial of two dose levels of cyclophosphamide, methotrexate, and fluorouracil chemotherapy for patients with metastatic breast cancer. J Clin Oncol 6:1377-1387

43. Carmo-Pereira J, Costa FO, Henriques E, et al (1986) A randomized trial of two regimens of cyclophosphamide, methotrexate, 5-fluorouracil, and prednisone in advanced breast cancer. Cancer Chemother Pharmacol 17:87-90

44. Hortobagyi GN, Bodey GP, Buzdar AU, et al (1987) Evaluation of high-dose vs standard FAC chemotherapy for advanced breast cancer in protected environment units: A prospective randomized study. J Clin Oncol 5(3):354-364

45. Norton L (1991) Personal Communication, CALGB Trial #85-41

46. Boni C, Cocconi G, Lottici R, et al (1990) Conventional vs high dose-intensity Cisplatin in advanced ovarian cancer, preliminary report of a randomized trial. Proc Am Soc Clin Onc 651(9):168

121

47. Colombo N, Pittelli MR, Marzola M, et al (1990) Randomized study of two Cisplatin (P) dose-intensity regimens in patients with stage II/IV epithelial ovarian cancer (EOC). Proc Am Soc Clin Onc 619(9):160

48. Ngan HYS, Choo YC, Cheung M, et al (Hong Kong Ovarian Carcinoma Study Group) (1989) A randomized study of high-dose vs low-dose cisplatinum combined with cyclophosphamide in the treatment of advanced ovarian cancer. Chemotherapy 35:221-227

49. Hryniuk WM (1991) Randomized Trial of Escalated (E) vs Standard (S) BACOP (Bleomycin-Adriamycin-Cyclophosphamide-Oncovin*-Prednisone) for intermediate grade lymphoma (IGL). Proc Am Soc Clin Onc 10(943):272

50. Frei E, Spurr CL, Brindley CO, et al (1965) Clinical studies of dichloromethotrexate (NSC 29630). Clin Pharm & Ther, 160-171

51. Hortobagyi GN, Hryniuk WM, Frye D, et al (1989) Dose-intensity (DI) analysis of high-dose (HD) chemotherapy for metastatic breast cancer (MBC). Proc Am Assn Can Res 30(1004):252

52. Mortimer JE, Chestnut J, Higano CS (1988) High-dose Cisplatin in metastatic melanoma: Comparison of two schedules. Proc Am Soc Clin Onc 7:254

53. Hrushesky WJM (1985) Circadian timing of cancer chemotherapy. Science 228:73-75

54. Speyer JL, Green MD, Kramer E, et al (1988) Protective effect of the bispiperazinedione ICRF-187 against doxorubicin-induced cardiac toxicity in women with advanced breast cancer. N Engl J Med 319(12):745-752

55. Peters WP, Shpall EJ, Jones RB, et al (1990) High-dose combination Cyclophosphamide (CPA), Cisplatin (cDDP) and Carmustine (BCNU) with bone marrow support as initial treatment for metastatic breast cancer: Three-six year follow-up. Proc Am Soc Clin Onc 9(31):10

56. Crawford J, Ozer H, Stoller R, et al (1991) Reduction by granulocyte colony-stimulating factor of fever and neutropenia induced by chemotherapy in patients with small-cell lung cancer. N Engl J Med 7:164-170

57. Hryniuk WM (1987) Average relative dose intensity and the impact on design of clinical trials. Semin Oncol 14:63-74

58. Goldie JH, Coldman AJ (1983) Quantitative model for multiple levels of drug resistance in clinical tumours. Cancer Treat Rep 67:923-931

59. Skipper H (1987) Southern Research Institute Booklet. 27:36

Epirubicin in lung cancer

M.E. Blackstein, R. Feld

Department of Medicine, University of Toronto, The Mount Sinai and Princess Margaret Hospitals, Toronto, Ontario, Canada

INTRODUCTION

Epirubicin was first described in 1975 and reported to have equal in vitro activity to doxorubicin with less in vitro damage to cardiac cells. (1) Early phase I studies concluded that the maximum tolerated dose (MTD) of the drug given as a single bolus was 90 mg/m2. (2,3,4) These studies usually reported epirubicin to be well tolerated and with clinical activity about equal to or slightly less than for doxorubicin.

A randomized phase III study in patients with small cell lung cancer compared cyclophosphamide (C) 1000 mg/m2, vincristine (Vx) 1.4 mg/m2 and either doxorubicin (A) or epirubicin (E) 50 mg/m2 every three weeks in patients with no prior treatment with local or extensive small cell lung cancer.(5) One hundred and twenty one patients were entered on the CEV arm (80 males and 41 females, mean age 62, 45 with limited disease) and 106 patients to the CAV arm (69 males and 41 females, mean age 61, 39 with limited disease). Ninety-three patients on CEV and 91 patients on CAV were considered evaluable. No significant difference in ECOG grade III-IV haematological toxicities were noted; however in non-haematological toxicities fever, stomatitis and malaise were significantly higher on the CAV arm. The overall response rate was 14 complete (11%) and 39 partial (32%) v 19 (16%) and 35 (32%) respectively. There were no differences in the response duration, time to progression or survival between the two groups. The authors conclude that epirubicin can be substituted for doxorubicin at equal dosage with an improvement in toxicity without sacrificing response or survival.

HIGH DOSE EPIRUBICIN IN SMALL CELL LUNG CANCER

In 1986 Adria Laboratories (Canada) conducted a series of phase I-II studies to re-examine the MTD for epirubicin. These studies in non small cell lung cancer and previously treated breast cancer concluded that 165 mg/m2 and 150 mg/m2 respectively represent the MTD of this drug. (6, 7). Dose limiting toxicities were usually febrile neutropenia often accompanied by stomatitis.

Small cell lung cancer (SCLC) is one of the solid tumours most responsive to cytotoxic drugs. The use of combination chemotherapy improves survival - particularly in the limited form of the disease. (8,9). However, despite high rates of partial and complete response, relapse occurs in the vast majority of cases and many such tumours display resistance to further drug treatment (10). SCLC is a model for the study of the biology and therapy of multiple drug resistance.

The evaluation of investigational drugs in this disease has been somewhat difficult. Patients who relapse after their first line treatment are likely to have resistant tumours precluding the appropriate evaluation of new agents, especially analogues.

In 1986, before the final phase I-II data became available, the National Cancer Institute of Canada (NCIC) began a phase II trial of single agent epirubicin in patients with extensive SCLC who had received no prior therapy. The intent was to study high doses of epirubicin in this group of patients and in the absence of the recently phase I data mentioned, 100 mg/m2 was selected as a starting dose. When, after the first 8 patients were enroled, it became apparent that higher doses of epirubicin could be given safely, the standard dose was increased to 120 mg/m2 for the remainder of the study. The objective was to assess the activity (as measured by objective responses) of epirubicin in this disease with secondary objectives to document the response to second-line therapy and to measure the survival of patients treated in this manner.

Eligibility criteria included: histological or cytological proof of small cell lung cancer with evidence of dissemination beyond one hemithorax; no prior chemotherapy; life expectancy > 12 weeks; ECOG performance status < 3; at least one bidimensional measurable lesion; > 18 years of age; adequate one marrow renal and liver reserve functions; Ineligibility criteria were: evaluable disease only; history of myocardial infarction; a radionuclide ejection fraction (MUGA scan) > 10% below the normal limits of the institution; uncontrolled cardiac arrhythmia. As well, any patient who had a prior malignancy within the previous five year period other than basal or squamous cell carcinoma of skin was ineligible. Patients may have received prior radiotherapy to non-indicator lesions but it mush have been to <

25% of the adult red bone marrow.   Finally, patients with active infections were not entered.

Blood counts were determined on days 7, 8, or 9 and days 14, 15 and 16. Doses were adjusted in retreatment cycles to maintain the nadir neutrophil count between 0.2-1.0 x 10-9/L and the nadir platelet count between 40-70 x 10/L.

After the first course of chemotherapy history, physical, and tumour measurements were repeated.   Only patients who demonstrated tumour regression continued epirubicin treatment. After the second course patients must have exhibited a partial response to continue to receive the drug. Patients who went into complete remission after four courses continued treatment up to a maximum of six courses.   Treatment with VP-16 and cisplatin was recommended for patients who failed to fulfil any of the above criteria.

Between April 29, 1986 and July 29, 1987, 41 patients were entered from 12 participating institutions.   One patient was ineligible because of a history of a prior myocardial infarction. The remaining 40 patients are evaluable for response and toxicity. Four patients had received prior radiotherapy (all for brain metastasis).   Seventy-seven percent of the patients had ECOG performance status < 2.   The majority of patients had more than two metastatic sites.

Non-haematological toxicity was generally mild or moderate and included nausea or vomiting (17 of 40 patients), hair loss (30 of 40) and stomatitis (9 of 40). Three patients are recorded as having cardiotoxicity. All three had an asymptomatic fall in LVEF but none fell below 49%. Haematologic toxicity included a dose related fall in nadir granulocyte counts although the number of courses at the highest dose is limited. Thrombocytopenia was also seen but was not as frequent or severe as neutropenia.   In the group of 34 patients evaluable for haematologic toxicity (having at least one cycle with blood counts done day 14,   15 or 16), 82 achieved at least grade 3 granulocytopenia (< 1.0 x 109/L) and 71% grade 4 granulocytopenia (< .5 x 109/L) during their time on epirubicin.   There was one chemotherapy related death from sepsis. There were five other episodes of febrile neutropenia requiring hospitalization.

Three complete and 17 partial responses were seen producing an overall response rate of 50%.   Eight additional patients demonstrated stable disease over a six week period. The study design required patients to respond early by definition; nevertheless, half (10 of 20) of the responding patients achieved their "best response" after only one cycle of epirubicin. The median duration of response is 212 days (range 49-468).

Patients who did not respond to epirubicin were encouraged to be switched to combination therapy with VP-16 and cisplatin. This was not mandatory, however, and of the 20 responders only 15 received this second line regimen. Five of these patients achieved PR status, while 7 had SD and 3 progressive disease. Those patients who were not in CR after four courses were encouraged to receive VP-16 and cisplatin until best further response. However, only 9 of the 17 patients in whom a PR was recorded went on to receive this therapy. Only one of these converted from PR to CR. Of the eight remaining patients in partial response two had no further therapy while six continued on epirubicin. Thus the overall design of this study (ie. first line epirubicin with VP-16/cisplatin for treatment failures) led to four complete and 21 partial responses for an overall response rate of 25/40 (62.5%). The median survival was 8.3 months.

The primary objective of this study was to determine whether or not epirubicin was effective in producing objective responses in patients with small cell carcinoma of the lung. The observed response rate of 50% (95% confidence intervals 33-66%) is one of the highest reported for single agent chemotherapy in this disease. The early reports of single agent doxorubicin in small cell lung cancer showed it produced response rates of 20-28%. (13-15) However, as we did not carry out a comparative trial we cannot make valid judgments about the relative efficacy of these two drugs.

The secondary objective of this study was to assess response to "salvage" therapy and to develop a sense of the safety of this approach by documenting the overall survival of the study group. The use of early salvage therapy with a VP-16/cisplatin combination improved the overall response rate to 62.5%. The median survival of 8.3 months in this group is comparable to that observed in a recent NCIC combination chemotherapy trial in extensive SCLC comparing CAV to CAV alternating with VP-16/cisplatin. Median survival times were 8.1 and 9.6 months in the 2 arms respectively. (17)

The problems of how to evaluate new drugs in small cell lung cancer and how to assess the impact of testing them in untreated patients have been discussed in several recent publications. (11,12,18). Concerns have been raised that first line investigational therapy may result in our overall decrease in survival and that, if the agent being tested was ineffective, the response rate to subsequent "standard therapy" might be less than expected. The trial of oral idarubicin by Cullen and co-workers is an example.(18) Of the 12 patients who failed to respond to oral idarubicin, only 3 responded to salvage combination chemotherapy with etoposide, cyclophosphamide and vincristine. The overall response rate to idarubicin and salvage treatment was 29% (6 of 21). The median survival of the entire group was 6.2 months.

At the present time we are continuing to test new agents in non-randomized phase II trials (19).

In summary, epirubicin in this study was well tolerated and produced a high response rate in small cell lung cancer patients. Thus we feel this drug is worthy of further study in combination with other agents. The use of first line single agent chemotherapy in this study with early salvage therapy using VP-16 and cisplatin therapy did not appear to compromise survival. This design allowed the identification of an analogue with substantial activity but whether or not it is safe to use this approach in general is uncertain as many new agents will not be active in this disease. Ongoing randomized and non-randomized studies should help to resolve this controversy.

A similiar study in Eastern Europe was conducted simultaneously which yielded response rates almost equal to the NCIC study.(26)

PHASE I - II STUDY OF HIGH DOSE EPIRUBICIN IN ADVANCED NON-SMALL CELL LUNG CANCER

Non small cell lung cancer (NSCLC) continues to be one of the commonest causes of cancer related death. A few cytotoxic drugs have shown response rates of approximately 15-20% as single agents in patients with advanced (extensive disease) NSCLC These include ifosfamide, vindesine, cisplatin, mitomycin-C and VP-16 (etoposide). Adriamycin (doxorubicin), one of the most useful antineoplastics, has only modest activity relative to even these agents against NSCLC(13). A recent NCIC trial comparing two chemotherapy combinations, n (CAP) v. vindesine and cisplatin, to best supportive care showed a survival advantage with either combination (20). In addition, the survival benefit seemed to be cost effective (21). These results suggest that chemotherapy must be considered as an option in the treatment of patients with advanced NSCLC. Nonetheless, current treatment results are disappointing and there is a need to identify new active agents that can be combined with other active agents in order to improve the outcome of patients with advanced disease, and for possible use in the adjuvant or neoadjuvant situation.

Single agent epirubicin has shown an overall response rate of only 5 - 9% in Phase II studies in advanced non-small cell lung cancer at standard doses (60 - 90 mg/m2) (22).

With the aim of determining the efficacy of high dose epirubicin in advanced NSCLC, in view of its mild to moderate toxicity in standard dosage, we decided to redefine the maximum tolerated dose (MTD) of epirubicin when given as a three day course every three weeks. The objective of the subsequent Phase II study was to determine the activity of high dose epirubicin in NSCLC.

Phase I Study: The purpose of this multicentre Canadian trial was to determine the maximum tolerated dose (MTD) of epirubicin when given on three consecutive days, every three weeks, to previously untreated patients with advanced NSCLC (Stage III & IV). Patients with either measurable or evaluable disease were eligible for treatment during this phase of the trial. Patients with unresectable, limited disease, non-amenable to potentially curative radiotherapy were eligible also, although only a very small number of such patients were entered. Eligibility criteria were otherwise similar to those used in the small cell study.

At least four patients were to be entered at each dose level starting at 35 mg/m2 of epirubicin i.v. given on three consecutive days (105 mg/m2 total dose), and escalating by 5 mg/m2 per injection at each dose level (15 mg/m2 total dose). Treatment was repeated every three weeks. If the first four consecutive patients qualified for an escalation from dose level 0 to 1, four subsequent patients were to be entered at level one. This escalation strategy was followed until the maximum tolerated dose (MTD) was reached. The MTD was defined as the dose level at which three of four patients developed nadir granulocyte counts of ≤ 0.2 x 10⁹/L or white blood counts of ≤ 1.0 x 10⁹/L and/or platelets $\leq$ 40 x 10⁹/L. If two out of four patients developed the above nadirs at a certain dose level, four additional patients were entered for a total of eight patients at that dose level. If three or more of eight patients developed the nadir counts specified above, dose escalation was stopped and this was considered the MTD. In addition, when three of four patients developed nadirs or granulocytes of ≤ 0.2 x 10⁹/L and/or platelets of $\leq$ 40 x 10⁹/L and/or recovery of granulocytes to $\geq$ 0.5 x 10⁹/L and platelets $\geq$ 70 x 10⁹/L lasted longer than seven days, this was considered the MTD. Febrile neutropenia and non-haematologic toxicity $\geq$ ECOG grade 3 were also used as criteria to establish the MTD. If two of four patients developed infection or bleeding, i.e. complications secondary to myelosuppression, this was an indication not to go to the next higher dose of epirubicin. A minimum of two courses and at least one follow-up assessment was required for a patient to be considered as having received an "adequate trial" to evaluate efficacy, unless the patient had rapid disease progression (greater than 25% increase in tumour size after the first treatment course) or death occurred. Chemotherapy was to be continued for a total cumulative dose of 900 mg/m2 or until disease progression. <u>Phase II Study:</u> Once the maximum tolerated dose was determined, a dose one level lower (150 mg/m2 every 3 weeks) was chosen to treat patients with the same eligibility requirements as in the Phase I portion of the study, except that the patients were required to have bidimensionally measurable disease. Patients with known brain metastases and those with non-measurable disease were excluded, although included in the Phase I portion of the trial.

Standard response criteria (WHO) were used to assess efficacy.
Thirty-five patients entered on this study between April, 1986 and October, 1988, two were considered ineligible after pathology review leaving 33 patients evaluable for response and 35 evaluable for toxicity. There were 19 males and 16 females with a median age of 58 years (36-75 years). Thirty-two of these had a performance status < 3. Most patients had adenocarcinoma (18) or large cell carcinoma (6). Patients were escalated on this part of the study up to a maximum dose of 60 mg/m2 daily times

three (180 mg/m2) every three weeks. A dose related reduction in WBC and granulocytes was noted. Dose limiting nadir granulocyte count of $\leq$ 0.2 x 109/L was seen with an epirubicin dose of 165 mg/m2 and above. However, the majority of these patients recovered their blood counts in $\leq$ 7 days. There was no suggestion of cumulative myelosuppression following multiple courses of therapy. Non-haematological toxicity was relatively mild with significant stomatitis seen only at 180 mg/m2. There were no treatment related deaths.

Seven partial responses were observed among 33 evaluable patients (21.2%) in the phase I study (95% confidence interval: 9 - 39%). No complete responses were noted. Five of the seven responses were observed at doses of 150 mg/m2 or greater. The median duration of follow-up of this patient group was 589 days (range 58 - 915 days). The median duration of response of the seven responders was 157 days (range 100 - 685 days) with a median survival of 147 days. The phase I data suggested that high dose epirubicin might be an active agent for the treatment of advanced non-small cell lung cancer, but the data needed confirmation in a phase II trial. Based on the results of this phase I trial, the MTD was determined to be 55 mg/m2 daily times three (165 mg/m2) given every three weeks.

During the phase II portion of the study, patients were treated with epirubicin in a dose of 50 mg/m2 daily times three (150 mg/m2) every three weeks with no dose escalation, but dose reduction was allowed according to criteria defined previously. Eligibility criteria were similar to the phase I portion of the study except that patients were required to have bidimensionally measurable disease, and patients with known brain metastases and those with non-measurable disease were excluded. Thirty patients were entered on the phase II portion of the study between December 1987 and December 1988. Four patients died within 7-10 days of the first course of therapy due to complications of rapidly progressive disease and were considered inevaluable for toxicity. With intent to treat analysis, all 30 patients were evaluated for response. Thirty patients with a median age of 61 years were entered, of whom 23 were males. All 30 patients had an ECOG performance status of two or less. At the planned epirubicin dose of 150 mg/m2, a median nadir WBC of 2.75 x 109/L and an absolute granulocyte count of 0.445 x 109\L was observed.

11/30 (37%) of the patients required dose reduction. The serious non-haematologic toxicity (Grade 3 or more) noted in the phase II study (Table 7) was similar to that seen in the phase I study, with remarkably little stomatitis.

There were five episodes of febrile neutropenia including one proven case of E coli bacteraemia requiring hospital admission. Because of the significant number of episodes of febrile neutropenia during the phase I portion of this study, the phase II study used prophylactically; a quinolone (norfloxacin) 400 mg twice daily from day 8 - 18 of each course, the period during which patients were susceptible to neutropenia. All but one patient with febrile neutropenia was on norfloxacin prior to developing fever, suggesting that it did not have a beneficial effect. There were no treatment related deaths.

When analyzed by intent to treat basis, 5/30 (17%) of patients on the Phase II study achieved a partial response. For evaluable patients who received at least two full courses of therapy, 5/23 (21.7%) of patients achieved a partial response.

The criteria for eligibility and response were virtually identical on the two phases of the trial. Since the two study populations were so similar, the two studies were combined to increase the cohort size, and the overall data analyzed for response; 12/63 evaluable patients achieved a partial remission, but no complete remissions were noted, for an overall response rate of 19%.

The response rate analyzed by histology in the two phases of the study revealed only 1 of 17 (6%) of patients with squamous histology responded as compared to 11 of 46 (24%) with non-squamous histology. This difference did not reach statistical significance (P=0.15), but the trend was present in both studies.

In this phase I-II study with high dose epirubicin, we observed an overall response rate of 19% (12/63 patients) with 95% confidence intervals of 10 - 31%. The patients had extensive stage predominantly measurable, non-small cell lung cancer, with good performance status and no previous treatment with chemotherapy.

This data suggests that high dose epirubicin is an active agent that can be used in the treatment of patients with NSCLC. Similar data have been seen by others (23-11). Interestingly, when standard doses of epirubicin were used (60 - 90 MG/M2) little activity was observed.   Although Adriamycin (doxorubicin) has commonly been used in the treatment of this disease, in fact, its activity is relatively limited with an overall response rate of only 9% (range 0%-24%) (2).

Epirubicin was remarkably well tolerated in these studies and stomatitis was relatively uncommon. The main toxicity was myelo-suppression. None of the patients on this study died as a result of toxicity; however, a significant number, 5/26 (20%), required hospitalization for febrile neutropenic episodes.   A pathogen was only identified in one case. From the phase I data, it was determined that the maximum tolerated dose was 165 mg/m2, but we recommended that a dose of 150 mg/m2 be utilized in the phase II portion of the trial.   Based on data from studies in different sites by administering high dose epirubicin as a single injection every three weeks rather than daily times three, we have not seen any obvious differences in toxicity to clearly recommend the three day approach over the single day treatment which is obviously more convenient for patients.

In view of the activity of high dose epirubicin in patients with non-small cell lung cancer and its reasonable tolerability, we recommend future studies be undertaken to combine it with other active agents to explore its role in the management NSCLC. Perhaps by combining high-dose epirubicin with other relatively non-myelosuppressive agents higher response rates and extended survival could be obtained.

Epirubicin would appear to be more than simply a doxorubicin analogue whose value lies in lower toxicity. At eqitoxic dosage epirubicin may well be a superior agent and clearly worthy of prospective trials to determine its value as well as the role of dose-intensity in lung cancer.

REFERENCES

01.   Casazza AM Giuliani FC: Preclinical Properties of Epirubicin
      Advances in Anthracycline Chemotherapy: Epirubicin. ed G.
      Bonadonna Masson Italia Editori Milano 1984. pg 31-40
02.   Schauer PK, Wittes RE, Gralla RJ, et al. A phase I trial
      of 4'-epidoxorubicin. Cancer Clinical Trials 1981 4:433-437.
03.   Bonafante V, Bonadonna G, Villani F. et al. Preliminary
      study of 4'-epidoxorubicin. Cancer Treat Rep 1979 6:915-918.
04.   Robert J, Vrignaud P, Nguyen-Ngoc T, Iliadis A, Mauriac L,
      and Hurteloup P: Comparative Pharmacokinetics and Metabolism
      of Doxorubicin and Epirubicin in Patients with Metastatic
      Breast Cancer. Cancer Treatment Reports, 1985 69(6):633-640.

05. Colajori E, Carr BI, Luce JK, Lyman GH, et al. A Multicenter Clinical Study comparing Cyclophosphamide, Epirubicin and Vincristine to cyclophosphamide Doxorubicin and Vincristine in the Treatment of Small Cell Bronchogenic Carcinoma. Proc Annu Meet Am Assoc Cancer Res 1987 28:A852.

06. Feld R, Wierzbicki R, Walde D, et al: High Dose Epirubicin given as a daily X 3 schedule in patients with untreated extensive non-small cell lung cancer (NSCLC). A Phase I-II Study. Proc Annu Meet Am Assoc Cancer Res 1988 29:A826.

07. Blackstein ME, Wilson K, Meharchand J, et al: Phase I Study of Epirubicin in metastatic breast cancer. Abst # 81 Proc Annu Meet American Soc of Clinical Oncology. 1988.

08. Klastersky J. Therapy of Small Cell Lung Cancer: Anything New? Eur J Cancer Clin Oncol 1988 24:107-112.

09. Jackson DV, Case, LD, Zekan PJ, Powell BL, et al Improvement of Long-Term Survival in Extensive Small-Cell Lung Cancer. Journal of Clinical Oncology 1988 6:1161-1169.

10. Cantwell BMJ, Bozzino JM, Corris P, Harris al. The multi-drug resistant phenotype in clinical practice; evaluation of cross resistance to ifosfamide and mesna after VP16-213, doxorubicin and vincristine for small cell lung cancer. Eur J Cancer Clin Oncol 1988 24:123-129

11. Cullen MH, Hilton C, Stuart NSA: Evaluating New Drugs as First Treatment in Patients with Small-Cell Carcinoma: Guidelines for an Ethical Approach with Implications for Other Chemotherapy-Sensitive Tumours. Cancer Treatment Reports 1987 71:Correspondence, pp. 1356-1357.

12. Aisner J: Identification of New Drugs in Small Cell Lung Cancer: Phase II Agents First? Cancer Treatment Reports 1987 71:1131-1133.

13. Cortes EP, Takita H, Holland J: Adriamycin in advanced bronchogenic carcinoma. Cancer 1979 34:518-525.

14. Blum RH: An overview of studies with Adriamycin (NSC-123127) in the United States. Cancer Chemother Rep 1975 6:247-251.

15. Krakoff IH: Adriamycin (NSC-123127) studies in adult patients. Cancer Chemother Rep 1975 6:253-257.

16. Blum RH, Carter SK: Adriamycin: A new anticancer drug with significant clinical activity. Ann Intern Med 1974 80:249-259.

17. Evans WK, Feld R, Murray N, et al: Superiority of alternating non-cross resistant chemotherapy in extensive small-cell lung cancer. A multicenter randomized clinical trial by the National Cancer Institute of Canada. Ann Intern Med 1987 107:451-458.

18. Cullen MH, Smith SR, Benfield GF, et al: Testing new drugs in untreated small cell lung cancer may predjudice the results of standard treatment: A phase II study of oral idarubicin in extensive disease. Cancer Treat Rep 1987 71:1227-1230.

19. Eisenhauer EA, Evans WK, Blackstein M. New Agent Testing in Untreated patients with Extensive Small Cell Lung Cancer: The NCI Canada Experience. Sixth NCI-EORTC Symposium on New Drugs in Cancer Therapy. March 7-10, 1989, Amsterdam, A458, 1989.

20. Rapp E, Pater JL, Willan A, et al: Chemotherapy can prolong survival in patients with advanced non-small cell lung cancer -Report of a Canadian multicenter randomized trial. J Clin Oncol. 1988 6(4):633-641.

21. Jaakkimainen L, Goodwin PJ, Pater J, et al: The costs of chemotherapy in a National Cancer Institute of Canada randomized trial in nonsmall-cell lung cancer. J Clin Oncol. 1990; 8(8):1301-1309.
22. Joss RA, Hansen HE, Hansen M, et al: Phase II trial of epirubicin in advanced squamous, adeno-and large cell carcinoma of the lung. Eur J Cancer. 1984; 20(4):195-199.
23. Meyers FJ, Cardiff RD, Quadro R, et al: Epirubicin in non-oatcell lung cancer - response rates and the importance of immunopathology: A Northern California Oncology Group Study. Cancer Treat Rep. 1986; 70:805-809
24. Henss H, Fiebig HH, Holdener EE, Kaplan E: Phase II study of high dose epirubicin in non-small cell lung cancer: Contrib Oncol. 1989; 37:136-140.
25. Martoni A, Melotti B, Guaraldi M, et al: High dose epirubicin for untreated patients with advanced tumours: A phase I study. Eur J Cancer. 1990; 26:1137-1140.
26. Eckhardt S, Kolaric K, Vukas D, et al: Phase II study of 4'-epi-doxorubicin in patients with untreated, extensive small cell lung cancer. Med Oncol and Tumour Pharmocother. 1990; 7(1):19-23.
27. Wils J, Utama I, Sala L, Smeets J, and Riva A: Phase II study of high-dose epirubicin in non-small cell lung cancer. Eur J Cancer. 1990; 26:1140-1141.
28. Blackstein M, Eisenhauer EA, Wierzibicki R, Yoshida S: Epirubicin in extensive small-cell lung cancer: A phase II study in previously untreated patients: A National Cancer Institute of Canada Clinical Trials Group Study. J Clin Oncol. 1990;8(3):385-389.
29. Macchiarini P, Danesi R, Mariotti R, et al: Phase II study of high-dose epirubicin in untreated patients with small-cell lung cancer. Am J Clin Oncol. 1990 13(4):302-307

Dose intensive chemotherapy for lung cancer

Masaaki Kawahara, Kiyoyuki Furuse, Masahiro Fukuoka

Department of Internal Medicine, National Kinki Central Hospital for Chest Diseases, Osaka Prefectural Habikino Hospital, Osaka, Japan

INTRODUCTION

Recently a concept of dose intensity (DI) has been proposed to address the impact of dose on outcome of breast, ovarian or lymphoma [1][2][3][4][5]. A standard calculation to convert all drug doses to mg/m^2/week for the duration of the treatment has been devised[6]. DI is the amount of drug given per unit of time , regardless of the schedule employed.

SMALL CELL LUNG CANCER (SCLC)

We treated extensive disease (ED) SCLC patients with intensive chemotherapy and also studied whether DI can be increased by recombinant human granulocyte-colony stimulating factor (rhG-CSF)[7]. This randomized study was initiated from May 1989 to Sep. 1991 at the Osaka Habikino Hospital and National Kinki Central Hospital.

Entry criteria. The criteria for eligibility were histologically or cytologically confirmed SCLC; ED; 15 to 75 years old; performance status (PS) of 0-2 in ECOG scale; no prior chemo- or radiation therapy; measurable or evaluable disease; normal bone marrow, liver and renal functions; no serious complications and no concomitant active malignant diseases; and informed consent.

Treatment schedule.   CODE regimen [8] (Fig 1) consisted of cisplatin, oncovin, doxorubicin and etoposide. CODE is intended to deliver a chemotherapy DI about 1.9 times that of cyclophosphamide, doxorubicin and vincristine, alternating with cisplatin and etoposide (CAV/PE regimen)[9]. The patients were randomly assigned to receive

Drug	Dose (mg/m²)	1	2	3	4	5	6	7	8	9
					Week					
Cisplatin (iv)	25	X	X	X	X	X	X	X	X	X
Oncovin (iv)	1	X	X		X		X		X	
Doxorubicin (iv)	40	X		X		X		X		X
Etoposide (iv)	80X3	X		X		X		X		X
rhG-CSF (sc)	50μg/m²	--								

Fig. 1. Schedule of CODE regimen
Patients were randomized to receive chemotherapy with or without rhG-CSF.

CODE chemotherapy with or without rhG-CSF (Kirin Brewery Company). The rhG-CSF was given 50 μg/m^2 subcutaneously daily except on the day of chemotherapy. If white blood cell count was less than 1000/μl or platelet count less than 30,000/μl, the treatment was postponed for recovery until the next week. The patients responding to therapy received 9 cycles of chemotherapy. Thoracic irradiation after chemotherapy was optional in this study.

<u>Results.</u>   Sixty-four patients were entered into this trial. Fifty-four patients were evaluable for analysis.   Twenty-seven patients were treated with rhG-CSF, and 26 patients were treated without rhG-CSF. Twenty-four (89%) of 27 patients treated with rhG-CSF, and   17 (65%) of 26 patients treated without rhG-CSF received a total of 9 cycles of CODE regimen. The number of patients who received chemotherapy within 10 weeks were 19 in the CODE with rhG-CSF group (71%) and 9 in the CODE alone group (34%). There was a statistically significant difference between the two groups (p<0.01). Use of rhG-CSF thus facilitated an improvement in actual DI of CODE (TABLE I).

TABLE I

Duration of CODE therapy

Duration (wks)	CODE with rhG-CSF n=27 (%)	CODE without rhG-CSF n=26(%)
9	11 (41)	5 (19)
10	8 (30)	4 (15)
≥11	5 (18)	8 (31)
Incomplete	3 (11)	9 (35)

    p<0.01

Table II shows other findings obtained from this study.

It is suggested that rhG-CSF helped bone marrow recover much faster   and   allowed the scheduled dose to be given weekly with little delay. The median survival of rhG-CSF group was statistically superior to   that of the CODE alone group. The major factors which contributed to these survival results will   be further clarified   by multivariate analysis.

NON-SMALL CELL LUNG CANCER (NSCLC)

Regarding cisplatin for NSCLC, Klastersky[10] and Gandara[11] reported that there were no dose response or dose survival relationship. It might be said that the drugs we use are   marginally active   against NSCLC, and   using these kind of drugs   may make the evaluation and analysis of DI difficult and immature.

TABLE II

RESULTS OF RANDOMIZED STUDY FOR SCLC

		CODE with rhG-CSF	CODE without rhG-CSF	Total
Sex	Male	2 1	2 6	4 7
	Female	6	1	7
		p<0.05		
PS (ECOG)	0,1	1 6	1 4	3 0
	2	1 1	1 3	2 4
Response to CODE				
	CR	8(31%)	7(29%)	15(30%)
	PR	18(69%)	15(63%)	33(66%)
Median		59wks	35wks	46 wks
Survival		p<0.05		
Leukopenia				
	Grade 3	8(30)	4(15)	1 2
	4	15(56)	22(85)	3 7
		p<0.05		
Median nadir		900/μl	600/μl	800/μl
		p<0.05		
Median duration		3days	9.5days	5.0days
of Grade 4		p<0.01		
No. of febrile		10(37)	20(77)	3 0
Neutropenia		p<0.01		

DISCUSSION

As a conclusion, rhG-CSF enabled us to significantly increase the actual DI of CODE regimen againt SCLC. However, the hypotheses generated by retrospective analyses regarding DI have not been proven for lung cancer. Klasa[12] et al. reported about DI meta-analysis of chemotherapy regimens in SCLC. They analyzed CAV (cyclophosphamide, adriamycin, vincristine), CAE (cyclophosphamide, adriamycin, etoposide) and CAVE (CAE+vincristine) regimens. No firm conclusions, either for or against DI effect, could be drawn from their analyses. There are many problems inherent in retrospective DI calculation or analysis: 1. planned DI or actual DI. 2. the setting of the treatment duration (unit of time) 3. the assumption that all the component agents have equivalent activity against the tumor. 4. drug-schedule dependency and drug interaction have been ignored. 5. the narrow range of relative DI in many regimens. 6. the variation of patient population. 7. difficulty to differentiate between total dose and DI. 8. the factors which determine actual DI. To increase DI, many studies use chemotherapeutic agents on a weekly basis. From the standpoint of time schedule, the weekly administration may allow a rapidly dividing tumor like SCLC little time to regrow between chemotherapy cycles, regardless of DI.

TABLE III
INTENSIVE WEEKLY CHEMOTHERAPY FOR SCLC

Author	n	Extent	Chemotherapy	CR(%)	Response Rate(%)	Median Survival (wks)
Taylor[13]	76	34LD	Adr,Cy(1) Mtx,Vcr(2)	47	82	LD 71,ED 49
(SWOG)		42ED	Cis,Vp(3)Vcr(4)			
Miles[14]	70	45LD	Cis,VP(1)Ifo,Adr(2)	51	91	LD 58,ED 42
		25ED		48	92	
Murray[15]	48	ED	CODE	58	95	ED 61
Our data	27	ED	CODE with rhG-CSF	31	100	ED 59
	27	ED	CODE without rhG-CSF	29	92	ED 35
Crawford[16]	82	32LD	Cis,Mtx,Vcr(1)	18	77	LD 58
		50ED	Cy,Adr(2)			ED 30

Adr:Adriamycin,Cy:Cyclophosphamide,Mtx:Methotrexate,Vcr:Vincristine
Cis:Cisplatin,Vp:Etposide,Ifo:Ifosphamide

TABLE III lists the recent studies of intensive weekly chemotherapy for SCLC.

Of these, the only regimen which resulted in more than 1 year survival in ED SCLC was CODE. This regimen is going to be compared with the conventional one (CAV/PE) in Japan. Despite limitations of the DI model as described above, these efforts have increased awareness of the importance of individual drugs in each regimen, and made it easier to present data and compare various regimens using these common methods.

ACKNOWLEDGEMENT

We gratefully acknowledge the many doctors who participated in this study.

REFERENCES

1.Frei E, Canellos GP (1980) Dose: a critical factor in cancer chemotherapy Am J Med 69:585-593

2.Hryniuk W, Bush H (1984) The importance of dose intensity in chemotherapy of metastatic breast cancer. J Clin Oncol 2:1281-1288

3. Levin L, Hryniuk WM (1987) Dose intensity analysis of chemotherapy regimens in ovarian carcinoma J Clin Oncol 5: 756-767

4. Kwak L, Olshen R, Halpern J, Horning SJ (1988) Dose intensity:
relationship to prognostic factors for diffuse large cell lymphoma Proc ASCO 7:226

5. Green JA, (1980) Measurement of drug dosage intensity in MVPP therapy in Hodgkin's disease Br J Clin Pharmacol 9:511-514

6.Hryniuk WM, Figueredo A, Goodyear M (1987) Application of dose intensity to problems in chemotherapy of breast and colorectal cancer Semin Oncol 14: 3-11

7. Morstyn G, Campbell L, Souda LM et al. (1988) Effect of granulocyte colony stimulating factor on neutropenia induced by cytotoxic chemotherapy. Lancet 26:667-671

8. Osoba D, Shah A, Murray N. et al. (1990) Improved survival in extensive stage small cell lung cancer on CODE chemotherapy. Pcoc. ASCO 9:225

9. Fukuoka M, Furuse K, Saijo N (1991) Randomized trial of cyclophosphamide, doxorubicin, and vincristine versus cisplatin and etoposide versus alternation of these regimens in small-cell lung cancer J Natl Cancer Insti 83: 855-861

10. Klastersky J, Sculier JP, Ravez P (1986) A randomized study comparing a high and a standard dose of cisplatin in combinaton with etoposide in the treatment of advanced non-small-cell lung carcinoma. J Clin Oncol 4:1780-1786.

11. Gandara DR, Tanaka MT, Crowny J (1991) Comparison of standard dose cisplatin, high dose cisplatin, and high dose cisplatin plus mitomycin in metastatic non small cell lung cancer Proceedings of ASCO 10: 246 (abstract).

12. Klasa RJ, Murray N, Coldman AJ (1991) Dose-intensity meta-analysis of chemotherapy regimens in small-cell carcinoma of the lung J Clin Oncol 9:499-508

13. Taylor CW, Crowley J, Williamson SK (1990) Treatment of small-cell lung cancer with an alternating chemotherapy regimen given at weekly intervals: A Southwest Oncology Group pilot study J Clin Oncol 8:1811-1817

14. Miles C, Harper P, Earl H (1989) Intensive weekly chemotherapy for good prognosis patients with small cell lung cancer Proc ASCO 8:225

15. Murray N, Shah A, Osoba D (1991) Intensive weekly chemotherapy for the treatment of extensive-stage small cell lung cancer J Clin Oncol 9: 1632-1638

16. Crawford SM, Parker D, Glaser MG (1989) Treatment of small cell lung cancer by eight weeks chemotherapy Med Oncol & Tumor Pharmacother 6: 279-283

Discussion

Professor Robert C. Bast, Jr (Duke Comprehensive Cancer Center, Durham, North Carolina, USA): Professor Hryniuk, how do you combine dose intensity and total dose in breast cancer, for example? Clinically, how do we start to factor in multiple treatments, which we probably could do even with autologous bone marrow support?

Professor Hryniuk: There are two ways to do it. One would be to use just sub-transplant doses, but administer each 2 or 3 times. For example, if the transplant dose is X and you used 2/3 X, but you gave it 3 times, then you would have 2 times as much total dose without ever having to transplant the patient. That increase in total dose might translate into an improved outcome. The other way is by doing a double or triple transplant, depending on the patient's tolerance; that will result in 2 or 3 times as much total drug and we can examine whether it makes a difference.

Dr Masahiro Fukuoka (Osaka Prefectural Habikino Hospital, Osaka, Japan): You showed that there are correlations between the outcome and dose intensity in the analysis of trials for small cell lung cancer. What kind of regimens or drugs are included for calculation of dose intensity?

Professor Hryniuk: In the retrospective study, it was cytoxan, doxorubicin, vincristine, and etoposide. In the 6 prospective studies, which were all unidirectional, every drug used in small cell lung cancer was included, including cyclophosphamide, methotrexate, cisplatin, etoposide, and vincristine. Those are the 6 prospective tests commonly quoted in the literature testing dose in small cell lung cancer.

Professor Bast: Dr Blackstein, have studies of *mdr* P170 expression been done prior to the administration of epirubicin to patients with small cell lung cancer? As a follow-up to that, is there any difference in P170 expression between squamous carcinomas and other non-small cell types?

Dr Blackstein: I cannot tell you, except to say that in the studies of drug resistance I have been aware of, P-glycoprotein expression in lung cancer does not seem to be a major factor in drug resistance. It seems to be the glutathione accumulation pathways and perhaps topoisomerase 2, which is a very difficult system to measure.

Dr Yasutsuna Sasaki (National Cancer Center, Tokyo, Japan): You mentioned that 10 years ago the maximum tolerated dose of epirubicin was thought to be 90 mg/m². What is the difference between your and earlier studies?

Dr Blackstein: I think there are several differences. The bottom line is that we did ours more carefully. The maximum tolerated dose had not been reached in either Milan or New York and it is not clear to me why they stopped. Certainly they had no significant amount of myelosuppression, nor did they have significant problems with

140

nonhematological toxicities that would have led to the ending of those studies. I have seen the raw data, but I do not know why they stopped.

Dr Sasaki: If there is a dose-response relationship in the treatment of lung cancer, what do you think about bone marrow support or support with G-CSF or GM-CSF to allow an increase in the maximum tolerated dose?

Dr Blackstein: At the present time, certainly in non-small cell lung cancer, I think that our responses would have to make that a very strict clinical trial, done in a small number of centers. In terms of small cell lung cancer, autologous bone marrow transplant has been tried. I believe that autologous bone marrow transplant with massive doses of chemotherapy is a very useful approach in patients who have had a complete response rate. It is not clear to me whether the marrow must be purged in small cell lung cancer because of the heavy probability of marrow involvement in that disease. It is also not clear to me that the drugs chosen for final consolidation in bone marrow transplantation are the drugs that I would necessarily choose as the most efficacious agents in the cancers that are being treated. In those small number of series for small cell lung cancer, however, it has not made a significant difference, even when patients who achieved complete response were treated. Probably the patients were not selected very well. I am sure that if you treated patients who had the most limited disease early on, perhaps even patients whose mediastinum was positive only at mediastinoscopy and not on CT, you might make a case, but I think by the time the disease becomes bulky, whatever the drug resistance factor is in small cell lung cancer has become expressed.

On the question concerning antibiotic support, I did not mention that in one of the Canadian studies we did use a quinolone because febrile neutropenia is the dose-limiting toxicity. It did not work, but I suspect that was because the quinolone we chose—norfloxacin, which was the first one available—was the wrong one. I suspect that had we stayed with co-trimoxazole or ciprofloxacin, we would have had much better results. I believe that with the use of GM-CSF or G-CSF we will be able to push the maximum tolerated dose for epirubicin to well over 200 mg/m^2. That now gives us one of the few drugs that has a dose range of response in treatment that is an order of 4 times. There are not many drugs we deal with that have that sort of a wide window with which to look at dose response and whether it is of benefit clinically.

Dr Nagahiro Saijo (National Cancer Center, Tokyo, Japan): In relation to Dr Sasaki's question, you decided that the maximum tolerated dose of epirubicin was 150 mg/m^2. If you want to combine other drugs with epirubicin under such circumstances, at what dose do you start?

Dr Blackstein: It depends on the agent you are going to combine it with. The toxicity of epirubicin is primarily on the granulocytes. The platelets are seldom seen to go below 100 000. In Canada we are running a study in adjuvant breast cancer utilizing a modified CEF regimen with C at 75 mg/m^2 by mouth for 14 days, 5-FU at 500 mg/m^2, and epirubicin at 50 mg/m^2 on days 1 and 8. So that is 100 mg/m^2 in the 28-day cycle compared to the classic Bonadonna regimen and that has been very well tolerated. There have been very few admissions to hospital for febrile neutropenia. That is a fairly aggressive regimen, but it would appear that you can combine these drugs by backing down to perhaps 2 dose levels below the maximum tolerated dose.

Dr Fukuoka: Do you consider that further studies are needed to evaluate the role of the dose intensity of epirubicin in small cell or non-small cell lung cancer? If so, how do you design such trials?

Dr Blackstein: I could not think of a safe way to do it in small cell lung cancer. We are in fact doing that study in breast cancer. In patients who have failed CMF chemotherapy, a well-defined group of women, the median survival is considered to be about 8.5 months after failure of CMF, and we are carrying out a randomized study comparing epirubicin 75 mg/m² to epirubicin 135 mg/m². That study should be completed by the end of 1991 and I have a strong feeling that that study will be positive for survival in favor of the high-dose arm, but I do not know the code yet.

Professor Hryniuk: Dr Kawahara, in the CODE regimen, the dose intensity was 1.86 higher than CAV alternating with PE. The duration was also shorter. What were the total dose differences between CAV/PE and CODE? I think that a mathematical correction for the difference in total doses must be introduced.

Dr Kawahara: We repeated the regimen 4 times, so both the CAV and PE regimens were given twice per patient. Maybe the total dose in the CODE regimen for 12 weeks is a little higher than in the CAV/PE regimen.

Professor Hryniuk: So for doxorubicin it may be higher and for cyclophosphamide it is, of course, much higher than the CAV/PE regimen, and for the other drugs it is higher or the same as in CODE. Is it higher in CODE?

Dr Kawahara: I think so, but cyclophosphamide is not included in CODE.

Dr Fukuoka: Six cycles of the CAV/PE alternating regimen are almost the same as the CODE regimen.

Dr Atsuya Karato (National Cancer Center, Tokyo, Japan): Do you have any data on the incidence of side effects, such as fever or susceptibility to infection, in patients treated with the CODE regimen, with or without G-CSF?

Dr Kawahara: We have data on leukocytopenic fever; the incidence was significantly lower in the CODE regimen with CSF.

Professor Bast: Clearly with the CSFs there are new opportunities for exploring dose escalation. One difficult question is, where are we on scale? Where does dose escalation beyond the intensive programs that we have heard described during this session really show promise either in terms of being able to "cure" more patients, ie, provide prolonged survival, or at least provide increased disease-free survival that would justify the increased toxicity we are seeing, even with the CSFs?

Professor Hryniuk: There is a relation between received dose intensity and survival, but it is very shallow. I think that in breast cancer, increases of 2-fold would be necessary to pick up differences in survival that were clinically meaningful. Three target tumors should be investigated. Two are already under investigation: one is the group of stage III breast cancer patients with many positive nodes. In this group, retrospective analysis of dose intensity and relapse-free survival shows a continuous rise rather than a plateau. We did see the plateau in 1–3 node-positive patients. So I think that the approach being used in heavy node-positive patients is correct and also in young women with metastatic disease. I would like to suggest that patients with bone metastases only are also a target for dose intensification, and they have not been included in all of our studies because they are difficult to evaluate. However, I suspect that they are a curable subset, if we could just evaluate them. Everything that we believe we know about breast cancer is distorted by selective deletion of this subset of potentially curable patients, and when we finally include them I believe we will have a much better picture. In terms of small cell lung cancer, I think that a 2-fold increase may be necessary and I would not be willing to go past that.

Dr Blackstein: I think that this area of cancer biology is the one in which it is probably most appropriate to go from the bedside back to the laboratory. With the techniques of PCR and immunohistochemistry that Dr Chan has demonstrated in the sarcomas, we should know in advance what we are dealing with in terms of possible resistance, so tailoring chemotherapy to the patient is becoming more of a reality. I do not know whether it is worth setting out with a massive hammer if you are going to fail. If a patient's tumor is a 5-node-positive for P-glycoprotein, should it be treated with massive doses of anthracyclines? The answer is, we do not know the correlation, but the data that Dr Chan has shown from pediatric tumors are very suggestive. It might be appropriate to channel these patients away from these sort of dose intensity studies and into those in which P-glycoprotein inhibitors are used.

Professor Hryniuk: I would challenge that. The dose intensity hypothesis is equally applicable to MDR-positive tumor cells if you use drugs to which they are sensitive. I have not heard that they are resistant to all drugs, only a group of drugs.

Dr Blackstein: That is true, but I think that the cancers in which phase-specific agents are effective are the ones that are probably curable anyway, such as the leukemias. So I think that the bulk of cancers which are going to be sensitive to the MDR testing are large and they are probably the common ones, with the exception of lung cancer, which does not seem to be clear at present.

Dr David P. Lane (University of Dundee, Dundee, Scotland, UK): Professor Hryniuk, I formed the impression from your presentation that more was better. Also,

I did not see any clear evidence of toxicity from the animal models according to your analysis. It seemed that in most of the treatment regimens we have seen we were still obtaining better results with higher doses.

Professor Hryniuk: The analyses that I showed in the human tumors were for response rate. I think that the data are not in yet for survival. In the animal model the endpoint used was the LD_{10}. Here and for moderately sensitive tumors, the total dose was more important than dose intensity in terms of antitumor effect. So there was a matrix combination of total dose and dose intensity in the moderately sensitive tumors. In the fast-growing leukemias, with the alkylating agents as test agents, dose intensity is the most important factor. Thus a combination of the tumor growth rate and the specific drugs must be taken into account in planning the optimum treatment.

III. CANCER THERAPY BASED ON BIOLOGY

Biological basis for modifying radiotherapy and chemotherapy

H. Rodney Withers

Department of Radiation Oncology and JCCC, UCLA Medical Center Los Angeles, California, USA

STANDARD FRACTIONATED DOSE RADIATION THERAPY

Standard radiotherapy is administered as a series of equal doses usually 5 per week for several weeks, a process termed fractionation. Each equal dose "fraction" kills the same proportion of cells. A common daily dose is 200 centiGray (previous terminology was 200 rad) which reduces tumor cell survival to about 50%. A similar dose administered the next day will further reduce survival by 50%, that is to 25% of the original population. This equal proportionate effect results in a logarithmic decline in total cell number with increase in number of dose fractions. Breaking the total dose into a series of dose fractions amplifies the therapeutic differential between normal tissues and tumors for several reasons, easily remembered as the 4 R's: repair of cellular injury, repopulation by surviving cells, redistribution within the division cycle, and reoxygenation of the tumor. Additional modifications of fractionation aim at increasing the advantage already gained from standard fractionation.

Biology of Dose Fractionation

Repair: X-irradiation produces breaks in the DNA. Single strand breaks are of little consequence because the cell has highly efficient mechanisms for repairing them, presumably evolved to protect us from accumulating injury from environmental radiations and other toxins. With increase in X-ray dose there is an increasing probability of interaction between two or more lesions in the DNA, each of which, if

147

independent, could be repaired but when present coincidentally in time and place are prone to non-repair or misrepair. This increasing potential for interactive injury causes a curve relating cytotoxicity and dose to bend progressively downwards. Dividing a dose into multiple small fractions permits cells to repair sublethal injury before it interacts with other sublethal injury to become lethal, diminishing the curvature of the dose survival relationship.

The repair of DNA damage is completed over a few hours, but the extent of repair is not equal in all tissues. In general, slowly-responding normal tissues (e.g. connective tissues, kidney, spinal cord) are capable of more repair than are malignancies (1,2). Thus, by spacing dose fractions by at least 6 hours, usually 24 hours, the recovery in slowly-responding normal tissues is relatively more than that in tumors. Because cell killing is logarithmic rather than linear, the difference in each day's effect is amplified exponentially (3). For example, if the greater repair occurring in critical "target" cells of a slowly-responding normal tissue leads to 60% of them surviving each dose fraction compared with only 50% of the cancer cells, then, after 30 dose fractions, the relative survival will be $(60/50)^{30} = 237$, a major therapeutic differential.

Repopulation: Repopulation by surviving cells in proliferative normal tissues occurs as a homeostatic response to injury, providing an important reason for extending treatment over several weeks. This regenerative response allows acutely-responding tissues (e.g. mucosa) to tolerate an escalation of the dose given to the tumor.

Recently, treatment-induced accelerated growth has also been identified and quantified in some cancers (4,5,6). Fortunately, the rate of repopulation in the average tumor is less than in acutely-responding normal tissues. Thus, there is still a therapeutic advantage from protracting treatment, proven in head and neck cancer and likely in all

148

but very rapidly-growing cancers. Previously, it was reasonable to prolong a course of radiotherapy to minimize acute toxicity. Now it is not. Since rapid regeneration is not a factor in the therapeutic differential between late-responding normal tissues and the tumor, the desired dose (without reduction) should be given in as short an overall time as compatible with acceptable acute toxicity (2).

Redistribution within the mitotic cycle: Cells exhibit large changes in their radiosensitivity as they progress through the division cycle. Only a small dose to the tumor is necessary to kill preferentially most of the cells in more radio-sensitive phases of the division cycle. The selective killing of the more radio-sensitive cells leaves the surviving cell population partially "synchronized" in more radioresistant phases of the cycle immediately after each daily dose fraction. By stopping the dose and waiting for some hours, those cells in radioresistant phases of the division cycle progress into more radiosensitive phases and ultimately return to asynchrony because of the wide spectrum of division cycle times in most tumors. A population of asynchronous cells is more radiosensitive, on average, than the population immediately surviving a dose of 200 cGy. This self-sensitizing effect of cell cycle redistribution affects the response of tumors and acutely-responding normal tissues to multi-fraction radiotherapy, but not that of late responding normal tissues whose cells are essentially static within the division cycle (in a phase which permits a great deal of repair, as described earlier). Thus, division cycle redistribution between successive doses in a course of radiotherapy enhances the differential in response between the critical late-responding normal tissues and the cancer. This was the original rationale for instituting hyperfractionation (7).

Reoxygenation: Solid tumors often outstrip their blood supply and develop areas of hypoxia and necrosis. Hypoxic cells are 2 to 3 times as radioresistant as euoxic cells (for radiochemical, not metabolic reasons). Hence, even a small proportion of hypoxic cells could limit radiocurability of the tumor. When multiple small doses of X rays are given over a period of days or weeks, the euoxic cells, being more radiosensitive, are killed selectively by each dose fraction. During the interfraction intervals sterilized euoxic cells are eliminated, providing better access of previously hypoxic cells to oxygen (8). This process of reoxygenation minimizes the influence of hypoxic cells on radiocurability.

Therefore, major reasons why standard fractionation achieves better results than large single doses are:

a.   Cells in late-responding normal tissues repair more damage than do tumor cells, maximized by using small doses per fraction.

b.   Repopulation in acutely-responding normal tissues outstrips that in the average tumor.

c.   The net sensitizing effect of cell cycle redistribution and reoxygenation have a greater effect on tumors than on normal tissues.

MODIFIED FRACTIONATION STRATEGIES

Current conventional (e.g. 2 Gy/fraction) treatment regimens have been arrived at because, when given 5 times per week, they permit the administration of a "tolerance" dose for late effects with acceptable, almost comfortable, acute toxicity.

The two primary advantageous departures from this standard treatment involve reducing the dose per fraction (hyperfractionation) and shortening the overall treatment duration (accelerated treatment). Obviously it is possible to incorporate both into a modified strategy.

Hyperfractionation

Hyperfractionation is dividing the treatment into smaller than conventional doses per fraction, without change in overall treatment duration. The goal is to further increase therapeutic differential between late-responding normal tissues and the tumor by maximizing the differentials in repair, redistribution, and reoxygenation. In a comparison with a 2 Gy per fraction standard regimen, a hyperfractionated regimen would be 1.15 Gy given twice daily. The increment in "biologically-effective" dose to the tumor can be calculated to be about 10% (9).

In clinical trials in head and neck cancer, control rates averaged 15 percentage points higher (10-12), representing a 25% to 50% reduction in recurrence rates, with no significant increase in sequelae in slowly-responding tissues.

Accelerated Treatment

It was thought until relatively recently that tumors did not accelerate their growth rate during a course of fractionated irradiation. There is now abundant experimental (5,13,14) and clinical evidence (4,5,6,15,16) for an acceleration in tumor growth as a result of radiation insult.

Maciejewski et al (4) estimated that accelerated tumor clonogen growth in squamous carcinomas of the head and neck reduced the efficacy of radiotherapy by about 0.6 Gy per day during the latter weeks of treatment. Analysis of similar data for head and neck cancer from published time-dose scattergrams, also showed a value of 0.6 Gy per day to be within the 95% confidence limits of 95% of the studies (6). This reflects a clonogen doubling time of 3 to 4 days, which resembles the values for T_{pot} estimated for these tumors (17) and contrasts with a pretreatment doubling time of 45-60 days (18,19). Thus, a decrease in clonogen doubling time from 2 months to about 3 or 4 days must occur at some time during radiotherapy. From analysis of published results of treatment regimens varying in length from 10 days to more than 8 weeks it has been suggested that the average lag time between the start of treatment and the onset of accelerated growth is between 3 and 5 weeks for head and neck cancer (6).

The therapeutic ratio between acutely-responding normal tissues and most cancers increases as the duration of treatment is extended because repopulation in normal mucosa begins earlier and is more efficient than that by surviving tumor clonogens (9). However, a limit is imposed on the total dose by slowly-responding normal tissues which show little or no repopulation over the period of treatment. Given that limit, the maximum therapeutic ratio is achieved by giving radiotherapy at the fastest rate consistent with sufficient repopulation in the mucosae to avoid unacceptable acute toxicity. in recurrence rates, with no significant increase in sequelae in slowly-responding tissues.

Accelerated Treatment

It was thought until relatively recently that tumors did not accelerate their growth rate during a course of fractionated irradiation. There is now abundant experimental (5,13,14) and clinical evidence (4,5,6,15,16) for an acceleration in tumor growth as a result of radiation insult.

Maciejewski et al (4) estimated that accelerated tumor clonogen growth in squamous carcinomas of the head and neck reduced the efficacy of radiotherapy by about 0.6 Gy per day during the latter weeks of treatment. Analysis of similar data for head and neck cancer from published time-dose scattergrams, also showed a value of 0.6 Gy per day to be within the 95% confidence limits of 95% of the studies (6). This reflects a clonogen doubling time of 3 to 4 days, which resembles the values for T_{pot} estimated for these tumors (17) and contrasts with a pretreatment doubling time of 45-60 days (18,19). Thus, a decrease in clonogen doubling time from 2 months to about 3 or 4 days must occur at some time during radiotherapy. From analysis of published results of treatment regimens varying in length from 10 days to more than 8 weeks it has been suggested that the average lag time between the start of treatment and the onset of accelerated growth is between 3 and 5 weeks for head and neck cancer (6).

The therapeutic ratio between acutely-responding normal tissues and most cancers increases as the duration of treatment is extended because repopulation in normal mucosa begins earlier and is more efficient than that by surviving tumor clonogens (9). However, a limit is imposed on the total dose by slowly-responding normal tissues which show little or no repopulation over the period of treatment. Given that limit, the maximum therapeutic ratio is achieved by giving radiotherapy at the fastest rate consistent with sufficient repopulation in the mucosae to avoid unacceptable acute toxicity.

b. In concomitant boost therapy, the "boost" dose is delivered to a reduced volume during the same overall time the larger field is being treated, rather than afterwards (22,23). The boost is given as a second treatment (using a 6 hour fractionation interval) on 5-10 days late in the course of treatment. In principle, they could also be delivered on weekend days. The biological basis for using this technique is an increased tolerance by the patient when the area of severe mucosal reaction is smaller. The overall duration of therapy can be shortened by a week or more.

c. In the CHART regimen, 54 Gy is given in three 1.5 Gy fractions per day over 12 days (24). It has the advantages of both hyperfractionated and accelerated treatment. The disadvantage is that the total dose is significantly reduced because the therapeutically advantageous differential in repopulation between the mucosal stem cells and tumor clonogens is not exploited. Such a rapid treatment would be predicted to be of special benefit to those patients in whom tumor clonogens grow quickly even before treatment, and to those who manifest an early tumor repopulation response.

MODIFICATIONS TO CHEMOTHERAPY

The radiobiology principles underlying fractionation of radiotherapy can be applied to chemotherapy but not with the same confidence as to radiotherapy.   Some speculative comparisons are worthwhile.

Bolus versus Slow Infusion

Part of the success of fractionation of radiotherapy derives from the self-sensitization of the tumor through progression of surviving cells through the division cycle between doses. The same should apply to tumors treated with chemotherapy. If a drug which only kills S phase cells is given as a bolus then regardless of the dose it will not affect the majority of the tumor cell population. If 20% of the tumor clonogens were in S phase, then even a 1000-fold escalation of dose would not increase cell killing above 20%. If, however, a small dose were given several times at regular intervals throughout the cycle time of the tumor, or if the blood levels were maintained by a constant infusion, then close to 100% of the clonogens could be sterilized by a total dose only slightly higher than the bolus dose required to kill 20% of the cells. The ultimate tumor cytotoxicity would be determined more by tumor kinetics than by dose. The limitation to the exploitation of tumor kinetics is the tolerance of acutely-responding tissues, but, as with radiotherapy, there are ways to reduce this problem.

Overall Treatment Time

Administering cytotoxic drugs spaced by time intervals for even 6 months, let alone 2 years, makes no sense now that the accelerated regrowth of treated tumors has been documented. As with radiotherapy, the intensity of dose should be maximized, administering tolerable doses as quickly as possible and modifying upwards the tolerance e.g. by growth factors, autologous bone marrow storage and re-infusion, etc. For example, if cardiac toxicity imposes an ultimate upper limit of Adriamycin dose then that limit should be reached as quickly as possible consistent with acceptable acute toxicity.

Neoadjuvant Chemotherapy

Neoadjuvant chemotherapy before radiotherapy also makes no sense if it is protracted over several weeks. By analogy with the acceleration resulting from radiotherapy, neoadjuvant chemotherapy lasting 3 to 4 weeks for head and neck cancer will transform the cancer from one which doubles every 45 to 60 days to one which doubles every 3 days by the time radiotherapy is begun. This leads to loss in efficacy equivalent to about 400 cGy of the 1000 cGy usually given per week. Whilst this normally happens after about 4 weeks of radiotherapy, it would be in progress at the outset after neoadjuvant chemotherapy, resulting in a loss of efficacy of radiotherapy equivalent to a decrease in total dose by about 1600 cGy. Thus, to be any advantage, the net depletion of clonogens by drugs needs to exceed the extra repopulation which would occur during chemotherapy and the first 4 weeks of radiotherapy, equivalent to at least 1600 cGy of radiotherapy. Furthermore, if neoadjuvant chemotherapy is suspended during radiotherapy, then the subclinical metastases beyond the radiotherapy fields will accelerate their regrowth and may regain or surpass their former cell numbers by the time chemotherapy is resumed. Thus, the patient's drug tolerance is reduced with little potential for gain and a significant possibility of loss.

The Illusion of Tumor Regression as a Prognosticator

The macroscopic behavior of the cancer being treated with neoadjuvant chemotherapy is not a reliable indicator of the changes in the clonogenic cell number over time. For example, the accelerated repopulation of tumor clonogens which is in full swing after 4 weeks of radiotherapy to a head and neck cancer involves, at the maximum, only 1 in 10,000 of the cells in the regressing tumor mass. Most of the mass consists of sterilized and differentiating cells with the accelerated growth of the small number of surviving cells having no impact whatever on the visible tumor volume. Contrary to the state of satisfaction usually gained from watching a tumor regress there should be alarm and urgency in the minds of both medical and radiation oncologists.

ACKNOWLEDGEMENTS

Supported in part by PHS grant number CA-31612 awarded by the National Cancer Institute.

REFERENCES

1.   Thames HD, Withers HR, Peters LJ, Fletcher GH (1982) Int J Radiat Oncol Biol Phys 8:219-226

2.   Withers HR (1985) Cancer 55:2086-2095

3.   Withers HR (1986) Int J Radiat Oncol Biol Phys 12:693-698

4.   Maciejewski B, Withers HR, Taylor JMG, Hliniak A (1989) Int J Radiat Oncol Biol Phys 16:831-843

5.   Trott K, Kummermehr J (1985) Radiother Oncol 3:1-9

6.   Withers HR, Taylor JMG, Maciejewski B (1988) Acta Oncologica 27:131-146

7.   Withers HR (1975) Radiology 114:199-202

8.   Kallman, RF (1972) Radiology 105:135-142

9.   Withers HR (1989) Radiat Res 119:395-412

10. Horiot JC, LeFur R, Nguyen T et al (1990) Europ J Cancer 26:779-780

11. Horiot JC, van den Bogaert W, Ang KK, van der Schueren E, Bartelink H, Gonzalez D, dePauw M, van Glabbeke M (1988) In: Vaeth, J.M., Meyer, M. (eds) Frontiers of Radiation Therapy and Oncology, vol 22. Karger, Basel, pp. 149-161

12. Million RR, Parsons JT (1988) Front Rad Ther Oncol 22:79-92

13. Hermens, AF, Barendsen GW (1969) Europ J Cancer 5:176-181

14. Kummermehr J, Trott KR (1982) In: Karcher, KH, Kogelnik HD, Reinartz G (eds) Progress in Radio-Oncology II. Raven Press, New York, pp. 299-307

15. Allen EP (1984) Australas Radiol 28:156-160

16. Hliniak A, Maciejewski B, Trott KR (1983) Brit J Radiol 56:596-598

17. McNally NJ (1989) In: McNally, NJ (ed) British Institute of Radiology Report 19: The Scientific Basis of Modern Radiotherapy. British Institute of Radiology, London, pp. 120-123

18. Charbit A, Malaise EP, Tubiana M (1971) Europ J Cancer 7:307-315

19. Steel GG (1977) Cell Population Kinetics in Relation to the Growth and Treatment of Cancer. Clarendon Press, Oxford

20. Wang CC (1987) In: Withers, HR, Peters, LJ (eds) Innovations in Radiation Oncology. Springer-Verlag, Heidelberg, pp. 239-243

21. Begg AC, Hofland J, Moonen L et al (1990) Int J Radiat Oncol Biol Phys 19:1449-1453

22. Knee R, Fields RS, Peters LJ (1985) Radiother Oncol 4:1-7

23.   Ang KK, Peters LJ, Weber RS, Maor MH, Morrison WH, Wendt CD,
      Brown BW (1990) Concomitant boost radiotherapy schedules in
      treatment of carcinoma of the oropharynx and nasopharynx.   Int J
      Radiat Oncol Biol Phys 9:1339-1346

24.   Saunders M, Dische S, Fowler JF, Denekamp J, Dunphy EP, Grosch E,
      Fermont D, Ashford R, Maher J, desRochers C (need year) 22:99-
      104

Discussion

Professor Franco Muggia (Kenneth Norris Cancer Center, University of Southern California, Los Angeles, California, USA): I was interested in your provocative statements about dose intensity of chemotherapy, on which I think we are in agreement with regard to breast cancer. What is the biology underlying the rapid repopulation? Does that also occur at distant sites when you treat with radiation therapy? Certainly with chemotherapy it should be a generalized phenomenon, but during radiation therapy do you think there is stimulation of other distant sites?

Professor Withers: No, I do not think there is any evidence for that. I am not quite sure how you would establish that that phenomenon occurs. I do not think there is any obvious evidence for it in experimental animals.

Professor William M. Hryniuk (Ontario Cancer Treatment and Research Foundation, Hamilton Regional Cancer Center, Hamilton, Ontario, Canada): You showed rapid regrowth, as a small nodule in the middle of a sea of necrosis, and mentioned thousands of cells. Over how many days did this occur?

Professor Withers: It occurred over 14 days.

Professor Hryniuk: From one cell at day zero, while the treatment was progressing, did you observe rapid regrowth?

Professor Withers: Yes. That was a mouse mammary carcinoma with a doubling time of 4 days which was exposed to a large single dose. I think that the trigger to repopulation, which presumably is depopulation, would be much quicker after a large single dose than after a series of small doses. Therefore that tumor was not exposed to fractionated radiation, but to a very large injury. The repopulation in human tumors occurred during a course of repeated daily doses.

Professor Hryniuk: Presumably the cell that produced that nodule survived that large dose. If you had given a larger dose, that cell would not have emerged, but some other cell might have from that moment on.

Professor Withers: I am not sure I understand your point. Certainly it was a sub-curative dose. It did not sterilize the tumor. That tumor would have recurred.

Professor Hryniuk: There is a distribution of cells in that tumor with respect to sensitivity to the tumor treatment at the time you start. Your dose did not kill that cell, so that cell apparently produced that nodule. That is not rapid regrowth, that cell simply survived.

Professor Withers: It survived the single dose, and then instead of doubling every 4

159

days as the tumor did before treatment, it doubled about twice per day. So the point is that had that cell continued to grow at the preradiation rate, it would have only had an opportunity to go though 4 doublings.

Professor Hryniuk: So there was some restraint on that cell at the time you started and the restraint was removed?

Professor Withers: Yes. Before radiation the tumor was doubling every 4 days, so the clonogenic cells on average doubled every 4 days. To produce such a large mass of cells in 14 days, it clearly had to have accelerated its growth rate. If it had continued to grow with a doubling time of 4 days, it would have undergone 4 doublings, so there would have only been 16 cells there.

Professor Hryniuk: When did it start to grow? On day zero? Did the treatment itself do that?

Professor Withers: It happened as a result of treatment, but I am not sure whether it began at day zero. Dr Kummermehr, Institut Strahlenbiologie, GSF, Munich, has done some studies looking at repopulation in these tumors using the increment in dose per day to achieve the same control rate, and there is only a short lag period in this rapidly growing mouse tumor.

Professor Hryniuk: Do you have any advice for us chemotherapists about how we would delineate the relative importance of total dose and dose intensity in the clinical arena? Do you have a parsimonious clinical trial design in mind that will involve fewer than 10 000 patients?

Dr Withers: I do not think that adjuvant chemotherapy that extends longer than 3 months is going to achieve very much, because I think by that time the injury to the metastases will have stimulated even faster growth and they will "escape." So the best dose intensity involves delivering the maximum dose possible in some reasonable, short overall time. I do not know what that time is. It will certainly vary with different tumor sites and from patient to patient, but on average, if head and neck cancer is an example, there are about 4 weeks before the accelerated growth begins when it is treated every day. I think that if chemotherapy can be given in a short burst in less than 3 months, there is a greater likelihood of improving the results. Extending treatment over 6 or 12 months, in view of this accelerated tumor growth, does not make much sense any longer, and because the tumor begins to accelerate its growth at 4 weeks, this does not mean that treatment must be completed in 4 weeks to get the maximum advantage, since normal tissues are repopulating even more efficiently than that. The bowel and mouth mucosae are replaced at least once a day, so that they repopulate much more quickly than tumor cells. Nevertheless, the total dose is limited by the late responding tissues, so the shorter the treatment can be made the better, but it does not have to be less than 4 weeks to gain a therapeutic advantage by further protraction.

160

Dr Martin E. Blackstein (Mount Sinai Hospital, Toronto, Ontario, Canada): The rate of growth of transplantable tumors is inversely proportional to their initial volume. If what you are telling us is true, this should be clonal. If those skin cells are salvaged and regrown, their rate of growth should continue at the same level, and the tumor should have a doubling time in the future of one day or less than one day. When it reaches the same volume as the time you irradiated it, does it then become genetic?

Professor Withers: No, I think you are correct. What you are doing with your treatment is pushing the cell back down along a gompertzian curve and it will bounce back quickly and then progressively slow its regrowth rate as it gets larger.

Dr Blackstein: Are you postulating that a volume change causes this and not a change in the cells?

Dr Withers: It is not due to any change in the genetics of the cell whatsoever. It is purely an environmental factor. It could be due to the release of growth factors from all the dead cells, or maybe just to better access to metabolites. I do not know what the real mechanism is, but it is not a genetic change in the cell.

Dr Norio Suzuki (University of Tokyo, Tokyo, Japan): We might do better to define the volume doubling time versus potential doubling time; 3 days of potential doubling time of tumor stem cells versus 2 months of volume doubling that we observed. After treatment, we are talking about simple comparison of the stem cell potential doubling time before and after the treatment, instead of the volume doubling time.

Professor Withers: Yes. When the tumor is large, if you can assume that the growth fraction is not changing significantly, then the volume doubling time is also the clonogenic cell doubling time. The potential doubling time reflects the cycle time and the growth fraction; the doubling time reflects the cycle time as modified by both the growth fraction and the cell loss. We can talk about the doubling time of clonogenic cells being 2 months when the volume doubling time is 2 months when the tumor is large, even though the potential doubling time as measured by various techniques might be only 3 or 4 days. So there has been a lot of speculation that the regrowth of the tumor will accelerate to the potential doubling time. I do not think there is any real biological basis for selecting the potential doubling time, because that is a parameter determined by the physiology of the tumor when it is large, and it may not be the same when the tumor has regressed to a smaller size. However, as you say, potential doubling time is a better predictor of accelerated growth rate than is the volume doubling time.

Dr Nagahiro Saijo (National Cancer Center, Tokyo, Japan): I would like to ask you about the cross resistance of radiation and chemotherapy. Inherently chemoresistant cells are usually also resistant to various oncotherapies, and inherently radioresistant cells are also resistant to chemotherapy. However, cells that have acquired resistance, such as MDR cells and cisplatin-resistant cells, are not resistant to radiation therapy.

What kind of biological basis exists for this discrepancy?

Professor Withers: I am not sure that there is any consistent evidence that chemoresistant cells are intrinsically more radioresistant than they were before they became chemoresistant. I think that recurrent tumors or tumors that have recurred in vivo due to drug resistance may exhibit other characteristics that make them less easy to cure by radiation. For example, they may have a higher growth rate, or a higher proportion of clonogenic cells when they recur than in the first instance. This is just speculation, however.

To answer the first part of your question, I think that there is no consistent evidence that a genetic change or an expression of MDR in a cell confers radioresistance or radiosensitivity in vitro in a consistent manner.

Dr Eisuke Matsui (Gifu University School of Medicine, Gifu, Japan): When is the optimal timing for giving chemotherapy after irradiation?

Professor Withers: That is a very interesting question. We must always be concerned about the therapeutic ratio. When a course of radiotherapy is completed, the mucosae and other acutely responding tissues are regenerating at their maximum rate, and therefore I think administering chemotherapy immediately at the end of treatment may exacerbate the acute response a little too much. It does not take very long in terms of days, however, for repopulation in those normal mucosae and skin to be sufficient that drug administration would not disturb it unduly. If at the end of radiotherapy the surviving malignant cells are doubling every 2 or 3 days, that is a perfect time to give chemotherapy. I think it makes more sense to give it at the end of radiotherapy, when you have tumor cells fully in cycle and well vascularized with plenty of access to the drug, than to give it at the beginning of treatment, when you have a low growth fraction and possibly problems in perfusion of drug into the tumor, into parts of the tumor remote from the blood vessels.

IV. COMBINED MODALITIES FOR LUNG CANCER

Chemoradiation

Combined chemotherapy and radiotherapy in the treatment of lung cancer

Martin Wolf

Philipps-University Hospitals, Department of Internal Medicine, Division of Hematology/Oncology, Baldingerstrasse, Marburg, Germany

1.   Introduction

In the past decade the prognosis of patients with locally advanced lung cancer has not been altered significantly. In both small cell and non small cell lung cancer cure rates are poor and the 5 year survival rate still has not exceeded the 5 % borderline.

Despite of initially high response rates, the vast magority of patients suffers from tumor progression within two years after the start of treatment. Sites of tumor progression are either the primary tumor or the occurrence of distant metastases. Therefore, improvements of both local and systemic tumor control are necessary to increase the long term survival rate in lung cancer. Combined chemo- and radiotherapy may be an appropriate treatment approach to reach these aims. In patients with locally advanced lung cancer combined chemo-radiotherapy aims at overcoming radio- and chemotherapy resistance as a cause of local treatment failure and at early eradication of distant micrometastases as a cause of systemic treatment failure.

Theoretically, different typs of interactions between chemo- and radiotherapy may exist. First, there may be an independent way of action of each treatment modality resulting in additive effects with respect to the antineoplastic activity and toxicity. This way of interaction can be described by the term of spatial cooperation. Second, there may be a direct interaction of radio- and chemotherapy resulting in an increased activity within the radiation field. This way of interaction can be described by the term of radiosensitization.

These different typs of interactions between chemo- and radiotherapy provide the theoretical basis for 2 different clinical approaches in the treatment of locally advanced lung cancer:

a)   Concurrent chemoradiotherapy is based on the concept of spatial cooperation. Chemotherapy and radiotherapy are given in nearly full dose to achieve additive effects in local and systemic tumor control. This treatment approach is clinically employed in NSCLC as well as in SCLC.

b)   Radiosensitizing is based on the concept of increased activity within the irradiation field. Practically, low dose chemotherapy is given simultaneously to irradiation in order to enhance the irradiation effects without a substantial increase of toxicity. This treatment approach especially focusses on improvement of local tumor control and therefore is used clinically predominantly in the treatment of locally advanced NSCLC.

2. Preclinical experiments of combined chemoradiotherapy in human lung cancer cell lines

In addition to clinical investigations, in our laboratories several preclinical experiments were performed to confirm the theoretical considerations of chemo- and radiotherapy interactions and to identify drugs with radiosensitizing properties.

Two small cell lung cancer (SCLC) and two non-small cell lung cancer (NSCLC) cell lines were involved in these experiments. The cell lines were established several years before either at the NCI-Navy Medical Oncology Branch in Bethesda (1) or at the Philipps-University in Marburg (2). In order to test various histological subtypes, one classic SCLC-, one variant SCLC-, one squamous cell-, and one on large cell lung cancer cell line was used. The drugs employed were cisplatin, carboplatin, vincristine, vindesine, etoposide, ifosfamide, ACNU and 5-FU. Each drug was tested in 6 different concentrations adjusted to the peak blood level which can be achieved when a conventional dose is applied.

The investigations were performed by using the colony forming assay (3). A single cell suspension was exposed to increasing drug concentrations for 1 hour. During this drug incubation time, the cell suspensions were irradiated with a single dose of 4 Gy given by a cobalt 60 source. Then the cells were plated in a 0,3 % agarose containing medium. After 2-3 weeks of incubation, the number of colonies were counted and the surviving fraction calculated by dividing the colonies on the treated plates with the number of colonies on the untreated control plates.

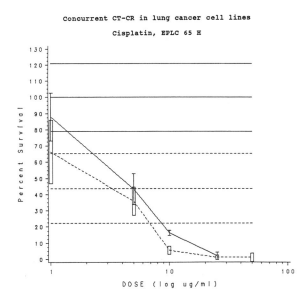

Concurrent CT-CR in lung cancer cell lines

Cisplatin, EPLC 65 H

Fig. 1

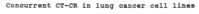

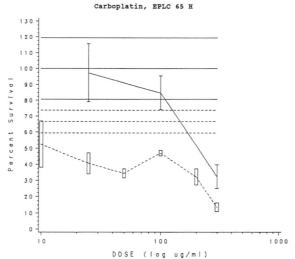

Fig. 2

DOSE (log ug/ml)

Table 1

Combined Chemoradiation in Lung Cancer
Cell Lines – Summary

	SCLC 22H	NCI-SCLC H82	EPLC 65H	LCLC 97TM1
Cisplatin	(+)	+	+	+
Carboplatin	(+)	+	+	+
Vincristin	–	–	–	(+)
Vindesin	–	(+)	(+)	(+)
Etoposide	–	–	–	–
Ifosfamide	–	(+)	+	(+)
ACNU	–	–	(+)	–

+ : increased activity by CT-RT (>20%)
(+) : slightly increased activity by CT-RT (10-20%)
- : no increasaed activity by CT-RT (<10%)

Figure 1 shows the results of these experiments for cisplatin and the cell line EPLC 65 H. The 100 % survival line indicates the no treatment control with the standard deviation. Irradiation alone reduces the number of surviving cells to about 50 % and as its is shown, the combination of cisplatinum and irradiation is slightly superior to cisplatinum treatment alone. Figure 2 shows the corresponding results for carboplatin. This platin analoque also exerts radiosensitizing properties which may be slightly superior to the parental drug, but the sole cytostatic activity was less pronounced. The results for the other cell lines and drugs are summarized on Table 1. In summary, cisplatin and carboplatin were effective in nearly all cell lines, whereas a minor degree of activity was seen for vindesin and ifosfamide and no or only marginal activity was noticed for vincristine, etoposide and ACNU.

3. Non randomized trials with cisplatin as a radiosensitizer in NSCLC

Based on the preclinical experiments showing an enhancement of radiation effects by cisplatin, most investigators used this drug for radiosensitizing in locally advanced NSCLC. In our institution we performed a phase II trial including 30 patients. Irradiation was given in single daily dosis for 2 Gy 5 days a week for 3 weeks and after a two week intervall for an additional 2 weeks. Total irradiation dose was 50 Gy. Cisplatin was given in a dose of 20 mg/m² on the first day of every treatment week. Irradiation started about 1 hour after cisplatin short time infusion. The main characteristics of the patient population were 3 females, 27 males, 93 % had a good performance status with a Karnofsky score of 80-100 %, and 40 % had stage IIIa and 60 % stage IIIb disease. The response rates were 5 CR, 15 PR, 6 NC and 4 PD. Thus, the overall response was 67 %. As expected the response rates were higher in stage IIIa than in stage IIIb patients. All CR's were seen in stage IIIa disease. Median survival was 14 month, the 2 year survival rate 20 %.

Comparable results were seen in several phase II trials performed by other investigators. These trials are listed up in Table 2. In the studies of Soresi et al. (4) and Schaake-Koning et al. (5) cisplatin was given once a week in dosis of 10-35 mg/m², the investigations of Trovo et al. (6), Bowen et al. (7) and Bedini et al. (8) used daily cisplatin application in a dose of 6 mg/m². Irradiation was given in daily dosis of 2-3 Gy 4 or 5 days a week up to total doses of 30-50 Gy. Despite of these varying study protocols, response rates of all trials were in the range of 50-86 %. However, the number of patients included was small and often no survival data has been published.

Table 2   Phase II trials with Cisplatin and RT in NSCLC

Author	No	DDP	RT	CR+PR
Soresi	20	20mg/m2 d1 weeks 1-5	2,5 Gy d1-4 weeks 1-5	76%
Schaake-könig	20	10-35 mg/m2 d1-8	3 Gy d1-5, 8-12	80%
Trovo	56	6mg/m2 d1-5 weeks 1-3	3 Gy d1-5 weeks 1-3	50%
Bowen	33	6mg/m2 d1-4 weeks 1-2,5-6	3 Gy d1-4 weeks1-2,5-6	68%
Bedini	50	6mg/m2 24h inf d1-5 weeks 1-3,6-7	2Gy d1-5 weeks1-3,6-7	86%

4. Randomized trials with cisplatin as a radiosensitizer in NSCLC

Until now a few randomized trials are available comparing sole radiotherapy to radiotherapy plus cisplatin. A large clinical trial has been performed by the EORTC (9). This study group compared sole radiotherapy with 55 Gy to radiotherapy plus either weekly cisplatin application in a dose of 30 mg/m^2 or daily cisplatin application in a dose of 6 mg/m^2. Threehundert-thirtyone patients were included. A recently published analyses showed a statistically significant advantage with respect to response and survival for the patient population receiving daily cisplatin in comparison to the patients treated with sole radiotherapy. The weekly cisplatin administration had no statistically significant advantage compared to radiotherapy alone. A further study performed by Soresi et al. (10). also noticed an advantage of the combined modality approach. A total of 94 patients were randomized to receive sole radiotherapy with 50 Gy or radiotherapy plus weekly cisplatin in a dose of 15 mg/m^2. Median survival was statistically significant superior (16 mo vs 12 mo) for the combined treatment arm. On the other side, the study of Trovo et al. (11) comparing radiotherapy to radiotherapy plus daily cisplatin in a dose of 6 mg/m^2 failed to demonstrate a statistically significant advantage of the combined treatment modality. Also the study of Ansari et al. (12) noticed no significant difference in survival, but these authors applied DDP in a dose of 70 mg/m^2 every 3 weeks concurrent to RT. This may not be the optimal study design to test the concept of radiosensitizing. The treatment protocols and the results of these trials are summarized in Table 3.

Table 3
Randomized trials with cisplatin and RT in NSCLC

Author	No.	Treatment Plan	Results
Schaake-könig	331	A: RT 3Gy d1-5,8-12 2,5 Gy d29-33, 36-40 B: RT+DDP 30mg/m2 weekly C: RT+DDP 6mg/m2 daily	Rt+DDP daily superior to RT (3 year survival 10% vs 5%)
Soresi	94	A: RT 1,8Gy d1-5 weeks 1-5,5 B: RT+DDP 15mg/m2 weekly	RT+DDP weekly superior to RT (med. survival 16 vs 12 mo)
Trovo	107	A: RT 3Gy d1-5 weeks 1-3 B: RT+DDP 6mg/m2 daily	no difference
Ansari	209	A: RT 2Gy d1-5 weeks 1-6 B: RT+DDP 70mg/m2 d1,22,43	no sign. diff. 2year survival 9% vs 15%

5. Trials with other drugs as radiosensitizers in NSCLC

Although cisplatin is most often used for radiosensitizing, a few studies were performed with other drugs looking for radiosensitizing effects of these compounds.

Based on the previously described in-vitro experiments we performed a pilot study with carboplatin as a radiosensitizer. Radiotherapy was performed in the same way as in the study with DDP. A total dose of 50 Gy was given within 7 weeks including a 2 week interval. Carboplatin was given on day 1 of each treatment week in escalating dosis. Starting dose level was 100 mg/m², and the dose was escalated every 5 patients in steps of 10-20 mg/m² up to a dose of 200 mg/m². Until now, 39 patients have entered the protocol. 33 patients were males, 5 females and most patients had a good performance status according to the WHO scale. Only 8 patients had stage IIIa disease, whereas 31 had stage IIIb disease. The median age was 60 years. Of 35 ovaluable patients, 1 achieved a complete remission, 18 a partial remission, 10 a no change and 6 had progressive disease despite of treatment. Thus, the overall response rate was 54 %. Of the 8 patients with stage IIIa disease, 6 had a major response. In stage IIIb the response rate was 48 %. Deviding the patients in those receiving low carboplatin dosis in the range of 100-130 mg/m² and those receiving higher dosis in the range of 140-180 mg/m², we observed a higher response rate in the latter group (75 % vs 48 %). These results indicate that carboplatin plus irradiation is an achive treatment approach in locally advanced NSCLC, but a longer follow up is necessary to assess survival.

Two other drugs tested as radiosensitizers in NSCLC are ACNU and vindesin. In the study of the Japan Radiation-ACNU Study Group (13) sole radiotherapy with 50-60 Gy was compared to the same radiotherapy plus ACNU in a dose of 30 mg/m² weekly for 4 weeks. Despite of a statistically significantly higher CR rate (51 % vs 21 %), the comparison of the survival curves was not significantly superior with a median survival of 48 vs. 38 weeks and a 2-year survival rate of 19 % vs. 5 %. The large trial of Johnson et al. (14) compared vindesine alone to radiotherapy alone and combined radiotherapy and vindesine. There was no difference in response (31 % vs. 33 %) and survival (2-year survival rate 13 % vs. 13 %) between radiotherapy and radiotherapy plus vindesine.

Thus, the currently available results of radiosensitizing in the treatment of NSCLC can be summarized as follows:

a) in in-vitro systems there is a superiority of the combined modality treatment.
b) most active drugs seem to be platin analogues
c) in clinical practice this treatment is well tolerated, can be performed on an outpatient basis, and seems to be slightly superior to radiotherapy alone.

6. Trials with concurrent chemo-radiotherapy in NSCLC

The second principal approach of combined chemoradiation is the application of concurrent full dose chemotherapy and radiotherapy. This concurrent chemo-radiotherapy can be used as a definitiv treatment for stage III a/b patients, or can be given as a neoadjuvant approach to reduce tumor burden and to enable a surgical resection of the remaining tumor. These different aims cause different treatment strategies especially with respect to the radiation protocol. Neoadjuvant protocols usually use total irradiation doses of 30-50 Gy, definitiv treatment strategies total doses of about 60 Gy.

Frequently used chemotherapy protocols are cisplatin/etoposide or cisplatin/5-FU or cisplatin/vindesine or 3-drug combinations mostly consisting of the afore mentioned drugs. Table 4 shows

Table 4

Concurrnt Chemo-Radiotherapy in NSCLC
Trials with DDP/Etoposide

Author	No	CT(mg/m2)	RT	CR+PR
Friess	20	DDP 50 d1,8x4q4w	60 Gy	80%
		ETO 50 d1-5x4q4w	w1-8	
Weitberg	44	DDP 25 ci d1-4,22-25	52 Gy	71%
		ETO 50 d1-5x4q4w	w1-6	
Wozniak	37	DDP 4 ci d1-5 x5	45 Gy	57%
		ETO 12 ci d1-5 x5	w1-5	
Albain	65	DDP 50 d1,8 x2q4w	45 Gy	57%
		ETO 50 D1-5 x2q4w	w1-5	

Table 5

Concurrnt Chemo-Radiotherapy in NSCLC
Trials with 3 drug combinations

Author	No	CT(mg/m2)	RT	CR+PR
Strauss	29	DDP 100 d1,29	30 Gy	62%
		VDS 3 d1,3,29,39	w1-3	
		5-FU 30 mg/kg ci 1-3,29-31		
Rowland	57	DDP 60 d1	40 Gy	
		ETO 60 d1-4	w1,4,7,10	
		5-FU 800 ci d1-4x4q4w		
Redischung	65	DDP 20 d1-4	48 Gy	75%
		5-FU 600 ci d1-4	w1,4,7,10	
		VDS 0.6 ci d1-4x4q4w		
Kubota	50	DDP 100 d1,29	50 Gy	86%
		VDS 3 d1,8,29,36	w1-3,6-7	
		MMC 8 d1,29		

trials with cisplatin and etoposide given concurrent to irradiation in NSCLC. Friess et al. (15) and Albain et al. (16) used bolus cisplatin and etoposide injection, Weitberg et al. (17) applied cisplatin as continuous infusion and Wozniak et al. (18) both drugs as continuous infusion. Radiotherapy dose varied from 45 to 60 Gy. These trials noticed response rates of 57 % to 80 % (Table 4).

Three drug combinations represent an a little more aggressive approach to improve response rates. The schedules for drug administration are comparable to those for 2 drug regimens. Strauss et al (19) applied DDP and vindesine as bolus injection and 5-FU as continuous infusion. Similar approaches have been performed by Rowland et al. (20) with DDP and etoposide bolus injection and continuous infusion of 5-FU and Redischung et al. (21) with DDP bolus administration and continuous infusion of 5-FU and vindesine. In the study of Kubota et al. (22) mitomycine C was added to DDP and vindesin. Total irradiation dose in these studies was 30-50 Gy and the overall response rates were 62 % to 86 % (Table 5). An assessment of survival is difficult because most of the studies were performed as neoadjuvant trials. Furthermore, until now, no randomized comparison has been published comparing this concurrent to a sequential treatment strategy. Such comparisons of concurrent chemo-radiotherapy to chemotherapy followed by radiotherapy are necessary to assess the efficacy of this treatment modality definitively.

7.   Concurrent chemo-radiotherapy in SCLC

In small cell lung cancer, there is an increasing number of trials testing concurrent chemo-radiotherapy to improve survival in limited stage patients. Important phase II trials are shown on Table 6. Irradiation is usually given during chemotherapy with cisplatin and etoposide. In the study of Murray et al. (23) chemotherapy consisted of CAV and PE and irradiation was given concurrent to PE. The trials of McCracken et al. (24), Johnson et al. (25) and Turrisi et al. (26) applied irradiation concurrent to 2 initial PE cycles, which were followed by alternating chemotherapy of CAV and PE or MEV. Johnson et al. (27) and Tamura et al. (28) used 4 cycles of PE chemotherapy. In all these trials high 2 year survival rates were noticed in the range of 32 % to 65 % (Table 6). However, these trials are relatively small phase II studies including patients with favorable prognostic features and none of the treatment protocols has been tested in a randomized fashion.

The only randomized trial dealing with concurrent chemo-radiotherapy in SCLC has been performed by the NCI-Canada (29). This group compared early radiation concurrent to the first PE cycle to late radiation concurrent to the last PE cycle. Chemotherapy was identical in both arms and consisted of CAV alternating PE. The early irradiation was superior to the late initiation with respect to median survival (20 mo vs. 15 mo) and 3-year survival rate (32 % vs. 22 %). This result indicate that the early concurrent use of CT-RT may have some advantage in comparison to CT followed by RT.

However, there is no doubt that the concurrent treatment approach

Table 6   Concurrnt Chemo-Radiotherapy in SCLC
Non-randomized trials

Author	No	Treatment	med surv	2 ys
Murray	67	CAV alt. PE x 6	18 mo.	32%
Canada		RT 30 Gy during 1.PE		
McCracken	154	PEV x2, +MEV/CAV	17.5 mo.	43%
SWOG		RT 45 Gy w1-5		
Turrisi	40	PE x2, +5x CAV/PE	20 mo.	54%
ECOG		RT 45 Gy bid w1-3		
Johnson	31	PE x2, +6x PE/CAV	27 mo.	65%
NCI USA		RT 45 Gy bid d5-24		
Johnson	34	PE x4q3w	24 mo.	40%
ECOG		RT 45 Gy bid w2,5,8		
Tamura	66	PE x4q3w	16 mo.	
Japan		RT 50 Gy w 1,2,4-6		

is connected with a higher degree of toxicity. Most relevant toxicities include myelosuppression, esophagitis and pneumonitis. The frequencies of severe grades of these side effects varied in the above mentioned phase II trials. The rate of treatment related fatalities seems to be in the range of 3 to 10 %.

8.   Conclusions

The use of combined chemo-radiotherapy in the treatment of lung cancer has been extended in the last years. Several phase II trials have provided clinical experiences with this treatment approach. Although the toxicity is increased in comparison to a sequential approach, the performance of combined chemoradiotherapy is feasible and side effects are tolerable. The results of phase II trials are promising and seem to be superior to those for conventional treatment, but large randomized comparisons are necessary to confirm this impression and to establish this strategy as a standard treatment procedure in lung cancer.

References

1.   Carney DN, Gazdar AF, Bepler G et al.: Establishment and identification of small cell lung cancer cell lines having classic and variant features. Cancer Res. 1985, 45:2913-2923.

2.   Bepler G, Kochler A, Kiefer P, et al.: Characterisation of the state of differentiation of six newly established human non small cell lung cancer cell lines. Differentiation 1988, 37:158-171.

3.   Salmon SE, Hamburger AW, Söhnlen B, et al.: Quantitation of differential sensitivity of human tumor stem cells to anti-cancer drugs. N. Engl. J. Med., 1978, 298:1321-1327.

4. Soresi E, Borghini U, Bongiovanni P, et al.: Radiotherapy (RT) plus low dose cis-platinum (CP) once-weekly for unresectable non small cell lung cancer (NSCLC). IV World Conference on Lung Cancer, Toronto, 1985, p. 112, abs. 442.

5. Schaake-Koning C, van Zandwijk N, Schuster-Uitterhoeve L, et al.: Radiotherapy (RT) combined with cisdiammine-dichloro-platinum (cDDP) as radioenhancer in a dose escalating way, in non small cell lung cancer (NSCLC). IV World Conference on Lung Cancer, Toronto, 1985, p. 22, abs. 356.

6. Trovo MG, Roncadin M, Bortolus R, et al.: Radiotherapy (RT) enhanced by cis-platinum (DDP) in stage III non small cell lung cancer (NSCLC). IV World Conference on Lung Cancer, Toronto, 1985, p. 113, abs. 488.

7. Boven E, Tierie AH, Stam J., et al.: Combined radiation therapy and daily low-dose cisplatin for inoperable, locally advanced non-small cell lung cancer: Results of a phase II trial. Seminars in Oncology, Vol. 15, No. 6, Suppl. 7 (December), 1988, pp. 18-19.

8. Amedeo V, Bedini MD, Luca Tavecchio MD, et al.: Prolonged venous infusion of cisplatin and concurrent radiation therapy for lung carcinoma. Cancer, 1991, 67:357-362.

9. Schaake-Koning C, van Zandwijk N, Dalesio O, et al.: Radiotherapy and cisdiammine-dichloro-platinum (II) as a combined treatment modality for the inoperable non-small cell bronchogenic carcinoma. A randomized phase III study by the eortc radiotherapy and lung cancer cooperative groups. Sixth International Symposium on Platinum and other Metal Coordination Compounds in Cancer Chemotherapy, San Diego, 1991, p. 36, abs. 0-15.

10. Soresi E, Clerici M, Grilli R, et al.: A randomized clinical trial comparing radiation therapy. Radiation therapy plus cis-dichlorodiammine-platinum (II) in the treatment of locally advanced non-small cell lung cancer. Seminars in Oncology, Vol. 15, Suppl. 7, 1988, pp. 20-25.

11. Trovo MG, Minatel E, Innocente R, et al.: Radiotherapy (RT) versus RT enhanced by cisplatin (DDP) in stage III non-small cell lung cancer: Randomized study. Proc. ECCO 5, 1989, abs. 14.

12. Ansari R, Tokars R, Fisher W, et al.: A phase III study of thoracic irradiation with or without concomitant cisplatin in locoregional unresectable non small cell lung cancer (NSCLC): A hoosier oncology group (H.O.G.) protocol. Proc. ASCO 10, 1991, p. 241, abs. 823.

13. Japan radiation-ACNU study group: A Randomized prospective study of radiation versus radiation plus ACNU in inoperable non-small cell carcinoma of the lung. Cancer 63, 1989, pp. 249-254.

14. Johnson DH, Einhorn LH, Birch R, et al.: Vindesine (DVA) versus radiotherapy (RT) versus vindesine plus radiotherapy in

locally advanced non-small cell lung cancer (NSCLC). Proc. ASCO 7, 1988, p. 212, abs. 821.

15. Friess G, Baikadi M, Harvey W, et al.: Concurrent cisplatin and etoposide with radiotherapy in locally advanced non-small cell lung cancer (NSCLC). Proc. ASCO 6, 1987, p. 176, abs. 695.

16. Albain K, Rusch V, Crowley J, et al.: Concurrent cisplatin (DDP), VP-16, and chest irradiation (RT) followed by surgery for stages IIIa and IIIb non-small cell lung cancer (NSCLC): A southwest oncology group (SWOG) study. Proc. ASCO 10, 1991, p. 244, abs. 836.

17. Weitberg A, Posner M, Yashar J, et al.: Combined modality therapy for stage IIIa non-small cell carcinoma of the lung (NSCCL). Proc. ASCO 9, 1990, p. 226, abs. 872.

18. Wozniak A, Kraut M, Herskovic A, et al.: Treatment of locally advanced non-small cell lung cancer (NSCLC) with continuous infusion (CI) VP-16 and cisplatin (DDP) and concurrent radiation therapy (RT). Proc. ASCO 9, 1990, p. 252, abs. 975.

19. Strauss G, Sherman D, Mathisen D, et al.: Concurrent chemotherapy (CT) and radiotherapy (RT) followed by surgery (S) in marginally resectable stage IIIa non-small cell carcinoma of the lung (NSCLC): A cancer and leukemia group B study. Proc. ASCO 7, 1988, p. 203, abs. 783.

20. Rowland K, Bonomi P, Taylor IV SG, et al.: Phase II trial of etoposide, cisplatin, 5-FU and concurrent split course radiation in stages IIIa and IIIb non-small cell lung cancer (NSCLC). Proc. ASCO 7, 1988, p. 203, abs. 784.

21. Rebischung JL, Vannetzel JM, Dartevelle P, et al.: Cyclic concomitant chemo-radiotherapy (CCCR) for primary inoperable non small cell lung cancer (INSCLC). Proc. ASCO 10, 1991, p. 254, abs. 874.

22. Kubota K, Furuse K, Kawahara M, et al.: Phase II trial of cisplatin (C), vindesine (V), mitomycin-C (M) and concurrent split course radiotherapy (RT) for inoperable locally advanced non-small cell lung cancer (NSCLC). Proc. ASCO 10, 1991, p. 256, abs. 883.

23. Murray N, Shah A, Band P, et al.: Alternating chemotherapy and thoracic radiotherapy with concurrent cisplatin for limited stage small cell carcinoma of the lung (SCCL). IV World Conference on Lung Cancer, Toronto, 1985, p. 85, abs. 118.

24. McCracken JD, Janaki LM, Crowley JJ, et al.: Concurrent chemotherapy/radiotherapy for limited small-cell lung carcinoma: A southwest oncology group (SWOG) study. Journal of Clinical Oncology, Vol. 8, No. 5 (May), 1990, pp. 892-898.

25. Johnson BE, Salem C, Nesbitt J, et al.: Limited (LTD) stage small cell lung cancer (SCLC) treated with concurrent bid chest radiotherapy (RT) and etoposide/cisplatin (VP/PT) followed by chemotherapy (CT) selected by in vitro drug

sensitivity testing (DST). Proc. ASCO 10, 1991, p. 240, abs. 818.

26. Turrisi A, Wagner H, Glover D, et al.: Limited small cell lung cancer (LSCLC): Concurrent bid thoracic radiotherapy (TRT) with platinum-etoposide (PE): An ECOG study. Proc. ASCO 9, 1990, p. 230, abs. 887.

27. Johnson DH, Turrisi AT, Chang AY, et al.: Alternating chemotherapy (CT) and thoracic radiotherapy (TRT) in limited small cell lung cancer (LSCLC): A test of the looney hypothesis. Proc. ASCO 10, 1991, p. 243, abs. 829.

28. Tamura T, Fukuoka M, Furuse K, et al.: Concurrent platinum (CDDP)-etoposide (VP-16) chemotherapy plus thoracic radiotherapy (TRT) for limited stage small cell lung cancer (SCLC): A japanese lung cancer chemotherapy group (JLCCG) study. Proc. ASCO 10, 1991, p. 242, abs. 826.

29. Murray N, Coy P, Pater J, et al.: The importance of timing for thoracic irradiation (TI) in the combined modality treatment of limited stage small cell lung cancer (LSCLC). Proc. ASCO 10, 1991, p. 243, abs. 831.

Combined modality treatment of chemotherapy and thoracic radiotherapy for limited-stage small cell lung cancer

Tomohide Tamura

Division of Internal Medicine, National Cancer Center Hospital, Tokyo, Japan

Small cell lung cancer differs from the other types of lung cancer in its more agressive clinical course and in its superior responsiveness to chemotherapy and radiotherapy. Median survival of patients with unresectable limited disease was reported only 3 months by supportive care alone(1). Small cell lung cancer was treated by surgery in 1950s, but the result was disappointing. In a British study in the 1960s, radiotherapy proved to be superior to surgery in survival(2). However, most patients treated thoracic radiotherapy alone died of distant metastases with median surival of 5-9 months, indicating the need for primary systemic treatment. After combination chemotherapy began to be used as main treatment for small cell lung cancer in the 1970s, the high response rate and improved survival led an idea that thoracic radiotherapy added only toxicities with no therapeutic advantage in chemotherapy-treated patients. However, considering the fact that 80% of patients treated chemotherapy alone relapsed in primary sites, and that radiotherapy achieved a response in 90% of limited disease patients, it is reasonable to attempt to combine systemic chemotherapy and thoracic radiotherapy to improve therapeutic results for this disease.

In 1980s, several radomized trials comparing chemotherapy alone versus the same chemotherapy with thoracic radiotherapy were conducted to clarify the role of thoracic radiotherapy in combination with chemotherapy for limited stage small cell lung cancer. The results of eight mature trials with at least 80 patients are shown in table 1(3-10). Radiation schedules are far from uniform in these trials. Concurrent method is defined as administration of chemotherapy and radiotherapy simultaneously. In alternating method, radiotherapy is administered between chemotherapy without any delay in chemotherapy cycle. Sequential

Table 1. Randomized Trial of Combined-Modality Therapy versus Chemotherapy
Alone in Limited-Stage Small Cell Lung Cancer

Reference	Chemotherapy	Thoracic Radiotherapy	No of patients	Median Survival (months)		Survival Differences
				CT	CMT	
Bunn	CML/VAP	40Gy/CONC/Cont	96	11.6	15.0	p=0.035
Perry	CAEV	50Gy/CONC/Cont	399	13.6	13.1	p=0.009
					14.6	
Perez	CAV	40Gy/ALT/Split	291	11.2	14.0	p=0.030
Fox	CAV	40Gy/SEQ/Cont	84	12.7	16.5	p=0.003
Østerlind	CMVL	40Gy/CONC/Split	125	11.5	10.5	p=0.240
Souhami	AV/CM	40Gy/SEQ/Cont	130	*12.0	13.0	p>0.05
				**7.0	8.5	p>0.05
Kies	VMEAC	48Gy/SEQ/Split	93CR	16.0	16.0	p=0.860
Creech	CML	50Gy/---/Cont	243	*14.2	17.2	p=0.003
				**12.4	16.0	

CT: chemotherapy, CMT: combined modality therapy,
C:CPA, M:MTX, L:CCNU, V:VCR, A:ADM, E:VP-16, P:PCB,
CONC: concurrent method, ALT: alternating method, SEQ: sequential method,
Cont: continuous course, Split: split course
*: responders, **: nonresponders, CR: complete response

method means administration of chemotherapy and radiotherapy
separately in time. These trials also differed in the chemotherapy
regimen used. Five of eight trials reported the superiority in
survival with combined modality treatment. Three of four trials
using concurrent or alternating method showed survival benefit in
radiotherapy. Only one of the three sequential trials did so.
Therefore, the timing of radiotherapy is one of the most important
issues for combined modality. The results of these trials suggested
superiority of concurrent method to sequential method. However, no
randomized trial of cuncurrent versus sequential method have been
reported.

On the other hand, thoracic radiotherapy added to toxicity in most
trials. In addition of hematologic toxicity, pulmonary and
esophageal complications are clearly increased with combined
modality, especially with concurrent regimens. In NCI trial
reported by Bunn et al. using concurrent method, 26% of patients
experienced severe pulmonary toxicity(3,11). So, increase of
toxicity was large problem for concurrent method.

Recently, platinum-based chemotherapy such as platinum/etoposide
which have less myelotoxicity and pulmonary toxicity has become
standard for small cell lung cancer, it has become easier to combine
with radiotherapy. Table 2 shows the results of pilot studies using
concurrent platinum-based chemotherapy plus radiotherapy(12-15). The
SWOG trial reported by McCracken used platinum, etoposide plus

Table 2. Pilot Studies of Concurrent Chemotherapy plus Thoracic Radiotherapy in Limited-Stage Small Cell Lung Cancer (1986-1987)

Reference	CT Regimen	TRT Schedule	No of Patients	Response CR/CR+PR (%)	MST (mo)	2-Year Survival Rate(%)	Unrelate Cancer Death(%)
McCracken	PEV	45Gy/25fr/5wk	40	57/82	17.3	43	-
Murray	CAValtPE	30Gy/10fr/2wk	70	76/93	18.0	32	2
Kwiatkowski	PEC	50Gy/25fr/5wk	50	57/88	14.0	-	4
Turrisi	PE	45Gy/30fr/3wk	23	91/91	22.8	57	4

CT: chemotherapy, TRT: thoracic radiotherapy, MST: median survival time,
CR; complete response, PR: partial response,
P: CDDP, E: VP-16, C: CPA, A: ADM, V: VCR, fr: fractions, wk: weeks, mo:
months

vincristine regimen and 1.8Gy daily radiation to total dose of
45Gy(12). The trial of Turrisi et al. used an accelerated
hyperfractination allowing 45Gy in 3 weeks in combination with
platinum/etoposide(15). These results were still preliminary, but
were encouraging with low incidence of severe complications.

Based on these results, Lung Cancer Study Group of JCOG(Japan
Clinical Oncology Group) conducted a trial of concurrent
chemotherapy plus thoracic radiotherapy for limited-stage small cell
lung cancer(16). The purposes of this study are to determine the
effects of concurrent platinum/etoposide plus thoracic radiotherapy,
with evaluation of objective response and long term survival rate,
and to evaluate the qualitative and quantitative toxicity of this
combined modality treatment. Eligibility criteria are;
histologically or cytologically proven limited-stage small cell lung
cancer, having measurable or evaluable disease, ECOG's performance
status of 0-2, age less than 75, and having adequate organ function.
Patients with stage I or stage II disease are excluded.
Chemotherapy regimen is consisted of cisplatin, 80mg/㎡ on day 1,
and etoposide 100mg/㎡ on day 1,2,3. Chemotherapy is repeated every
4 weeks for 4-6 courses in 6 months. Thoracic radiotherapy is given
by split course, 2Gy daily, 5 times per week, on day 2 to day 12 and
on day 29 to day 47. Total radiation dose is 40 to 50 Gy.
Prophylactic cranial irradiation is adminsterd in patients with CR
or good response. Of 59 eligible patients, 24(41%) acheved a CR,
and 32 achieved a PR. Overall response rate is 95%. Median
survival time is 15.1 months, and 1-year survival rate is 62% with
median follow up time of 12 months. First relapse sites of 39
relapsed patients are brain in 23%, and within radiation fields in

Table 3. Results of Combined Modality Treatment with Chemotherapy and Thoracic Radiotherapy Presented at 1991 ASCO

Reference	CT Regimen	TRT Schedule	No of Patients	Response CR/CR+PR (%)	MST (mo)	2-Year Survival Rate(%)
B.E.Johnson	PE	45Gy/CONC/Hyper	35	81/100	27	65
D.H.Johnson	PE	45Gy/ALT	34	59/97	23.5	40
Frytak	PEC	48Gy/CONC/Hyper	54	54/98	14	39
Trillet	EAI	51Gy/ALT	89	69/--	13	21
Tamura	PE	45Gy/CONC/Split	59	41/95	15	

CT: chemotherapy, TRT: thoracic radiotherapy, MST: median survival time, CR; complete response, PR: partial response, P: CDDP, E: VP-16, C: CPA, A: ADM, I: IFX, mo: months, CONC: concurrent method, ALT: alternating method, Hyper: accelerated hyperfractionation, Split: split course

21%. Although all patients experienced greater than grade 3 leukopenia, most patients could receive scheduled-treatment with almost planned interval. Esophageal complications are mild to moderate. Other non-hematologic toxicities are seem to be almost same as those in chemotherapy alone.

Table 3 shows main results on combined modality treatment with chemotherapy and radiotherapy for limited-stage small cell lung cancer presented at ASCO meeting in 1991(16-20). Bruce Johnson reported a CR rate of 90% and median survival of 27 months using concurrent twice daily radiation. D.H. Johnson reported a CR rate of 59% and median survival of 23.5 months using sequential method. The results of our study seem to be slightly inferior to these trials. One of the reasons may be that all our patients had stage-III disease, and other reason may be radiation schedule employed.

After completion of this trial, we changed the radiation schedule to accelerated hyperfractionation method by continuous course. A randomized trial of sequential versus concurrent platinum/etoposide plus continuous twice daily radiotherapy has started in our study group.

This work was supported by a grant-in-aid for Cancer Research and Comprehensive 10 Year Strategy from the Ministry of Health and Welfare. I thank Drs. N.Saijo, M.Fukuoka, K.Furuse, Y.Nishiwaki, H. Ikegami, Y.Ariyoshi, M.Oritsu, T.Shinkai, K.Eguchi, Y.Sasaki, Y.Ohe, M.Shimoyama, and K.Suemasu.

REFERENCES

1. Zelen M (1973) Cancer Chemother Rep 4:31-42.
2. Fox W, Scadding JG (1973) Lancet 2:63-65.
3. Bunn PA, Lichter AS, et al. (1987) Ann Intern Med 106:655-662.
4. Perry MC, Eaton WL, et al. (1987) N Engl J Med 316:912-918.
5. Perez CA, Einhorn L, et al. (1984) J Clin Oncol 2:1200-1208.
6. Fox RM, Woods RL, et al. (1980) Int J Rad Oncol Biol Phys 6: 1083-1085.
7. Østerlind K, Hansen HS, et al. (1986) Br J Cancer 54:7-17.
8. Souhami RL, Geddes DM, et al. (1984) Br Med J 288:1643-1646.
9. Kies MS, Mira JG, et al. (1987) J Clin Oncol 5:592-600.
10. Creech R, Richter M, et al. (1988) Proc Am Soc Clin Oncol 7:196.
11. Brooks BJ, Seifter EJ, et al. (1986) J Clin Oncol 4:200-209.
12. McCracken JD, Janaki LM, et al. (1986) Sem Oncol 13:31-36.
13. Murray N, Shah A, et al. (1986) Sem Oncol 13:24-30.
14. Kwiatkowski DJ, Propert KJ, et al. (1987) J Clin Oncol 5:1874-1879.
15. Turrisi AT, Glover DJ, et al. (1988) Int J Rad Biol Phys 15:183-187.
16. Tamura T, Fukuoka M, et al. (1991) Proc Am Soc Clin Oncol 10:242.
17. Johnson BE, Salem C, et al. (1991) Proc Am Soc Clin Oncol 10:240.
18. Johnson DH, Turrisi AT, et al. (1991) Proc Am Soc Clin Oncol 10:243.
19. Frytak S, Shaw E, et al. (1991) Proc Am Soc Clin Oncol 10:260.
20. Trillet V (1991) Proc Am Soc Clin Oncol 10:264.

Chemotherapy combined with interferons in lung cancer

Karin Mattson

Department of Pulmonary Medicine, Helsinki University Central Hospital, Helsinki, Finland

Interferon (IFN) can exert a wide range of regulatory actions on normal tissue cells, cancer cells, and host immune defence cells. Experimental evidence suggests that IFNs exert their antitumour activity by growth regulation not by immunostimulation. IFN gamma interacts with a distinct membrane receptor and differs from IFN alpha and IFN beta with respect to its antiproliferative and immunomodularory properties.

The presence of histocompatibility antigens on the cell surface is critical to the efficacy of cell-mediated cytotoxicity. SCLC cell lines express reduced levels of the class I HLA antigens (A B C $_2$-microglobulin). Treatment with IFNs may stimulate upregulation of these antigens and allow normal immune mechanisms to then eliminate these cells and prevent metastases. In preclinical studies it has been shown that 5/6 SCLC cells lines where inhibited by IFN alpha, beta or gamma but no growth inhibition was observed in 5/7 NSCLC lines.

Studies both in vitro and in laboratory animals have shown synergistic or additive interactions between IFNs on some cytotoxic drugs particularly alkylating agents and cisplatin on lung cancer cells. Although data on optimum scheduling of these two classes of antitumour agents and mechanisms of enhancement are not available in experimental systems clinical trials have been performed. They indicate that it is possible to give alpha interferons combined with cytotoxic drugs. To further test this concept of synergism clinically we performed several studies of combined treatment in patients with lung cancer.

CLINICAL STUDIES OF INTERFERON AND CHEMOTHERAPY PERFORMED BY THE HELSINKI UNIVERSITY LUNG CANCER STUDY GROUP

1. Very high dose natural alpha interferon as a single agent before chemotherapy in SCLC (1981).

In 1981 when only limited amounts of interferon were available for clinical use we performed a phase I-II study of natural alpha-IFN (Finnferon-alpha) in patients with previously untreated SCLC. Nine patients with limited disease received high-dose IFN followed by a low-dose regimen; and six patients had a low dose regimen from the beginning (Table I).

TABLE I

CLINICAL CHARACTERISTICS OF PATIENTS WITH SCLC RECEIVING nIFN ALPHA AS A SINGLE AGENT BEFORE CHEMOTHERAPY

	High-dose IFN	Low-dose IFN
Number of patients	9	6
Age, mean (range)	64 (53-75)	58 (39-70)
Performance, Karnofsky (%)	70-100	70-100
Clinical stage (1982)		
II T2N0M0	1	0
III T1N2M0	1	1
III T2N2M0	6	5
III T3N2M0	1	0
Weight loss before treatment		
< 10 kg	7	6
$\geq$ 10 kg	2	0
Histological subtype (WP-L classification)		
Lymphocyte-like 21	2	2
Intermediate 22	6	4
21 + 22	1	0

The high dosage of IFN consisted of 800×10^6 IU given as a continuous intravenous infusion for 5 days, followed by 6×10^6 IU i.m. three times weekly. If the first site of disease progression was local or in a central nervous system location, radiotherapy (55Gy/20 F/7 weeks locally and/or 30 Gy/10 F/2 weeks whole brain) was applied and IFN was continued. Chemotherapy was administered only if there was disease dissemination outside the chest. Tumour response and survival figures are shown in Table II. Three patients achieved minor response for as long as 20, 25 and 42 weeks, respectively, with IFN alone. Three of five complete responders to IFN-radiotherapy died 18, 33 and 41 weeks from the start of IFN treatment without chemotherapy. Autopsy did not reveal macroscopic or microscopic tumour at any site, but there was severe radiation pneumonitis. Four of nine patients were administered chemotherapy subsequent to IFN-radiotherapy because of disease dissemination. The median length of survival of the entire high-dose group was 41 weeks (18-162). On the low-dose regimen, one patient achieved partial response with IFN alone (duration, 12 weeks); of five evaluable patients three achieved complete remission and two partial remission to IFN-therapy, and one of the three complete responders to IFN-radiotherapy died of severe radiation pneumonitis at 21 weeks from the start of IFN treatment. No tumour was detected at autopsy. 4 of 6 patients were administered chemotherapy subsequent to IFN-radiotherapy. The median length of survival of the entire low-dose group was 78 weeks (12 - 348+) with one patient still alive at 8 years. The results derived from both our studies suggested a growth delaying effect of nIFN-alpha (Le) on SCLC. They also suggested potentiation of radiation by nIFN-alpha (Le). In contrast to other types of cancer therapy responses to IFN alpha (Le) were typically slow. Memory and psychomotor dysfunction, fatigue, and anorexia were dose limiting with both short-duration, high-dose and long-duration, low-dose nIFN-alpha (Le)-therapy (Ref. 3 updated).

2. Natural Alpha-interferon as maintenance therapy for small cell lung cancer. (1982-90)

A 3-armed phase III study was performed between 1982 and 1990 to evaluate low dose natural alpha-interferon (nIFNa, Finnferon-alpha) as a maintenance therapy in SCLC following induction chemotherapy (CT) and consolidation radiotherapy (RT). All patients received 4 cycles of CT (cyclophosphamide, vincristine, etoposide), followed by split-course RT (55 Gy/ 20F/ 7 wk). 410 patients entered the study. 237 patients who completed induction CT+ RT and were classified as responders (CR + PR) were randomly assigned to Arm 1: low dose nIFNa (91 patients); Arm 2: maintenance CT, 6 cycles CAP (cyclophosphamide,

TABLE II

RESULTS OF TREATMENT OF SMALL CELL LUNG CANCER WITH NATURAL INTERFERON-ALPHA ALONE FOLLOWED BY RADIATION THERAPY (RT) AND CHEMOTHERAPY (CT) AT TUMOUR PROGRESSION

Patient	Total dose during monotherapy		Maximal response	Duration of response (wk)	Site of first progression	Total dose (IU)/duration (WK) of IFN, partly in combination with RT	Tumour response to IFN + RT	Brain RT	Subsequent CT, 6 cycle	Survival (wk)	Current status TNM classification[a] (TN/M)
	I.V.	I.V.+I.M.									
High-dose HuIFN-$\bar{x}$ (Le)											
V.S.[c]	800	878	SD	5	Primary	878/5	CR	M_1 brain	Yes	55	PD/M_1
T.E.	700	1,024	MR	20	CNS (epidural)	1,420/44	CR	PBI/RT spinal cord	Yes	94	CR/M_1
H.A.	800	1,208	MR	25	-"-	1,382/38	CR	-	No	41	CR/M_1
E.B.[d]	425	1,263	MR	42	Primary	2,074/124	PR	PBI	Yes	162	PD/M_1
A.T.[c]	500	650	SD	10	Primary	794/18	CR	-	No	18	CR/M_0
A.W.[c]	800	974	SD	10	Primary	1,148/20	PR	M_1 brain	No	33	CR/M_1
A.N.[e]	800	920	SD	7	Primary	1,376/33	CR	PBI	No	33	CR/M_0
H.V.[c,d,e]	680	974	SD	20	CNS	1,061/29	Unevaluable	M1 brain	No	29	PD/M_1
E.K.[d,e]	800	860	SD	5	Primary	1,556/43	PR	PBI	Yes	78	PD/M_1
Low-dose HuIFN-$\bar{x}$ (Le)[f]											
	Daily	Daily+TIW									
T.K.	216	220	SD	8	Primary	354/20	CR	-	No	21	CR/M_0
V.O.	66	174	SD	8	Primary	810/53	PR	M_1 brain	Yes	77	PD/M_1
N.M.	150	306	SD	17	Primary	1002/80	CR	PBI	Yes	149	PD/M_1
R.K.	510	510	PR	12	Primary	828/30	CR	M_1 brain	Yes	80	AWD-PR/M_1
M.O.[g]	186	306	SD	11	Primary	789/55	PR	PBI	Yes	384+	PR/M_0
O.V.[g]	282	354	SD	7	Primary	354/8	Unevaluable	-	No	12	PR/M_0

AWD, alive with disease; CNS, central nervous system; TIW, three times weekly; PBI, prophylactic brain irradiation; CR, complete response; PR, partial response; MR, minor response; SD, stable disease; PD; progressive disease.

[a] Pathological stage (postmortem) or, if AWD, current disease status.
[b] High dose: 800 x 10^6 IU i.v./5 days followed by 6 x 10^6 IU three times a week; 55 Gy/20F/7weeks.
[c] Did not receive prophylactic prednisolone.
[d] Reduced radiation dose: E.B., 50 Gy; E.K., 44 Gy; H.V., no radiotherapy to the primary site.
[e] Received NK2-IFN (highly purified leukocyte IFN).
[f] Low dose: 6 x 10^6 IU I.M./day, followed by 6 x 10^6 IU two or three times a week; 44 Gy/40F/4 weeks.
[g] Received cimetidine along with IFN.
[h] IFN treatment stopped because of side effects.

187

adriamycin, cisplatin) (59 patients); or Arm 3: control arm (no maintenance treatment) (87 patients). Half way through the study the CAP arm was discontinued. The clinical characteristics of the 237 patients shows that the 3 groups were well balanced with respect to age, sex, disease status and performance status (Table III).

TABLE III

CLINICAL CHARACTERISTICS OF 237 PATIENTS WITH SCLC RANDOMISED TO RECEIVE MAINTENANCE THERAPY

	IFN arm	CAP arm	0 arm
N	91	59	87
Age, years, median	62	60	60
range	42-79	43-74	46-79
Sex, M/F	72/19	47/12	64/23
Clinical stage			
I-III, MO (LD), (%)	56 (62)	33 (56)	56 (64)
III, M1 (ED)	35	26	31
Performance status Karnofsky, (%)			
90-100, (%)	29 (32)	21 (36)	36 (41)
80	31	20	25
< 80	31	18	26
Tumour response to induction therapy			
CR, (%)	41 (45)	30 (51)	39 (45)
PR	50	29	48
Relapse pattern*			
Local only, (%)	9 (10)	8 (14)	5 (6)
Distant only, (%)	29 (32)	20 (34)	31 (36)
Both, (%)	15 (16)	14 (24)	25 (29)

LD = limited disease, ED = extensive disease
* Site of the first relapse, occurring at any time after completion of induction therapy

The response rates we achieved with our induction chemotherapy regime corresponded to those of other groups. We achieved an overall response of 78% after 3 cycles of chemotherapy, and of 90% after chemotherapy and radiotherapy.

Thoracic radiotherapy was combined with chemotherapy for all patients. This was valuable in that it increased the local response rate to 90%. However, in many cases the 11-12 week interruption in systemic treatment may have allowed metastases to develop at other sites, even when CR had been achieved at the primary site. By the time maintenance therapy was due to start many patients had therefore died or had progressive disease. The duration of maintenance therapy in 237 randomised patients is described in Table IV.

TABLE IV

DURATION OF MAINTENANCE THERAPY IN 237 RANDOMISED PATIENTS WITH SCLC

	IFN arm	CAP arm	O arm
No of patients alive 6 months after the start of the maintenance therapy study	53	36	44
No of patients completing 6 months in the maintenance therapy study	25	16	44
No of patients failing to start assigned maintenance therapy	27	14	0
Reasons for failing to start			
Death*	19	10	-
Patient refusal	4	4	-
Fall in performance status	4	0	-
No of patients leaving# the study within 6 months of starting	39	29	43
Reasons for leaving			
Disease progression	15	20	42
Patient refusal	7	4	-
Fall in performance status	5	1	-
Side effects of therapy	4	3	-
Acute myocardial infarction	1	1	-
Death	7	1	43(42+1)
Total randomised	91	59	87

* Death between randomisation and the start of the maintenance therapy programme.
# Patients who left the maintenance therapy trial continued to be monitored and were included in the statistics on relapse and surviv

The main reason for failing to start the maintenance therapy after randomisation was death (19 in the IFN arm and 10 in the CAP arm). 8 patients refused the treatment assigned to them, and the performance status of another 4 fell below acceptable levels. For those patients who left the study during the period of maintenance therapy disease progression was the most common reason (15 in the IFN arm, 20 in the CAP arm and 42 in the control arm). Other less common reasons were treatment refusal, a fall in performance status, minor side effects of therapy and death.

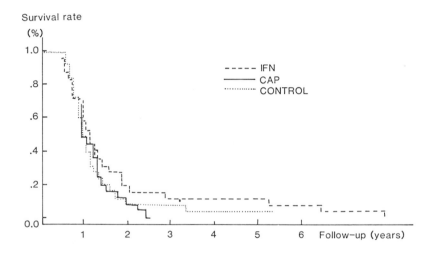

There was a very significant difference in the numbers of patients surviving for 2 years or more in the interferon group as compared to either the CAP or the control groups. 21% of patients in the interferon group survived for 2 years whereas only 8% survived this long in the CAP group and 6% in the control group. Similarly the figures for the 5 year survival rate are 11%, 0%, and 2%, for the interferon, CAP and control group respectively (Table V).

Haematological toxicity was more of a problem during induction therapy than during maintenance therapy. No patient discontinued maintenance therapy because of haematological toxicity, but there were 9 (2%) deaths due to myelosuppression during induction therapy. Some patients refused maintenance therapy because of peripheral polyneuropathy caused by vincristine. Some

TABLE V.

LONG-TERM SURVIVAL OF 237 PATIENTS WITH SCLC RANDOMISED TO
RECEIVE MAINTENANCE THERAPY

Treatment	N	1-year (%)	2-year (%)	3-year (%)	4-year (%)	5 year (%)
IFN	9 1	45/90 (50)	17/80 (21)	9/65 (14)	7/54 (13)	5/42 (11)
CAP	5 9	32/59 (54)	5/59 (8)	1/58 (2)	0/51 (0)	0/35 (0)
0	8 7	27/86 (31)	5/78 (6)	4/63 (6)	1/51 (2)	1/47 (2)

*p = 0.008___p = 0.008___p = 0.035___p = 0.005___p = 0.055_

* chi square test

patients treated with IFN suffered so severely from anorexia or fatigue that they did not wish to continue the treatment.

In retrospect, we believe that there were at least two major weaknesses in the design of this study: 1) The interferon therapy was started much too late - about 6 months after the patients had entered the study. This long delay, early randomisation and the decision not to continue maintenance treatmentwith nIFN-alpha to patients with progressive disease all meant that many patients assigned to the interferon arm in fact received no or only a few IFN injections. In those patients interferon obviously had no chance to show its potentially beneficial effects. 2) The interferon therapy was much too short. This was in part due to the shortage of interferon in 1981, when the present trial was designed. Even in malignancies such as hairy cell leukemia, which are highly responsive to interferon, very long treatment is required. It was also our impression that in many of our SCLC patients, relapse or recurrence began within a few months of cessation of interferon treatment.

It is encouraging that, in spite of the weaknesses of our trial, interferon therapy prolonged the life of a proportion of the patients. To exploit the therapeutic potential of interferon in SCCL more effectively, we have embarked on a new study in which interferon is a part of the induction therapy and interferon treatment is continued until the death of the patients (Ref. 4 updated).

3. Gamma and alpha interferon combined with chemotherapy in the treatment of non small cell lung cancer (NSCLC). (1991)

We are currently running a randomised phase II study of cisplatin-etoposide and interferon in NSCLC in which chemotherapy is combined with rIFN-alpha (alpha-IFN-2c Boehringer) and/or rIFN-gamma (Gamma-IFN-1B Boehringer).

Arm I chemo alone, Arm II chemo plus gamma-IFN, Arm III chemo plus gamma and alpha-IFN: cisplatin (P) 60 mg/m2 d 1 and etoposide (VP16) 100 mg/m2 d 1, d 3, d 5, q 28 d x 6; rgamma-IFN 0.2 mg/m2 s.c. TIW / alpha-IFN 6 x 106 IU s.c. TIW. Both IFNs were given from d 1 over 6 months. Preliminary results show the following: Arm I 5 PR/17 evaluable patients, Arm II 4 PR/16 evaluable patients, Arm III 3 PR/12 evaluable patients. Median time to progression for responders: Arm I 23 (15-27) weeks, Arm II 40 (24-104) weeks and Arm III 25 (24-27) weeks. Toxicity was mild in all treatment arms. Treatments are given on an outpatient basis and are readily accepted by the patients. The study is ongoing (Table VI).

4. High dose gamma interferon as a single agent in NSCLC. (1989)

In NSCLC we also treated fifteen patients with previously untreated, inoperable disease with high dose rIFN-gamma 2 mg/m2 i.v TIW (Bioferon, Biogen). At 12 weeks 7 patients were evaluable; one had PR, and 6 had SD (Table VII).

IFN-gamma treatment was discontinuation due to toxicity in 7/15 of patients. Main toxicities were the "flu"-like syndrome (in 15 patients) and cardiovascular events (in 13 patients).3 were withdrawn because of cardiotoxicity. We concluded that high-dose r-IFN-gamma as a single agent showed some biological activity in NSCLC. To our knowledge such activity had not been seen using other interferons. High i.v. doses of r-IFN-gamma in lung cancer patients exacerbated underlying cardiovascular disease. It should therefore be used with caution in elderly patients with chronic pulmonary disease. Close monitoring of ECG and electrolyte levels, particularly calcium, is recommended to further clarify the real spectrum of cardiotoxicity of high-dose rIFN-gamma (Ref. 5).

TABLE VI

CHEMOTHERAPY ALONE OR COMBINED WITH EITHER rIFN-GAMMA OR rIFN-ALPHA AND GAMMA IN THE TREATMENT OF INOPERABLE NSCLC

I   P-VP16
II   P-VP16 +rIFN GAMMA
III   P-VP16 + rIFN ALPHA+GAMMA

		I	II	III
N		73	23	25	25
F/M		19/54	9/14	5/20	5/20
Histology				
	Adeno	37	12	14	11
	Epid	29	8	9	12
	Large	7	3	2	2
Evaluable for response		48	17	16	15
	PR	13	5	4	4
	NC	21	7	6	8
	PD	14	5	6	3
WHO gr 3		2	2	10
	Leukopenia	-	-	-
	Trombopenia	4	6	5
	Nausea	-	-	-
	Fever	-	-	1

TABLE VII

TUMOUR RESPONSE TO HIGH-DOSE rIFN -GAMMA IN PATIENTS WITH NON-SMALL CELL LUNG CANCER (n = 15)

Time of assessment	Number of patients	Tumour response
rIFN-gamma		
4 weeks	10	1 MR, 8 SD, 1 PD
12 weeks	7	1 PR, 3 MR, 3 SD

CONCLUSIONS

Our results suggest:

- a role for nIFN-alpha in improving long-term survival in patients with SCLC
  by maintaining a clinically disease free status achieved with other
  treatments
- that the spectrum of toxicity is different for alpha and gamma interferons
- that new clinical studies are warranted with a different design concept: IFN
  should start early and continue long and be combined with other
  treatments that reduce tumour burden.

REFERENCES

1. Mattson K, Niiranen A, Iivanainen M, Färkkilä M, Bergström L, Holsti LR,
    Kauppinen H-L, Cantell K (1983): Neurotoxicity of interferon. Cancer Treatm
    Rep 67: 10 95-961.

2. Mattson K, Niiranen A, Laaksonen R, Cantell K (1984): Psychometric
    monitoring of interferon neurotoxicity. Lancet I: 275-276.

3. Mattson K, Holsti LR, Niiranen A, Kivisaari A, Iivanainen M, Sovijärvi A,
    Cantell K (1985): Human leukocyte interferon as part of a combined
    treatment for previously untreated small cell lung cancer. J Biol Resp Modif
    4: 8-17.

4. Mattson K, Niiranen A, Holsti LR, Pyrhönen S, Kumpulainen , Numminen S
    and Cantell K (1988): Natural alpha interferon as maintenance therapy for
    small cell lung cancer. The Biology of the Interferon System 1988, ISIR, .
    Kyoto, Japan, 213-218.

5. Mattson K, Niiranen A, Pyrhönen S, Cantell K (1991): Recombinant
    interferon gamma treatment in non-small cell lung cancer - antitumour effect
    and cardiotoxicity. Acta Oncol 30(5):607-610

6. Maasilta P, Halme M, Mattson K, Cantell K (1991): Pharmacokinetics of
    inhaled recombinant and natural alpha interferon. Lancet 337:371, Letter to
    the Editor.

7. Balkwill FR, Smyth JF, Cavalli F, Grossberg H, Huber C, Kimchi A, Kirchner H, Mattson K, Niederle N, Taylor-Papadimitriou J (1987): Interferon in cancer therapy: A reappraisal. Lancet 317-319.

8. Carney DN, Berendsen H, Berhg J,Doyle A, Ikegami H, Mattson K, Mulshine J, Wolf M and Woll P (1989). Third IASLC workshop on small cell lung cancer, Elsinore, Denmark. Biological response modifiers in the management of SCLC. Lung Cancer 5:143-145.

Discussion

Dr Kaoru Kubota (National Kinki Central Hospital for Chest Diseases, Osaka, Japan): Dr Wolf, in non-small cell lung cancer, how do you select the patients for sensitization or concurrent chemoradiotherapy?

Dr Wolf: This is a difficult question. We usually select the patients based on the feasibility of operability. If the patient's physical condition would allow us to perform surgery, but the tumor extent is too large to perform the surgery, we include these patients in trials with concurrent chemoradiotherapy. Patients with physical conditions that would not allow surgical resection of the tumor are included in radiosensitizing studies.

Dr Masahiro Fukuoka (Osaka Prefectural Habikino Hospital, Osaka, Japan): As you showed, in the trials of combined modality of cisplatin and etoposide plus concurrent radiotherapy reported by Drs A.T. Turrisi et al [*International Journal of Radiation Oncology, Biology, Physics* 1988;15:183–7] and B.E. Johnson et al [*Proceedings of the American Society of Clinical Oncology* 1991;10:240], the radiotherapy was administered as twice daily fractionations. Do you think the fractionations are important in improving the outcome of small cell lung cancer patients?

Dr Wolf: We have no experience with twice daily irradiation. We built up our study protocols in cooperation with a radiologist at our institution and we usually have done conventional fractionations in all the trials.

Professor H. Rodney Withers (Jonsson Comprehensive Cancer Center, UCLA Medical Center, Los Angeles, California, USA): If the problem is local control, as it sometimes is in non-small cell lung cancer, I think maximizing radiotherapy for local disease is worthwhile. I think radiotherapy has a minor role in the overall survival of patients with small cell lung cancer. You therefore must consider logistic problems, patient convenience, and cost before doing hyperfractionation just because it might be helpful in achieving local tumor control. In non-small cell lung cancer there has been shown to be an improvement in survival with radiation dose escalation. So in early stage non-small cell lung cancer you could envisage some advantage from modifying fractionation schemes either to hyperfractionation or accelerated treatment.

Dr Nagahiro Saijo (National Cancer Center, Tokyo, Japan): In your trial using cisplatin/vindesine with courses of concurrent radiation, you randomized patients to surgery and 20 Gy radiation. In these kinds of trials, all patients thus randomized are able to receive radiation therapy, but some who are randomized to surgery cannot be operated on. How do you correct this kind of bias?

Dr Wolf: Prior to this ongoing study we carried out a pilot study with concurrent chemoradiotherapy with cisplatin and vindesine and total irradiation dose of 30 Gy.

Given 30 Gy concurrent with 2 cycles of cisplatin and vindesine, the surgeons had no problems with surgical technique, even though we decided to increase the dose up to 40 Gy. This trial will now become a phase II trial to determine whether the study with 40 Gy irradiation dose is feasible. After we have done this we will decide whether to perform a randomized trial or not.

Dr Saijo: Dr Tamura, has any severe toxicity been reported in recent randomized trials of concurrent radiation plus chemotherapy?

Dr Tamura: Up to now only a few patients have been entered into the study and no severe toxicity has been reported.

Professor Withers: If you have a 20% local recurrence rate, as the sign of first recurrence, would the toxicities you currently observe allow you to increase your dose of radiation or increase the intensity of the dose of radiation?

Dr Tamura: In our ongoing phase III trials we changed the radiation schedule to twice daily radiation from conventional 2 Gy daily radiation by split course through interruptions in treatment.

Professor Withers: There is a problem in trying to escalate the dose intensity. If you exceed the tolerance of the acutely responding tissues in your field, you end up lessening the actual dose intensity.

Dr Saijo: In the previous study, radiation was given by split course, 2 Gy per day, but in recent randomized trials radiation therapy administered was 3 Gy × 2 per day, so the dose intensity of radiation was markedly increased.

Professor Withers: Are the complications causing you many interruptions in your treatment? Do you have any difficulty in completing such an intensive course of treatment?

Dr Tamura: There were no severe complications in this study. But in the CALGB trial, comparing chemotherapy alone versus chemotherapy plus early concurrent radiation versus chemotherapy plus late concurrent radiation, the late radiation arm tended to be superior to the early radiation arm. The reason given is that patients in the early radiation arm could not receive the full dose of chemotherapy after radiotherapy due to the toxicity.

Dr Saijo: So far I am not sure. Thirty patients have been included in this randomized trial to date. We have not yet done the interim analysis.

Dr Nobuyuki Hara (National Kyushu Cancer Center, Fukuoka, Japan): Dr Tamura, why were survival and response rates so different in the study you reported? Could this be because of some difference in chemotherapy or radiation or are the methods different?

Dr Tamura: The radiation schedule in this study was different from those in other studies. The difference in patient selection may have been the main reason, however.

Dr Saijo: Dr Mattson, in your current phase III trials on small cell lung cancer, do you include patients with limited and extensive disease, or do you treat only extensive disease patients?

Dr Mattson: We treat all patients aged less than 75 with a performance over 50% with the same radiotherapy and chemotherapy. When this trial started, it was believed that radiotherapy and local control of the tumor influence survival in SCLL so we used exactly the same induction treatment for all patients. If we analyze the relapse pattern, there are only 9% local relapses. Today, I would not include radiotherapy for extensive disease patients. In our new study we use 6 cycles of chemotherapy as induction treatment.

Dr Yatsusuna Sasaki (National Cancer Center Hospital, Tokyo, Japan): Dr Mattson, what is the major mechanism of antitumor activity of interferon in the treatment of small cell lung cancer? You mentioned that the mechanism may depend on the antimetastatic ability of interferon. Do you have any evidence that interferon can suppress metastatic ability in your animal model for small cell lung cancer?

Dr Mattson: I base my assumption on clinical results. If you treat stage III, limited disease small cell lung cancer with interferon alone and nothing happens for 40 weeks, then treat them with radiotherapy when the local tumor starts to grow, and at autopsy you have no metastases, there must be a slowing of the metastatic spread. We had 9 patients in the high-dose trial and 6 in the low dose, which clearly showed this. As to the mechanism of action, there are many possible hypotheses, one of which is the HLA theory.

Dr Sasaki: If you combine chemotherapy with interferon, how do you decide the optimal dose of interferon in combination with chemotherapy?

Dr Mattson: It is possible to give different doses, but I think from the hairy cell leukemia experience we have learned that it is sufficient to give a low dose but for a long time. So you can use just normal chemotherapy, the doses that you would use normally, and then add a small dose of interferon as frequently as possible (daily or every other day), but go on for a long time and start from the very beginning.

Dr Blackstein: In your study now under way why have you chosen to give cisplatin and etoposide on a q28 day schedule and thereby reduce the dose intensity of the regimen by a full one-third? Second, in the analysis of your results on the 3-armed study, could you present the results by intent to treat and not by the fact that 19 patients were able to complete the 6 months of interferon, because that in itself may confer a survival advantage that you select for patients who are going to live longer simply because they could survive 6 months of interferon. We must report these results by intent to treat and not by completion of treatment, as we must for chemotherapy in reporting these results to date.

Dr Mattson: The cisplatin dose of 80 mg/m^2 every 28 days should be safe and effective, but the dose and schedule of etoposide is not optimal. There is a moderate addition of hematological toxicity when you add interferon. We sometimes have postponed the next cycle 3–4 weeks. Do you think we will lose effect?

Dr Blackstein: Yes.

Dr Mattson: Then I think we should start all over again, because this is a very big trial. Maybe we should lower the interferon dose even more to 3 MU every second day and change the chemotherapy.

Professor Hryniuk: It seems that if you have positive results, you will not be able to interpret them, if Dr Blackstein is correct. The low dose intensity that allows you to give the interferon and therefore show a superiority for the interferon arm must be compared with better chemotherapy. You are in a difficult situation, and the addition of another arm with better chemotherapy would settle the issue.

Dr Mattson: That would certainly be feasible. We plan to accrue 300 patients, and our new study is in the very beginning.

Neoadjuvant chemotherapy

Neoadjuvant chemotherapy in non-small cell lung cancer

Nael Martini, Mark G. Kris

Departments of Surgery and Medicine, Memorial Sloan-Kettering Cancer Center, New York, New York, USA

Lung cancer has been the leading cause of cancer deaths in men for nearly three decades. In the United States it has become also the leading cause of cancer deaths in women for the past 5 years, and the incidence is still on the rise. Most are non-small cell lung cancers, and although their treatment includes surgery, irradiation or chemotherapy, the majority of the long-term survivors have had surgery as their main mode of therapy. Patients who present with stage I or II carcinomas of the lung are currently best treated by surgical resection. A significant proportion of the more advanced tumors have only locally advanced disease at presentation and are currently referred to as stage IIIa or IIIb disease. Some of the patients in this category benefit from surgery or from combined modality therapy that includes surgery as a treatment arm. In the absence of regional lymph node metastases, patients with tumors invading the chest wall and those in whom the T3 disease is due to the proximity of the tumor to the mainbronchus and carina, are best treated by surgical resection. However, despite a localized presentation, many stage III tumors are either unresectable or their resectability rate is low. Within this category are included patients who present with ipsilateral mediastinal lymph node metastases or N2 disease and patients who present with tumors extending to the mediastinum with or without regional nodal metastases. There has been a considerable interest over the past 8-10 years to treat this group of patients with neoadjuvants.

In earlier studies by us and by others, we had identified the patients with N2 disease that best benefit from surgery as their primary treatment (1-3). Those are patients that present with peripheral tumors (T1 or T2), a normal mediastinum on chest x-ray and at bronchoscopy, and a normal mediastinum on CT-scan or with a single but well encapsulated ipsilateral lymph node enlargement. In our experience, surgical resection combined with post-operative radiation therapy to the mediastinum, has proven to salvage 34% of these patients for 5 or more years (2). The resectability rate in patients with more advanced N2 involvement has been low, hence the interest in the use of neoadjuvant treatments.

Several centers are assessing the benefit of preoperative treatment by chemotherapy or by combined chemotherapy and radiation in locally advanced lung carcinoma that is unresectable and incurable at present by conventional treatments with surgery and irradiation. Regimens containing Cisplatin have had the highest and most reproducible response rates in non-small cell lung cancer (4-6). Of these, the MVP combinations (Mitomycin + Vinca alkaloid + Cisplatin) and regimens with 5-FU infusions plus Cisplatin are reported to have high response rates.

From 1984 to 1991, nearly 30 different neoadjuvant trials have been reported encompassing a total of over 1,000 patients. Major responses to treatment with neoadjuvant chemotherapy or combined chemotherapy and irradiation, have ranged from 38% to 86% with a median response of 62%. However most reports are viewed as feasibility studies because of the small number of patients entered but all demonstrate response to treatment with increasing resectability in responders. In our Center, MVP regimens have been primarily used as neoadjuvants and are the subject of this review.

Materials and Methods:

We initially reported on 41 patients evaluated by us in a surgical neoadjuvant program (7). All had stage IIIa disease and all had confirmation of N2 disease either by mediastinoscopy or at the time of thoracotomy. No patient with T3N0 or T3N0-N1 was included in the series. The chemotherapeutic regimen consisted of Cisplatin /m^2, Mitomycin and a Vinca alkaloid. An overall major clinical response of 73% (30/41) was achieved and only 1 patient had disease progress under therapy. Twenty-eight went to thoracotomy and 21 (75%) had a complete resection. All patients surgically explored received an additional 2 cycles of chemotherapy post-operatively. Those with tumor in the resected mediastinal nodes were also given radiation therapy post-operatively.

From 1984 to the present, we have treated with neoadjuvants over 120 patients with clinical N2 disease. Seventy-three of these cover the period of 1984 to 1989, and have been completely evaluated and analyzed (8). All patients had clinical evidence of bulky ipsilateral mediastinal lymph node involvement on chest x-ray or at bronchoscopy but no evidence of extrathoracic spread. Patients were required to have a creatinine clearance of greater than 65 ml/minute; leucocyte count of greater than 4,000/mm^3; platelet count greater than 150,000/mm^3; bilirubin less than 2 mg, and clinically normal auditory function. Patients with a medical contraindication to surgery due to severe obstructive pulmonary disease or significant cardiac disfunction were excluded from the study as were patients with stage IIIb disease.

All patients received 2-3 cycles of preoperative chemotherapy. Cisplatin was given with a strict program of hydration and diuresis. Patients received Cisplatin at a dose of 120/m^2 on days 1, 29 and 71. All patients received antiemetic therapy usually with metoclopromide plus dexamethasone (20 mg. IV) plus lorazepam or diphenhydramine. Mitomycin (8 mg/m^2) was administered on days 1, 29 and 71. Dexamethasone was always administered prior to each Mitomycin dose. Twelve patients received a 2 drug regimen (Cisplatin and

Vindesine) and 61 had a 3 drug regimen (Cisplatin, Vindesine or Vinblastine and Mitomycin).

Major response criteria to preoperative chemotherapy consisted of complete response (CR) or partial response (PR). Complete response was defined as total resolution of all radiographic findings following chemotherapy, partial response was recorded when the diameter of the tumor was reduced by half or more, and minimal response when reduction in tumor size was less than 50% of its diameter.

Patients who responded to chemotherapy were then surgically explored with intent to resect all disease at the original primary site and to perform a formal dissection of accessible ipsilateral and subcarinal mediastinal lymph nodes. After surgery, all patients were planned to receive 2 additional cycles of chemotherapy. Mediastinal irradiation was given after completion of chemotherapy to those patients found to have tumor in the resected mediastinal lymph nodes. Survival was calculated by the Kaplan-Meier Method and was measured as the elapsed time between the start of chemotherapy and death.

Pretreatment Patient Characteristics:

Eighty-three percent had a Karnofsky performance of greater than 70%. The median age was 53 years (range 31-71) with a male to female ratio of 1.7:1 (46 male, 27 female). The histologic diagnosis was squamous carcinoma in 23 patients (31%), adenocarcinoma in 40 (55%) and large cell carcinoma in 10 (14%). The initial primary tumor was a T1 lesion in 8 patients (11%), a T2 lesion in 46 (63%) and a T3 lesion in 19 (26%).

The median follow-up time was 60 months for all patients. The overall major response rate to preoperative chemotherapy was 77% (56 responses in 73 patients). Seven patients (10%) had a complete response and 49 patients (67%) had a partial response to chemotherapy (Table 1). Of the 7 patients with a complete response, 6 had thoracotomy and all 6 had a complete

TABLE 1

RESECTION BY CHEMOTHERAPY RESPONSE

Chemotherapy Response

	Complete	Partial	None	Total
Number	7	49	17	73
Explored	6	44	8	58
Complete Resection	6	33	5	44 (60%)
Path CR	4	5	0	9 (12%)

resection. Three of the 6 had no residual tumor in the resected specimen (pathologic CR). The patient who was not explored had a preoperative myocardial infarction and subsequently died with brain metastases 9 months after entry into the study. Of the 49 patients with partial response to chemotherapy, 44 had a thoracotomy (90%). Thirty-three of these (33/44 or 75%) were completely resected and in 4 patients a complete pathologic response with no residual tumor was noted. Of the 17 patients who had minimal or no response to chemotherapy, 8 were surgically explored and 5 had a complete resection. The overall complete resection rate was 60% (44/73) with a 70% (39/56) complete resection rate in patients with a major response to chemotherapy. There was one postoperative death and one chemotherapy death in this series.

TABLE 2

SURVIVAL BY RESECTION

	Extent of Resection		
Survival	Complete	Less than Complete	Overall
Alive	14/44	0/29	
Median	26 mos	12 mos	19 mos
1 yr	84%	52%	73%
2 yr	54%	7%	35%
3 yr	47%	0%	28%

The median survival for the 73 patients entered into the study is 19 months with a 1 year survival of 73%, a 2 year survival of 35% and a 3 year survival of 28% (Table 2). In the patients whose tumors were completely resected, the median survival was 26 months and the 3 year survival was 47%. The median survival of 29 patients who had an incomplete or no resection was 12 months with no survivor beyond 3 years. Thirty of the 44 patients rendered free of disease have since relapsed, mostly at distal sites (Tables 3-4).

TABLE 3

RELAPSE DATA

Number Patients Disease Free	44
Median Follow-Up (Range)	5 yrs (1.5-7.4)
No Evidence of Disese	14 (32%)
Relapsed	30 (68%)

Initial Relapse Sites:
-Local-Regional		10
-Distant		20
Bilateral Lung	8	
Brain	5	
Other Sites	7	

TABLE 4

STATUS OF PATIENTS WITH PATHOLOGIC COMPLETE RESPONSE

4	Alive Disease Free	at 54+, 61+, 79+, 89+ months
1	Alive With Disease	at 84+ months
1	Died Disease Free	at 3 months
3	Died With Disease	at 18, 42, 64 months

Discussion:

Our experience with neoadjuvants has been primarily centered on patients with stage IIIa clinical N2 disease as reported. Several other trials have investigated preoperative chemotherapy both alone and in combination with preoperative radiation therapy in stage III and IV non-small cell lung cancer. Many have included T3N0-N1 lesions as well as N2 lesions. Despite the differences among these trials, each has reported high response rates with chemotherapy when used in a preoperative setting and complete resection rates higher than historical controls. It has been our opinion from the outset that the merits of chemotherapy in this group of patients would be best assessed if used alone without combining with preoperative radiation therapy. Our results with preoperative chemotherapy without irradiation are essentially identical to results attained by other centers with the use of chemotherapy plus irradiation.

In a recent review by Drs. Faber and Bonomi (5), the results of 7 neoajuvant reports which have evaluated 30 or more stage III non-small cell lung cancers were analyzed (5-7,9-11). It was noted that no evidence of tumor was found in the resected specimen in up to 20% of the total patients entered into the trials. It also was noted that sterilization of the tumor was a most important treatment related prognostic factor for long-term survival. Complete resection was most frequently achieved when preoperative therapy was utilized and varied from 68-97% in these reported series. It was also pointed out that resections following neoadjuvant therapy can be extremely difficult due to fibrosis. The use of Cisplatin achieved relatively high response rates, resectability rates were increased, and morbidity and mortality were acceptable, and the tumor sterilized in 10-15% of responders.

Pulmonary problems consequent to Mitomycin toxicity have occurred with MVP regimens. However, with close monitoring of the pulmonary diffusion capacity and with the use of steroid therapy in the symptomatic patients, many of these pulmonary problems have been reversible. We have observed an improvement in the pulmonary diffusion capacity to 60-80% levels with the use of steroids permitting subsequent safe surgical treatment in some of these patients. In our opinion, MVP without irradiation remains the most effective chemotherapy regimen as neoadjuvant in locally advanced non-small cell carcinoma of the lung. More investigation is needed to clarify the role of Mitomycin with efforts directed to identify and treat patients at risk for respiratory complications. We prefer to find ways to lessen or prevent the toxicity of an effective chemotherapy drug rather than attenuating its dose or eliminating it all together.

Since a major goal of these preoperative trials is to increase the complete resection rates, it is important to look at resection rates by response. Of those patients who had a major objective response in our trial, 70% were able to undergo a complete resection. For those who did not have a major response, only 29% had a complete resection (p = 0.003). Moreover, of those patients who were able to undergo a complete surgical resection, 89% were chemotherapy responders whereas only 11% had no major response to chemotherapy. Our data clearly shows that only those patients who have complete surgical resection have long-term survival.

Outside study settings, the vast majority of physicians in the United States treat patients with mediastinal lymph node metastases by palliative irradiation. It is difficult to ascertain at this time whether this impressive response rate to chemotherapy regimens and the enhanced resectability in responders will eventually translate into prolonged survival in a sufficient number of patients as to impact on the overall survival of all those with stage IIIa carcinomas. A randomized study between conventional radiation treatment and the use of neo-adjuvants is necessary yet difficult to implement. Perhaps a carefully conducted cooperative study of multiple institutions might gather enough case material into such a randomized prospective study to answer this question. I sincerely doubt that a single institution can accomplish such a review.

It has been our experience that patients presenting with invasion of the mediastinum with or without lymph node metastases do also poorly. Recently 225 consecutive patients undergoing operation for non-small cell lung cancer were pathologically confirmed to have had mediastinal invasion at our Institution. The records of these patients were reviewed in an attempt to evaluate the role of surgery in these patients and the details of the report have since been published (12). Of note was the fact that the majority of the patients (68%) demonstrated mediastinal lymph node metastases. Although all 225 patients were surgically explored, complete resection was possible in 22% of the patients. The majority of the patients received some form of adjuvant therapy (postoperative radiotherapy 70% and postoperative chemotherapy 20%). The overall survival for these 225 patients was 22% at 2 years and 7% at 5 years. More importantly, the 5 year survival following complete resection was only 9%. It is clear that patients with mediastinal invasion have a poor prognosis when treated primarily by surgery and should also be included in neoadjuvant programs.

We conclude that MVP chemotherapy produces high major response rates in patients with stage IIIa clinical N2 non-small cell lung cancer. Although resections can be specially difficult in this group of patients due to fibrosis secondary to chemotherapy effect, the procedure can be performed safely with a reasonable expectation of a complete resection in 70% of the patients. The improved resection and survival rates justify further trials to compare this approach to other treatments.

ACKNOWLEDGEMENT

We gratefully acknowledge Miss Phyllis Byczek for her invaluable assistance in the preparation of the manuscript.

REFERENCES

1. Martini N, Flehinger BJ, Zaman MB, et al.: Results of Resection in Non-Oat Cell Carcinoma of the Lung with Mediastinal Lymph Node Metastases. Ann Surg 198:386-396, 1984.

2. Martini N, Flehinger BJ: The Role of Surgery in N2 Lung Cancer. Surg Clin N Amer 67:1037-1049, 1987.

3. Naruke T, Goya T, Tsuchiya R, et al.: The Importance of Surgery to Non-Small Cell Carcinoma of the Lung with Mediastinal Lymph Node Metastases. Ann Thorac Surg 46:603-610, 1988.

4.   Kris MG, Gralla RJ, Martini N, Stampleman LV and Burke
        TM: Preoperative and Adjuvant Chemotherapy in Locally
        Advanced Non-Small Cell Lung Cancer. Hem/Oncol Clin N.
        Amer 2:407-415, 1988.

5.   Faber LP and Bonomi PD: Neoadjuvant Treatment in Locally
        Advanced Non-Small Cell Lung Cancer. Sem Surg Oncol
        6:255-262, 1990.

6.   Burkes R, Ginsberg R, Shepherd, et al.:   Neoadjuvant
        trial with MVP (Mitomycin C + Vindesine + Cisplatin)
        Chemotherapy for Stage III (T1-3, N2, M0) Unresectable
        Non-Small Cell Lung Cancer. Proc Am Soc Clin Oncol 8:221,
        1989.

7.   Martini N, Kris MG, Gralla RJ, Bains MS, McCormack PM,
        Kaiser LR, Burt ME and Zaman MB: The Effects of
        Preoperative Chemotherapy on the Resectability of Non-
        Small Cell Lung Carcinoma with Mediastinal Lymph Node
        Metastases (N2M0).   Ann Thorac Surg 45:370-379, 1988.

8.   Pisters KMW, Kris MG, Gralla RJ and Martini N:
        Preoperative Chemotherapy in Stage IIIA Non-Small Cell
        Lung Cancer: An Analysis of a Trial in Patients with
        Clinically Apparent Mediastinal Node Involvement.   In:
        SE Salmon, M.D. (ed) Adjuvant Therapy of Cancer,
        Proceedings of the 6th Int'l Conference on the Adjuvant
        Therapy of Cancer. V:6. Philadelphia: WB Saunders, 133-
        137, 1990.

9.   Weiden P, Piantadosi S: Preoperative Chemoradiotherapy
        in Stage III Non-Small Cell Lung Cancer (NSCLC): A Phase
        II Study of the Lung Cancer Study Group (LCSG). Proc Asco
        7:197, 1988.

10.   Skarin A, Johchelson M, Sheldon T, et al.:   Neoadjuvant
        Chemotherapy in Marginally Resectable Stage III M0 Non-
        Small Cell Lung Cancer: Long Term Follow-Up in 41
        Patients.   J Surg Oncol 40:266-274, 1989.

11.   Eagan R, Ruud C, Lee R, et al.:   Pilot Study of Induction
        Therapy with Cyclophosphamde, Doxorubicin, and Cisplatin
        (CAP) and Chest Irradiation Prior to Thoracotomy in
        Initially Inoperable Stage III M0 Non-Small Cell Lung
        Cancer. Cancer Treat Rep 71:895-900, 1987.

12.   Burt ME, Pomerantz AH, Bains MS, McCormack PM, Kaiser LR,
        Hilaris BS and Martini N: Results of Surgical Treatment
        of Stage III Lung Cancer Invading the Mediastinum. Surg
        Clin N America 67:987-1000, 1987.

212

Neoadjuvant therapy for non-small cell lung cancer

Nobuyuki Hara, Yukito Ichinose, Mitsuo Ohta

Department of Chest Surgery, National Kyushu Cancer Center, Fukuoka, Japan

INTRODUCTION

Surgery is the most effective therapeutic modality for non-small cell lung cancer (NSCLC) because it offers a chance for long-term survival. Thoracotomy, therefore, has been offered to patients whose disease was considered sufficiently localized to permit surgical resection. However, curative resection for all lung cancer is possible in less than 40% of patients, and for advanced stage III patients only 20%.

Recently, in order to increase curative resection and to improve survival of stage III patients (approximately 30% of NSCLC), a new treatment modality, neoadjuvant therapy, has been introduced in the management of NSCLC. This treatment refers to chemotherapy or radiation administered before surgery when surgery is intended as the definitive local treatment (1).

We designed a phase II trial for locally advanced stage III NSCLC patients to determine whether neoadjuvant therapy could increase the resectability, improve local control and improve survival. In addition, we determined the safety of surgery after neoadjuvant therapy.

MATERIALS AND METHODS

Patients with cytologically or histologically proven stage III NSCLC were entered in the study. Patients were divided into two groups. The first group consisted of marginally resectable or unresectable stage III patients who were treated concurrently with chemotherapy and radiation therapy followed by surgery. The second group consisted of clinically resectable stage IIIA patients who were treated preoperatively with chemotherapy only.

Eligibility requirements for the first group included the following: measurable or evaluable disease; performance status 0 and 1; age <75 years old; adequate cardiopulmonary function (to allow for surgery) and hematologic, renal and liver functions. Ineligibility criteria included: prior chemotherapy or radiotherapy; other primary malignancies; pleural effusion caused by malignant disease. Patients who were considered technically unresectable but who had potentially resectable tumors if they responded to the induction chemoradiotherapy, were also entered in this study.

Clinical staging consisted of detailed history, physical examination, complete hematology and blood chemistry profiles, bone scan, computerized tomography (CT) of the chest, brain and upper abdomen to include liver, adrenal glands and kidneys, and bronchoscopy. Clinical N2 disease in this study was determined mainly by CT documentation (single node > 2.0 cm or multiple nodes > 1.5 cm) although histologic confirmation of mediastinal lymph nodal involvement was encouraged.

The protocol therapy is schematically represented in Fig. 1. Cisplatin 100 mg/m^2 was administered on day 1 and vindesine 3 mg/m^2 on days 1, 8 and 15. The thoracic radiation was given concurrently with chemotherapy. A total dose of 30 Gy was administered in 4 weeks, generally 5 days per week, 1.6 Gy per fraction. After completion of the induction therapy, patients were reevaluated to determine the response and resectability of the tumors. Patients with complete resection received one more cycle of chemotherapy, while those with unresectable disease were treated with a single cycle of chemotherapy and 30 Gy of radiation therapy.

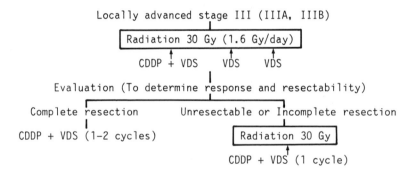

Fig. 1. Schedule of neoadjuvant therapy.

In the second group, patient eligibility was the same as the first group except that clinically resectable stage IIIA patients were selected. Patients received 2 cycles of chemotherapy followed by surgery. After surgery, patients were planned to receive 1 or 2 cycles of the same chemotherapy regimen. Chemotherapy consisted of PMV, cisplatin 80 mg/m^2 and mitomycin 8 mg/m^2 on day 1 and vindesine 3 mg/m^2 on days 1 and 8, and PV, cisplatin 100 mg/m^2 on day 1 and vindesine 3 mg/m^2 on days 1, 8, and 15. Of 10 patients, 8 patients received PMV regimens and 2 patients received PV regimens.

The response to induction therapy was assessed after completion of the initial chemoradiotherapy in the first group, and the initial two cycles of chemotherapy in the second group. Response categories included complete response, the complete disappearance of all evidence of disease; partial response, >50% reduction in the sum of the products of the greatest tumor diameter and its pendicular; no change, < 50% decrease in tumor size and progress disease, > 25% increase in tumor size or any new sites of disease.

Survival was calculated from the start of induction therapy using the methods of Kaplan and Meier.

RESULTS

Between April 1986 and August 1990 thirty six patients were registered in the first group and ten patients in the second group (Table I). Of the 36 stage III patients treated with induction chemoradiotherapy, 19 underwent thoracotomy. Sixteen of the 19 patients had resection and 3 had unresectable tumors. All of the 10 stage IIIA patients, treated with induction chemotherapy, underwent complete resection.

TABLE I

CLINICAL AND HISTOLOGIC FEATURES OF THE 36 PATIENTS

Characteristics		Types of Preoperative Therapy	
		Chemoradiotherapy (n=36)	Chemotherapy (n=10)
Sex	Male	28	9
	Female	8	1
Age (yrs)	Mean	58	62
	Range	42–73	54–70
Stage	IIIA	25	10
	IIIB	11	0
N factor	N0	6	0
	N1	4	2
	N2	24	8
	N3	2	0
Cell type	Adenoca.	18	3
	Squamous cell ca.	12	6
	Large cell ca.	6	1
Therapy	Thoracotomy	19(3)*	10
	No thoracotomy	18	0

* Unresectable.

Response to Induction Therapy

The response to the initial chemoradiotherapy was determined prior to surgery (Table II). The overall response rate for all 36 patients was 58%. Patients with thoracotomy demonstrated a higher response (68%) compared with that of patients without thoracotomy (47%). The overall response for the 10 patients with resectable stage IIIA was 80%. However, all patients achieved a partial response only.

215

TABLE II

EXTENT OF SURGERY ACCORDING TO RESPONSE TO INDUCTION THERAPY IN THE 36 PATIENTS

| Response to Induction Therapy | No Thoracotomy | Thoracotomy | | Total |
		Unresectable	Resectable	
Partial response	8	2	11	21
No response	7	1	5	13
Progressive	2	0	0	2
Total	17 (47%)	3 (8%)	16 (45%)	36 (100%)

Toxicity

Hematologic, esophagitis and gastrointestinal toxic effects were the most frequent findings in patients treated with chemoradiotherapy. Grade 3 and 4 leukopenia occurred in 81%, while anemia and thrombocytopenia occurred in only 8%, respectively. Mild to moderate esophagitis and gastrointestinal toxicities were observed in most patients, but these were well controlled. Temporally elevation of creatinine occurred in 5 patients. No patients, however, experienced major nephrotoxicity related to cisplatin. One patient with an unresectable tumor died of pneumonia 3 weeks after the second cycle of chemotherapy and radiotherapy. Hematologic and gastrointestinal toxicity in patients treated with chemotherapy only were mild compared to those who had chemoradiotherapy. All toxic effects from induction therapy were considered to be tolerable and acceptable in both treatment groups. There were also no deaths related to induction therapy.

Surgery

Nineteen of the 36 patients were considered resectable after chemoradiotherapy, and had thoracotomy. The types of resection performed at thoracotomy were pneumonectomy in 7, lobectomy in 5, lobectomy combined with chest wall resection in 3 and partial resection in 1. Three patients were unresectable. All but one patient had complete resection. One patient with incomplete resection (partial resection), however, showed no tumor cells in the resected specimen. On the other hand, all of the 10 patients with clinically resectable stage IIIA had complete resection after induction chemotherapy.

Of the 19 patients with induction chemoradiotherapy, 4 (21%) had pulmonary complications and 6 (32%) had cardiac complications. Types of complications included the following: pneumonia in 2; atelectasis in 1; empyema in 1; arrhythmia in 6. Complications in the 10 patients who received preoperative chemotherapy alone, included the following: respiratory failure in 1; empyema in

216

1; arrhythmia in 2; hepatitis in 1; gastric dilatation in 1. All patients
recovered from their complications and there were no postoperative deaths.

Survival

The median survival time (MST) for the 36 patients with induction chemoradiotherapy was 20 months, with 2- and 3-year survivals of 34% and 29%, respectively
(Fig. 2A). For the 16 resected patients, the MST was 20 months, with 2- and 3-
year survivals of 38%, respectively. Survival for the 10 resected patients with
induction chemotherapy was 48% at 3 years, with a MST of 16 months (Fig. 2B).

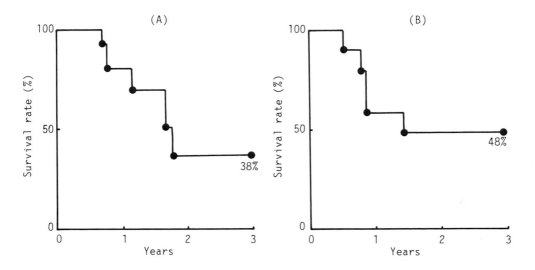

Fig. 2. Survival of all 36 patients (A) treated with chemoradiotherapy and 10
resected patients (B) treated with chemotherapy only.

Sites of Relapse

The sites of first relapse for the 26 resected patients in the two treatment
groups are shown in Table III. Of the 15 patients with relapse, 5 (33%) occurred
in intrathoracic sites and 10 (67%) in extrathoracic sites. The local relapse
rate was slightly higher in patients treated with chemotherapy only compared with
those treated with chemoradiotherapy.

Microscopic Findings in Resected Specimen

A higher pathological response was observed in the 16 patients treated with
chemoradiotherapy, demonstrating no residual tumor cells in 25% and microscopic
tumor cells in 50%. Pathological response to induction chemotherapy without
radiotherapy was lower. Only 30% of the 10 patients had microscopic cells; the
remaining 70% had gross residual tumor.

TABLE III

FIRST SITES OF POSTOPERATIVE RECURRENCE IN 16 RESECTED PATIENTS

Recurrence	Types of Preoperative Therapy		Total
	Chemoradiotherapy (n=16)	Chemotherapy (n=10)	
None	7 (44%)	4 (40%)	11 (42%)
Local	2 (12%)	3 (30%)	5 (19%)
Distant	7 (44%)	3 (30%)	10 (38%)
Bone	3	1	4
Lung	3	0	3
Liver	1	1	2
Brain	0	1	1

DISCUSSION

The rationale for neoadjuvant therapy is to increase the potential for curative therapy with radiation and/or surgery of the primary tumor plus to improve the cure rate by eradication of distant micrometastases.

In the first group, we attempted to clarify whether neoadjuvant chemoradiotherapy could increase the resectability rate without residual disease, thereby decreasing local relapse, and improve survival in patients with unresectable and marginally resectable stage III disease.

Sixteen (44%) of the 36 patients were successfully resected after neoadjuvant chemoradiotherapy. Although postoperative pulmonary complications occurred in 21% and cardiac complications in 36%, these incidences do not appear to have been increased by the preoperative therapy employed. There were also no postoperative deaths.

The response rate of 58% achieved in this study is similar to that of other published series, which vary from 43 to 78% (2-4). We added radiation therapy in combination with chemotherapy, but the advantages of this treatment modality are still controversial. Some investigators reported increased response rate but others did not. Eagan et al. (2) and Taylor et al. (3) demonstrated that radiation increased difficulty in performing surgery because of tissue fibrosis.

The resection rate of 44% in our study was slightly lower than that in other reports. The difference is probably due to the selection of patients as potential candidates for neoadjuvant therapy. However, this treatment modality appeared to improve chances of resection in selected patients.

The second study of neoadjuvant chemotherapy was planned to improve survival mainly by eradicating distant micrometastases, and in addition, to increase complete resection in patients with clinically resectable stage IIIA.

Since we selected clinically resectable stage IIIA patients, a response rate of 80% and a resection rate of 100%, without gross residual disease, was obtained in this study. Therefore, radiation therapy may not be a necessary part of the induction regimen when patients, with resectable disease, are selected in the trial. Similar results are also reported in other series (5-7).

The median survival was 20 months, with a 3-year survival of 29% in the first study. The median survival was 16 months with a 3-year survival of 48% in the second study. These results are encouraging even in selected patients, compared with those in patients treated with conventional therapy.

Following surgery, 9 of the 16 (56%) patients treated with neoadjuvant chemo-radiotherapy and 6 of the 10 (60%) patients treated with neoadjuvant chemotherapy without radiation, had relapses in intrathoracic and other thoracic sites. In addition, only 25% of patients treated with chemoradiotherapy showed, histologic-ally, an absence of tumor cells in the surgical specimen. There was no complete disappearance of tumor cells in patients treated with chemotherapy only.

Therefore, more effective chemotherapy will be required to improve the complete remission rate and also to reduce local relapse and distant metastases. However, phase III randomized trials are needed to determine whether neoadjuvant therapy is or is not beneficial for locally advanced stage III disease compared with radiotherapy and surgery alone.

REFERENCES
1. Frei E III (1982) Cancer 50:1979-1992
2. Eagan RT, Rirud C, Lee RE, et al (1987) Cancer Treat Rep 7:895-900
3. Taylor SG, Trybula M, Bonomi P, et al (1987) Ann Thorac Surg 43:87-91
4. Weiden PL, Piantadosi S (1991) J Natl Cancer Inst 83:266-272
5. Martini N, Kris MG, Gralla RJ, et al (1988) Ann Thorac Surg 45:370-379
6. Faber PL, Kittle CF, Warren WH, et al (1989) Ann Thorac Surg 47:669-677
7. Murren JR, Buzaid AC, Hait WN (1991) Am Rev Respir Dis 143:889-894

Discussion

Dr Martin E. Blackstein (Mount Sinai Hospital, Toronto, Ontario, Canada): Professor Martini, did you say that at Memorial Sloan-Kettering the stage IIIA surgery-alone survival was 28% in the past?

Professor Martini: No. In the past, stage IIIA was not assessed routinely by mediastinoscopy. Most patients in our historical review of stage IIIA patients treated surgically preceded the use of CT scanning and did not have routine mediastinoscopy if the chest X-rays and endoscopic findings did not indicate disease involving the mediastinum. In the group of patients who underwent surgery with a presumed clinical N0 or N1 disease, the overall resectability rate was 53%, and survival in the resected cases was 34% at 5 years. In this group, 224 patients were surgically explored and 119 patients had complete resection.

Dr Blackstein: As I remember, in the more modern era of the Lung Cancer Study Group, our disease-free survival in the stage III trials without chemotherapy approached 0 at 3 years, but was boosted slightly by CAP.

Professor Martini: Our original review had included 151 patients who had complete resections, all of whom were proven histologically to have had mediastinal nodes, usually at thoracotomy. All patients with few exceptions also received external radiation therapy to the mediastinum. That study was closed in 1981. The actuarial 5-year survival of all 151 patients who had resection was 30% at 5 years. There were 37 patients alive at 5 years, an absolute survival of 25%. When we analyzed the patients with bulky N2 disease, we found that the resectability rate dropped to 18% and despite a complete resection, the 3-year survival was only 9%. Of 32 patients who had complete resection in the face of bulky N2 disease, we had salvaged only 3 at 3 years, ie, 9% of 18%, which is nearly 1%. Our conclusion was that in patients presenting with bulky N2 disease, surgery plus radiation is not helpful.

Dr Blackstein: You have mentioned the Toronto Lung Group. After hearing the early results we began this study and closed it several years ago with 40 patients. The results are almost identical in terms of CR and PR to those you achieved in New York, with one exception: the morbidity and mortality of MVP chemotherapy was higher in the Toronto group, and patients who had complete obstructive pneumonitis were a major risk group for going on to developing abscess and death if they did not respond to the treatment.

Professor Martini: I am now reviewing the records of all patients who received neoadjuvant MVP, focusing specifically on the pulmonary complications that may be drug related. I recall 2 patients who had pulmonary problems similar to those observed with mitomycin toxicity. However, one had received only vindesine and platinum but not mitomycin and the other had candidiasis. We are trying to find out whether mitomycin toxicity is frequent enough to be excluded from our regimens or if we would be dropping an effective drug of which the toxicity is infrequent and manageable.

Dr Makoto Ogawa (Cancer Chemotherapy Center, Tokyo, Japan): I understand that you gave 2 or 3 cycles of chemotherapy prior to surgery. Were there any differences of major responses in patients receiving between 2 and 3 cycles? Also, you gave 2 cycles of chemotherapy after surgery. Do you belive that postadjuvant chemotherapy is necessary?

Professor Martini: Your second question is easier than the first. If you have a response to chemotherapy preoperatively, it stands to reason that adding 1 or 2 more cycles postoperatively may sterilize any residual microscopic disease. The answer to your first question, what is the magic number of cycles, I do not know. I know that 4 is too many, because we have observed many patients who recur after the 3rd cycle. It is our impression that one cycle is insufficient and that 2–3 cycles should be given. If you have no regression at the end of 2 cycles, you should interrupt treatment. If you have continued regression, a 3rd cycle is justified if the patient is tolerating the chemotherapy.

Professor William M. Hryniuk (Ontario Cancer Treatment and Research Foundation, Hamilton Regional Cancer Centre, Hamilton, Ontario, Canada): Dr Hara and Professor Martini, are these encouraging results due to patient selection or true activity of the treatment? Dr Hara called for a randomized trial to test this, however we are dealing with surgically nonresectable disease so it is hard to design a trial, and yet one has the feeling that one should do a randomized study to corroborate these encouraging, but phase II studies. What would be the design of such a randomized trial?

Dr Hara: According to the consensus report published on lung cancer this year [Klastersky J et al. *Lung Cancer* 1991;7:15], perhaps patients resistant to neoadjuvant therapy can be divided into 3 groups. One group consists of possibly resectable stage IIIA patients with resectable stage III, I mean T1, T2, and T3, with minimal N2 disease. The 2nd group consists of marginal resectable stage III with T1, T2, and T3 not with minimal, but large involvement of mediastinal lymph nodes. Perhaps we must divide the patients when we try randomized trials. The first group I consider to be candidates for surgery alone as a control and the 2nd group are candidates for radiotherapy as the control.

Professor Hryniuk: Certainly the experience in head and neck cancer, where chemotherapy has spectacular results, has not improved survival compared to local treatment alone.

Dr Hara: If we select the patients with clinically resectable IIIA, perhaps we should use only chemotherapy preoperatively.

Professor Martini: Professor Hryniuk, I would like to respond in a different fashion. We have no difficulty in getting patients to accept neoadjuvants in stage IIIA N2 disease using the following guidelines. Patients who at the time of diagnosis present with bulky, radiographically apparent ipsilateral lymph nodes form one subset; patients who have a normal mediastinum on routine X-rays, but who show multiple ipsilateral enlarged mediastinal nodes on CAT scan, form another. All patients are histologically documented to have N2 disease and receive chemotherapy first. We exclude patients with contralateral mediastinal metastasis. We also exclude patients found to have a single mediastinal node metastasis. In our experience, the resectability rate in this small subset is 60–90% without the use of neoadjuvants and the 5-year survival rate is as high as 46%.

The surgery is more difficult after chemotherapy. It is worse after chemotherapy and radiation. For a randomized study, I believe the only standard treatment to randomize against should be radiation therapy as usually used in most hospitals. For N2 patients, treatment at our center has never been radiation therapy alone. We have usually combined surgery with radiation, which is not the standard treatment offered at other insitutions.

Professor Hryniuk: I hope it can be done.

Professor Martini: There are 2 cooperative randomized trials currently under consideration. One is that of the Southwest Oncology Group (SWOG). Their control arm consists of cisplatin and etoposide plus radiation, assumed to be standard therapy. Responders are then randomized to either more radiation or surgery. Unfortunately, this study assumes the gold standard to be cisplatin/etoposide plus 3000 rads of radiation therapy. The Radiation Oncology Group (RTOG) currently has another study that assesses etoposide plus radiation against etoposide plus radiation plus surgery.

Dr Hara, I think your 2nd study is somewhat confirmatory of what we discussed concerning MVP therapy, but the number of patients is still very small. You are including only one dose of mitomycin, which we believe is insufficient to obtain complete response, and you are also considering in some of your 10 patients only one cycle of chemotherapy. I think you are undertreating them and therefore not obtaining enough complete responses, despite an impressive partial response. In your 1st study, two-thirds of your patients are stage IIIA, but one-third are stage IIIB, and in fact only two-thirds have N2 disease. So you have a mixed bag. It is an impressive response, consistent with the experience of others with neoadjuvants, whether with chemotherapy plus radiation or chemotherapy alone. The range of response with neoadjuvants reported in the literature is between 38% and 80%.

222

V. CLINICAL TRIALS BASED ON PHARMACOLOGY

Pharmacokinetics and pharmacodynamics

The relevance of the investigation of clinical pharmacokinetics and pharmacodynamics in medical oncology

Duncan I. Jodrell,[1] Merrill J. Egorin[2]

[1]Drug Development Section, Institute of Cancer Research, Sutton, Surrey, UK; [2]Division of Developmental Therapeutics, University of Maryland Cancer Center, Baltimore, Maryland, USA

Pharmacokinetic studies are now performed routinely in conjunction with the early clinical studies of new anti-cancer drugs. However, pharmacokinetic studies are costly to perform in terms of both time and money. Therefore it is important that the data generated by pharmacokinetic studies are used rationally, to guide both further clinical trial design and the routine use of anti-cancer drugs.

Cytotoxic anti-cancer drugs generally have a narrow therapeutic index (the ratio between the theoretical minimum effective dose and the maximum tolerated dose) and often there is also marked interpatient variability in drug handling. This leads to variability in the pharmacodynamic effects of a given dose of drug, i.e. an identical dose of drug given to three different patients may result in a therapeutic response with acceptable toxicity in one patient, unacceptable and maybe life-threatening toxicity in the second and no response and no toxicity in the third. It is only by developing a knowledge of the various factors affecting the pharmacokinetics of a given drug and the relationships between the drug's pharmacokinetic parameters and pharmacodynamic end-points (both toxicity and tumour response) that it will be possible to administer an optimum dosage of that drug. The optimum dosage is in effect that dosage which maximises the likelihood of response and simultaneously minimises the likelihood of toxicity in that particular patient.

A major concept that has become accepted during attempts to individualise drug therapy, is that physiological variables, genetic characteristics and environmental factors can alter the relationship between dose and the concentration versus time profile in plasma and tissues. As a result, there is commonly a better relationship between the area under the plasma concentration versus time curve (AUC) in plasma and the intensity of pharmacodynamic effects than there is between dose and these effects[1].

Several studies have now shown relationships between pharmacokinetic parameters (usually total body clearance or AUC) and haematological toxicity for a number of commonly used anti-cancer drugs such as; carboplatin[2][3], etoposide[4], doxorubicin[5], 5-FU[6] and vinblastine[7]. If it is found that a relationship also exists between the pharmacokinetic parameter and a physiological parameter, such as glomerular filtration rate (GFR), it is possible to individualise dosing of the drug by adapting to changes in that physiological parameter. Individualisation of dose, or adaptive control, can be performed using a dosing equation, such as those used in the administration of carboplatin[2][3]. The use of such equations has been shown to give more predictable, and therefore manageable, thrombocytopenia (the dose limiting toxicity of carboplatin). It is hoped that as other relationships between pharmacokinetic paramaters and measurable physiological variables are defined, more precise dosage recommendations will be possible for other drugs. Use of adaptive control also maximises drug exposure in each individual patient, and classical thinking suggests that this in turn should also maximise the likelihood of a therapeutic response.

However, a retrospective analysis of data from over 1000 patients has recently been completed at University of Maryland Cancer Center. This analysis compared both toxicity (myelosuppression) and tumour response in ovarian cancer to carboplatin exposure (AUC)[8]. Renal function (GFR) and carboplatin dosage were used to calculate the carboplatin AUC by rearranging the Calvert dosing equation[2], to the form;

$$AUC = Dose/(GFR + 25)$$

In previously treated and untreated patients, relationships were identified between carboplatin AUC and both the toxic and therapeutic pharmacodynamic end-points. These relationships could be fit by a sigmoidal model derived from the Hill equation;

$$E = \frac{(E_{max})(AUC)^H}{(AUC_{50}) + (AUC)^H}$$

In this model, E can represent response or toxicity and estimates are obtained for E_{max}, the maximum effect; AUC_{50}, the AUC giving 50% E_{max}; and H, the Hill factor, which describes the sigmoidicity of the curve. This sigmoidal model was used because it has been shown to be biologically relevant and is commonly used to model *in vitro* anti-tumour data[9]. It has also been found to be relevant in the analysis of clinical data[10].

The model fits showed that as the administered carboplatin AUC increased above 5-7 mg/ml•min, the likelihood of tumour response did not increase, in both previously untreated and treated patients (figure 1).

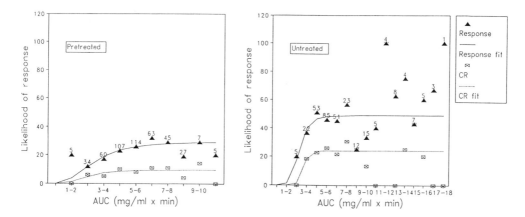

Figure 1.   The likelihood of tumour response in ovarian cancer with increasing carboplatin AUC. Numbers above symbols = patients in AUC subset

The maximum likelihood of response estimated by this fit for previously untreated patients was 49%. There was also no increase in the likelihood of a complete response above the same AUC, the maximum likelihood of complete response being 24%. In previously treated patients, the maximum likelihood of response was 29%, with a corresponding likelihood of complete response of 14%. It is of note that the modeled maximum likelihood of response for pretreated patients is identical to that previously reported from a study of high dose carboplatin in a similar group of patients with ovarian cancer[11]

The likelihood of thrombocytopenia was greater than the likelihood of leucopenia at any given carboplatin AUC (figure 2) and approached 100% above a carboplatin AUC of 10 mg/ml•min. The modeled likelihoods of W.H.O. grade 3 or 4 thrombocytopenia occurring at AUC 4-5, 6-7 and 8-9 mg/ml•min, were 4%, 20% and 48%. This demonstrates a clear increase in the likelihood of platelet toxicity over that range, in contrast to the tumour response data. Similarly, the modelled likelihoods of grade 3 or 4 leucopenia at AUC 4-5, 6-7 and 8-9 mg/ml•min, were <1%, 7% and 30%, respectively.

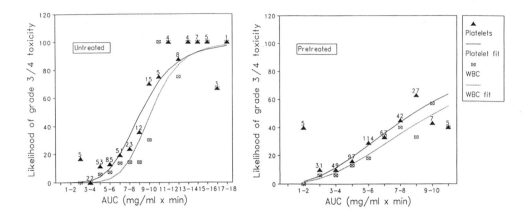

Figure 2.   The likelihood of myelosuppression with increasing carboplatin AUC.
Numbers above symbols = patients in AUC subset

Therefore, when the model fits for likelihood of response and toxicity, as a
function of carboplatin AUC, are combined (figure 3) the lack of significant increase in
the likelihood of response above an AUC of 5-7 mg/ml•min, despite an increased cost
in terms of toxicity, is clearly illustrated.

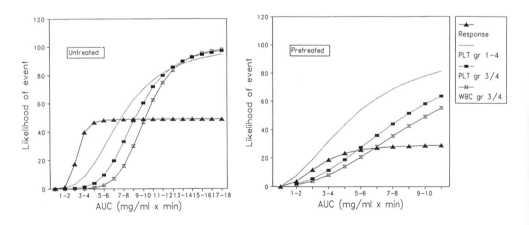

Figure 3.   Combination of computer generated fits for myelosuppression and tumour
response with increasing carboplatin AUC.

These data were also analysed using a multivariable regression approach, which
confirmed the findings of the Hill analysis. In addition to the relationships discussed

above, a clear relationship between W.H.O. performance status (PS) and likelihood of response was also observed. For previously untreated patients the odds ratios for response to carboplatin were 0.65 (PS = 1) and 0.27 (PS = 2) when compared to patients with PS = 0. Thrombocytopenia was also more likely to occur in patients with poor performance status.

It should be noted that this analysis was performed retrospectively and uses response as its therapeutic end-point. However it does draw attention to the need for carefully designed randomised studies to compare the cost/benefit consequences of administering high-dose carboplatin and to define the truly optimal carboplatin exposure in ovarian cancer, i.e. that which maximises the likelihood of response and minimises the incidence of toxicity. It is only by obtaining pharmacokinetic and pharmacodynamic data on large numbers of patients, that this type of analysis can be performed. In the case of carboplatin, it was possible to calculate the carboplatin AUC for such a large number of patients because of the demonstrated relationship between carboplatin clearance and the glomerular filtration rate.

In an effort to address the logisitic problems of obtaining pharmacokinetic data on large numbers of patients, attention has centred on the development of limited sampling strategies to minimise the resources required. One such approach has been developed at the UMCC, using output from a new computer program "PopIT" [a], which implements the iterative 2-stage approach[12] to population pharmacokinetic modeling. Data from a "PopIT" analysis can be used to derive a sampling strategy (using optimal sampling theory[13]) and to develop *maximum-a-posteriori* Bayesian priors which can be used in the analysis of sparse data sets. The application of the essence of Bayes hypothesis, that current data should be analysed in the light of prior expectations from all other sources, has been applied to pharmacokinetic modeling[14]. It is because this approach allows data from an individual to be fit whilst attention is paid to the population pharmacokinetics, that the meaningful analysis of sparse data sets is possible. Limited sampling strategies can also be developed without the requirement for a population pharmacokinetic model[15 16]. However, in general, these strategies provide

---

[a] Hawtof J.E., Jodrell D.I., Forrest A. and Egorin M.J. The development and validation of PopIT: a computer program used to implement the iterative 2-stage approach to population pharmacokinetic modeling. *submitted manuscript*

data on only a single parameter, usually AUC, in contrast to strategies based on optimal sampling theory, which are designed to approximate all parameters i.e. the whole model. Also the sampling strategies developed using stepwise regression approaches allow no flexibility with regard to sampling time as they are based on an equation of the form: $A(conc\ t_a) + B(conc\ t_b) + ...N(conc\ t_n) + z$ (where A, B, ...N, and z are constants and conc t = the plasma concentration at n sampling times a, b, ...n). It should also be noted that the regression-derived equation can only be applied to studies using the same administration schedule as the study from which the sampling strategy was developed. In contrast, optimal sampling theory predicts the optimal sampling times, and data is then analysed using a Bayesian algorithm. This approach can be used to develop sampling strategies for dosing schedules different from that used in the initial pharmacokinetic study. In addition, use of the Bayesian algorithm does allow variability in the times that samples are actually obtained, without invalidating the data set. Therefore, although more complicated to apply, the latter approach should lead to less waste of precious patient and sample resources. It is hoped that limited sampling strategies will be developed during phase I testing of a new anti-cancer drug and should facilitate the accrual of pharmacokinetic data on large numbers of patients in phase II testing.

Adaptive control principles can be extended to utilise data from an individual patient, gathered either following an initial course of therapy or early in a continuous infusion regimen. This approach can be refered to as adaptive control with feedback and an example of its application is the control of 5-FU infusions[6]. The 5-FU AUC administered during the first 3 days of a 5 day continuous infusion is measured. The dose of drug administered in the second half of the infusion is then modified to achieve a predetermined target AUC over the 5 days. The use of adaptive control with feedback has been reported to increase the therapeutic index of infusional 5-FU in head and neck cancer[6]. A similar approach has also been used in the early clinical development of the differentiating agent hexamethylene bisacetamide (HMBA). HMBA plasma concentrations at steady state were measured 24 hours after the start of an HMBA infusion and the infusion rate modifed in order to maintain the plasma concentration at 1.5-2 mM[17]. As a result of this study, the model has now been modified to incorporate a pharmacodynamic end-point (thrombocytopenia), and a MAP-Bayesian algorithm is used to analyse the sparse pharmacokinetic data available[18].

A population pharmacokinetic model and Bayesian estimator have also been developed for suramin, a drug which has recently been found to be an active anti-tumour agent[19]. This model is now used in the adaptive control of suramin dosing[20], where subsequent doses are calculated based on the apparent volume of the central compartment of a 2- or 3-compartment open linear pharmacokinetic model. Prior to the UMCC study, suramin was usually administered by continuous infusion, but its long terminal halflife of 50 days[21] made intermittent therapy more rational. In a phase I study of intermittent dosing, a target plasma concentration range was chosen and dose size and interval were individualised using a MAP-Bayesian estimator, based on peak and trough plasma suramin concentrations measured by HPLC[22]. Use of adaptive control with feedback has achieved the goal of maintaining plasma suramin concentrations within the desired range for >83% of treatment duration (37-92 days) in the first 12 patients to complete the study (a representative profile is shown in figure 4).

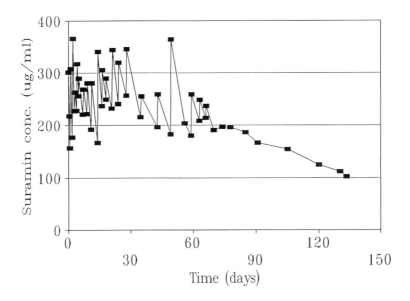

Figure 4.   Plasma suramin concentration profile in a representative patient. Treatment duration = 70 days, terminal halflife = 48 days.

Initial loading (daily administration) resulted in trough values within the desired range within 4 days in most patients, and the dose interval could then be increased gradually so that all patients eventually required treatment on only 1-2 days each week. A number of patients with hormone resistant prostate cancer have been included in the study. Of the first 12 evaluable for response, 5 had measurable disease and tumour responses were noted in all 5 (1 CR, 4 PR). In addition 9 of the 12 patients had a greater than 50% reduction in prostate specific antigen[23]. Therefore, preliminary clinical data from this study are very encouraging and support previous reports of activity of suramin in hormone resistant prostate cancer[24].

This paper has attempted to outline some of the recent developments arising from the application of a knowledge of the pharmacokinetics and pharmacodynamics of anti-cancer drugs. Carboplatin has been used as an example of adaptive control of dosing and it is also a drug where pharmacodynamic analyses are leading to the definition of an optimum drug exposure for individual patients. Suramin has been used as an example of the use of adaptive control with feedback to control precisely, plasma drug concentration in an individual patient. Incorporating such knowledge and techniques into the clinical development of new drugs will facilitate the early definition of the optimal drug exposure and the achievement of that exposure in individual patients.

1.   Gibaldi M. (1991). In Biopharmaceutics and Clinical Pharmacokinetics, 4th Edition, Pub; Lea and Febiger, Philadelphia, PA., 176-186.

2.   Egorin M.J., Van Echo D.A., Olman E.A., Whitacre M.Y., Forrest A., Aisner J. (1985). Prospective validation of a pharmacologically based dosing scheme for the cis-diamminedichioroplatinum (II) analogue diamminecyclobutane-dicarboxylatoplatinum. Cancer Res., 45: 6502-6506.

3.   Calvert A.H., Newell D.R., Gumbrell L.A., O'Reilly S., Burnell M., Boxall F.E., Siddik Z.H., Judson I.R., Gore M.E. and Wiltshaw E. (1989). Carboplatin dosage: Prospective evaluation of a simple formula based on renal function. J. Clin. Oncol., 17(11): 1748-1756.

4.   Ratain M.J., Schilsky R., Choi K.E. et al (1989). Adaptive control of etoposide dosing: Impact of interpatient pharmacodynamic variability. Clin Pharmacol. Ther. 45, 226-233.

5.   Ackland S.P., Ratain M.J., Vogelzang N.J., Choi K.E., Ruane M., Sinkule J.A. (1989). Pharmacokinetics and pharmacodynamics of long-term continuous-infusion doxorubicin. Clin. Pharmacol. Ther., 45, 340-347.

6.   Santini J., Milano G., Thyss A. et al. (1989). 5-FU therapeutic monitoring with dose adjustment leads to an improved therapeutic index in head and neck cancer. Br. J. Cancer, 59, 287-290.

7. Ratain M.J. and Vogelzang N.J. (1986). Phase I and pharmacologic study of vinblastine by prolonged continuous infusion. Cancer Res., 46, 4827-4830.

8. Egorin M., Jodrell D., Canetta R et al. (1991). Tumor response and toxicity in ovarian cancer correlates with carboplatin area under the curve. Proc. Am. Soc. Clin. Oncology, 10, 184.

9. Wagner J.G. (1968). Kinetics of pharmacological response I. Proposed relationships between response and drug concentrations in the intact animal and man. J. Theor. Biol. 20, 171-201.

10. Egorin M.J., Van Echo D.A., Whitacre M.Y., Forrest A., Sigman L.M. (1986). Human pharmacokinetics, excretion and metabolism of the anthracycline menogaril (7-OMEN, NSC 269148) and their correlation with clinical toxicities. Cancer Res. 46, 1513-1520.

11. Ozols R.F., Ostchega Y., Curt G., Young R.C. (1987). High-dose carboplatin in refractory ovarian cancer patients. J. Clin. Oncol., 5, 197-201.

12. Steimer J.L., Mallet A., Golmard J.L. and Boisvieux J.F. (1984). Alternative approaches to estimation of population pharmacokinetic parameters: Comparison with the non-linear mixed-effect model. Drug Metab. Rev., 15, 265-292.

13. D'Argenio D.Z. (1981). Optimal sampling times for pharmacokinetic experiments. J. Pharmacokinetics and Biopharm., 9, 6, 739-756.

14. Sheiner L.B., Beal S., Rosenberg B., Marathe V.V. (1979). Forecasting individual pharmacokinetics. Clin. Pharmacol. Ther., 26 (3), 294-305.

15. Ratain M.J. and Vogelzang N.J. (1987); Limited sampling model for vinblastine pharmacokinetics. Cancer Treat. Rep. 71, 935-939.

16. Egorin M.J., Forrest A., Belani C.P., Ratain M.J., Abrams J.S. and Van Echo D.A. (1989); A limited sampling strategy for cyclophosphamide pharmacokinetics. Cancer Research 49, 3129-3133.

17. Conley B.A., Forrest A., Egorin M.J. et al. (1989) Phase I trial using adaptive control dosing of hexamethylene bisacetamide (NSC 95580). Cancer Res., 49, 3436-3440.

18. Forrest A., Egorin M.J., Zuhowski E., Van Echo D.A. (1987). Development and validation of a unique adaptive control algorithm. Clin. Pharmacol. Ther., 41 (2), 178.

19. Stein C.A., La Rocca R.V., Thomas R., McAtee N., Myers C.E. (1989). Suramin: An anti-cancer drug with a unique mechanism of action. J. Clin. Oncol., 7, 499-508.

20. Jodrell D., Zuhowski E., Egorin M., Sinibaldi V., Forrest A., Eisenberger M. (1991). Intermittent bolus dosing with suramin: the use of adaptive control with feedback. Proc. Am. Soc. Clin. Oncology, 10, 92.

21. Collins J., Clecker R.W., Yarchoan R. et al (1986). Clinical pharmacokinetics of suramin in patients with HTLV-III/LAV infection. J. Clin. Pharmacol., 26, 22-26.

22. Tong W.P., Scher H.I., Petrylak D.P., Curley T., Vasquez J. (1990). A rapid HPLC assay for suramin in plasma. Proc. Am. Assoc. Cancer Res., 31, 381.

23. Eisenberger M., Jodrell D., Sinibaldi V. et al (1991). Preliminary evidence of anti-tumor activity against prostate cancer with long term treatment with suramin in a phase I trial. Eur. J. Cancer. (in press).

24. Myers C.E., La Rocca R., Stein C. et al (1990). Treatment of hormonally refractory prostate cancer with suramin. Proc. Am. Soc. Clin. Oncol., 9, 113.

Pharmacological approach to the platinum compounds

Yasutsuna Sasaki, Nagahiro Saijo

Department of Medical Oncology and Pharmacology Division, National Cancer Center, Tokyo, Japan

INTRODUCTION

The importance of pharmacological aspects in cancer chemotherapy has been well recognized in recent years. The factors which affect clinical response include chemosensitivity of the target cells, maximum tolerated dose or recommended dose of the anticancer agents in human and pharmacokinetic behavior of the drugs. For example, even if the same dose of the same drug were administered, clinical response would be different according to cell types. In addition to the dose, pharmacokinetic behavior is thought to be important. Not only peak plasma concentration or peak achievable plasma concentration, but also protein binding, elimination half life or area under the concentration vs. time curve (AUC) are critical pharmacological factors for prediction of clinical response and /or side effects.

Lung cancer is one of the most common neoplastic disease in Japan. The development of additional active anticancer agent is essential for the improvement lung cancer treatment because the majority of the patients die from disseminated disease. Chemotherapeutic strategy for lung cancer is different between small cell lung cancer (SCLC) and non-small cell lung cancer (NSCLC). SCLC is more responsive to chemotherapy than NSCLC with fifteen to twenty percent surviving more than three years by non-surgical approach. Although many kinds of anticancer agents have been tried for the treatment of NSCLC, it is known as one of the chemo-resistant tumors without identification of a standard chemotherapy. The development of new anticancer agents which have efficacy not only for SCLC but also NSCLC is necessary to improve the treatment results of lung cancer.

cis-Diamminedichloroplatinum (II) (cisplatin) is one of the key drugs in the treatment of solid tumors. cis-Diammine-1, 1-cyclobutanedicarboxylateplatinum (II) (carboplatin) and cis-diammine(glycolato)-platinum (254-S) are second-generation platinum-coordination complexes developed in recent years not only to reduce nephrotoxicity but also to have antitumor activity equivalent or superior to cisplatin. Indeed many platinum analogs including carboplatin and 254-S have been synthesized, but it has been difficult to predict whether these analogs will have superior antitumor activity against human cancers compared to their parent compound cisplatin before the clinical phase II and III trials are completed.

The objective of the present study was to establish a predictive model of clinical response of new platinum analogs against lung cancer by a bioassay using human lung cancer cell lines including SCLC and NSCLC. The biological pharmacology of the active state of platinum which was determined by ex vivo pharmacodynamics was investigated by colony inhibitory activity of the plasma of the patients who were receiving platinum compounds. And finally, a prospective evaluation of antitumor activity of an investigational new platinum, 254-S by this screening model was investigated. On the other hand, we investigated whether the same strategy could be applied to predicting myelotoxicity of 254-S as we used for carboplatin, for which we had developed an equation to predict the percent reduction in platelet count nadir from creatinine clearance.

In vitro activity:

The in vitro anticancer activity of cisplatin, carboplatin and 254-S against 6 SCLC and 6 NSCLC cell lines were compared with the IC50 values. Studies were performed utilizing twelve different established human lung cancer cell lines. The three SCLC cell lines, NCC-c-Lu-134, NCC-c-Lu-135 and NCC-c-Lu-139 were established at Pathology Division of National Cancer Center Research Institute and supplied by Dr. Shimosato [1] and other three SCLC cell lines NCI-H-69, NCI-N-231 and NCI-N-857/N-230 were kindly provided by Dr. J. D. Minna, National Cancer Institute-Navy Medical Oncology Branch, U.S.A [2]. PC-1, PC-3, PC-7, PC-9, PC-13 and PC-14 were derived from human NSCLC (adenocarcinoma, squamous cell carcinoma and large cell carcinoma of the lung) and were provided by Prof. Hayata, Tokyo Medical College [3]. The cells were propagated in 75-cm2 plastic flasks (Corning Glass works, Corning, New York) in RPMI 1640 medium supplemented with 10% fetal calf serum (FCS), 100 µg/ml of streptomycin and 100 U/ml of penicillin in an incubator under a humidified atmosphere at 37°C of 5% CO2 and 95% air. All the reagents for culture were obtained from Grand Island Biological Co. (Gland Island, New York).

Each of the cell lines was tested in a series of continuous drug exposure experiments by clonogenic assay. The colony forming assay devised by Hamburger and Salmon was modified and used for the evaluation of in vitro anticancer activity of the three platinum analogs against the human lung cancer cell lines [4]. Briefly, the cells to be tested were harvested from cell culture flasks and were washed with RPMI 1640 medium. The cells were made into

238

single cell suspension by mechanical dissociation and were counted by Coulter Counter Model ZB1 (Coulter Electronics, Inc. Florida). Viability of the tumor cells was confirmed by trypan blue dye exclusion test (>90% of cell viability). One ml of tumor cell suspension (1 x 105 cells/ml of PC series and NCI-H-69 and 3 x 105 cells/ml of the other SCLC cell lines) in 10% FCS and 0.5% Bacto-Agar (Difco Laboratories, Michigan) containing RPMI 1640 medium with or without appropriate concentration of the platinum compounds was pipetted on to 1 ml of under layer in a 3.5 x 1.0 cm tissue culture multi well plate (Linbro, Flow Laboratories, Inc., Virginia). The under layer contained 0.5% agar in enriched McCoy's 5A medium that was consisted of 400 ml McCoy's 5A medium (Grand Island Biological Company, New York), 40 ml 10% heat inactivated FCS, 20 ml 5% heat inactivated horse serum (Grand Island Biological Company, New York), 4 ml 2.2% Na pyruvate, 4 ml 200 mM glutamine, and 0.8 ml 2.1% serine (Wako Pure Chemical Industry, Osaka, Japan).

Table I. Differences of chemosensitivity between SCLC and NSCLC cell lines by mean IC50 values

Cell line	Cisplatin (μg/ml)	Carboplatin (μg/ml)	254-S (μg/ml)
[SCLC]			
NCC-c-Lu 134	0.27	0.80	0.27
NCC-c-Lu 135	0.25	0.90	0.27
NCC-c-Lu 139	0.20	0.70	0.33
NCI-H-69	0.07	0.90	0.08
NCI-N-231	0.09	0.34	0.25
NCI-N-857/N-230	0.25	1.45	0.29
Mean±SD	0.18±0.08 a)	0.84±0.31 b)	0.26±0.09 c)
[NSCLC]			
PC-1	0.85	4.33	0.84
PC-3	0.50	4.41	0.90
PC-7	1.80	4.42	1.90
PC-9	0.95	4.80	0.85
PC-13	0.90	5.42	1.20
PC-14	1.60	5.63	1.75
Mean±SD	1.10±0.45 a)	4.90±0.48 b)	1.13±0.40 c)

Mean IC50 values of human lung cancer cell lines were determined from the survival curves of three replicate colony assays and were compared between SCLC and NSCLC by using Student t-test.
a) p=0.0063 with cisplatin, b) p=0.0001 with carboplatin, c) p=0.0023 with 254-S

After plating, the tumor cells were inspected under the inverted microscope to confirm that each cell was separated into single cell in upper layer without making any tumor clumps in the dishes and then incubated at 37°C in 5% CO_2 in a highly humidified incubator for 9-21 days until maximum colony growth in control plates of each cell line was obtained. The target tumor cells were continuously exposed to different concentrations of each agent (0.1-100.0 μg/ml) in the soft agar. Each test was performed triplicate. After 9-21 days of incubation, the colonies larger than 60 μm in diameter were counted by an automatic particle counter (CP-2000, Shiraimatsu Instrument, Osaka, Japan). The percent colony survival was calculated from the following formula:

$$100 \times \frac{\text{Mean counts in test dishes}}{\text{Mean colony counts in three control dishes}}$$

The drug sensitivity of the lung cancer cell lines was compared by the IC 50 (50% colony inhibitory drug concentration) values which were determined graphically after obtaining a dose-response curve for each cell line.

The IC50 values for cisplatin, carboplatin and 254-S in SCLC cell lines were significantly lower than those in NSCLC cell lines. In addition, the IC50s for carboplatin were significantly higher than those for cisplatin and 254-S in both SCLC and NSCLC lines (Table I.). The IC50s for carboplatin were significantly higher than those for cisplatin and 254-S in both SCLC and NSCLC. This result indicated that both cisplatin and carboplatin have stronger in vitro anticancer effect than carboplatin in a same drug concentration. In addition, SCLC cell lines were proven to be more sensitive to the drugs, at least these 3 platinum compounds, than NSCLC cell lines.

Pharmacokinetics:

Fifteen patients entered in the pharmacokinetic study. To be eligible for this study, patients with lung cancer or other malignancies had to have failed conventional chemotherapy or have no available effective chemotherapy. No patients had received platinum compounds previously. A performance status of 0, 1 and 2 on the Eastern Cooperative Oncology Group scale was needed. Adequate bone marrow function (wbc counts >3000 cells/μl and platelet counts >100,000/ μl), liver function (bilirubin <2.0 mg/dl) and renal function (serum creatinine <1.5 mg/ml) were required before chemotherapy. Informed consent was obtained from all patients before treatment.

The does of cisplatin, carboplatin and 254-S were 80 mg/m^2 , 450 mg/m^2 and 100 mg/m^2, respectively. The dose of 254-S was the recommended dose for phase II study . These platinum compounds were each administered to five patients by intravenous (i.v.) drip infusion over 30 minutes in 150 ml of 5% glucose solution without diuretic agents. The patients who received cisplatin also received 3000 ml of normal saline before and after administration of the drug. An indwelling i.v. cannula was placed in the arm opposite to that receiving the drug. Blood samples were obtained before and just after the end of the drug infusion, and at 5, 15, 30, 60, 120, 240 and 480 min. Blood was collected by heparin containing syringe and plasma was separated immediately by centrifugation at 600 x g for 10 min. As soon as plasma was prepared, the part of it was passed through Amicon CF 25 filter (Amicon Corporation, Danvers) by centrifugation at 2000 x g for 30 min at 4°C to remove protein. Then protein free ultrafiltrate for chemical assay and aliquots of whole plasma for chemical assay and bioassay were stored at -70° C until analysis.

Total and ultrafilterable platinum in the plasma were assayed with a Hitachi (Tokyo, Japan) model 170-50A flameless atomic absorption spectrometer according to Takahashi et. al [5]. Following the end of the infusion a bi-exponential equation of the for $C = Ae-at + Be-bt$, where C is the concentration at time t and A, B and a, b are the concentration and rate constants, respectively, was fitted to the plasma platinum levels. The free platinum level of cisplatin was fitted to mono-exponential equation. These pharmacokinetic parameters were calculated by using a computerized non-linear least squares technique by the computer program of MULTI [6]. Concentration times time (C x T) for the curve of platinum in plasma was estimated by calculating the area under the curve (AUC) and AUCs were determined from the computer generated fit by the trapezoidal rule.

Table II. Pharmacokinetic parameters of ultrafilterable platinum in plasma of patients treated with platinum compounds

Drug	Dose (mg/sqm)	Peak plasma concentration (μg/ml)	T1/2α (min)	T1/2β (min)	AUC (μg/ml min)
Cisplatin	80	3.09	33	-	208
Carboplatin	450	19.90	34	145	3446
254-S	100	5.31	43	261	959

Plasma concentrations of total platinum by the atomic absorption method for the three compounds declined biexponentially. Ultrafilterable platinum declined biexponentially for carboplatin and 254-S, whereas the free platinum of cisplatin fitted to a monoexponential equation. The area under the concentration vs. time curves (AUCs) as an active compartment were 3,446, 959, and 208 μg/ml min for carboplatin, 254-S and cisplatin, respectively (Table II.). The concentration of free platinum or non protein binding platinum measured by atomic absorption spectrophotometry are thought to be critical for the drug effects. The peak plasma concentration and AUC of free platinum are highest in carboplatin, however, it is quite impossible to conclude that carboplatin has higher anticancer activity than cisplatin and 254-S.

The kidney is the major platinum excretion route in patients receiving 254-S, with more than 50% eliminated within the first 8 hours after administration of the drug. The urinary excretion of 254-S is similar that of carboplatin. Thus, carboplatin and 254-S have similar pharmacokinetic characteristic. On the other hand both agents have also similar pharmacodynamic characteristics. Although G-I toxicity and neurotoxicity are mild as compare with cisplatin, the dose limiting toxicity of both carboplatin and 254-S are thrombocytopenia.

Prediction of clinical activity by ex vivo pharmacodynamics:

It is one of the major endopoints in preclinical and clinical pharmacology for anticancer agents to predict clinical response of new anticancer agents or analogues. It may be more easy to predict side effect induced by anticancer agent than to predict clinical response. If we can determine the concentrations which are clinically effective for various kinds of cancers, it will be more easy to predict clinical response or to make adaptive control dosing not only to reduce side effects but also to maximize clinical response.

Bioassay was achieved by clonogenic techniques using NCI-H-69 (SCLC cell line) and PC-9 (NSCLC cell line) as target. Using the same plasma samples to determine the pharmacokinetics previously presented, bioassay was performed by using colony forming assay. Target cell lines used in this study were NCI-H-69 and PC-9, representing SCLC and NSCLC, respectively. After the target cell lines were incubated with whole plasma for 1 hour at 37°C, they were plated on to soft agar. The colony suppression rate were calculated by comparing the numbers of colonies formed in plasma obtained from patients treated with platinum compounds with those formed in plasma before the administration of platinum compounds. Percentage of colony suppression vs. time curves in plasma from 0 to 510 min after the beginning of drug administration are plotted in Fig. I.

When H-69 was used as the target cell, the peak percentage of colony suppression reached more than 75% for carboplatin and 254-S, and colony

242

suppressive activity for both agents was detected even after 510 min. in upper figure. If PC-9 was chosen as the target cell, antitumor activity could not be detected after 120 minutes and maximum colony suppression did not reach 50% in lower figure.

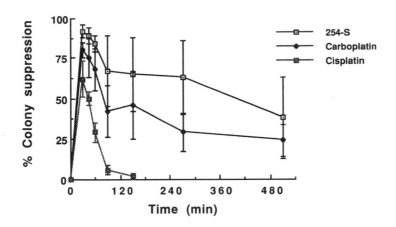

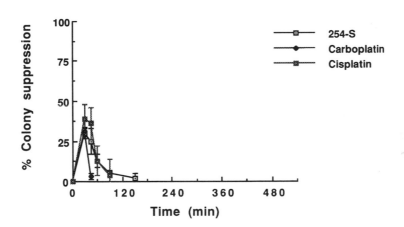

Fig. I. *Comparison of antitumor activity of platinum compounds in 5 patients treated with 80 mg of cisplatin, 450 mg of carboplatin or 100 mg of 254-S per m² by bioassay. Human lung cancer cell lines, NCI-H-69 (upper) and PC-9 (lower) were utilized as the target cells for bioassay. The points represent means ± SD of 5 patients.*

The area under the percentage of colony suppression induced in the patient's plasma from 0 to 510 minutes after beginning of the therapy was calculated by trapezoidal rule and was defined as the antitumor index ATI (Table III.).

Table III. Comparison of three platinum compounds by antitumor index (ATI)

Drugs	ATI/SCLC	ATI/NSCLC
Cisplatin	3202± 664	1634±667
Carboplatin	19004±5436 a)	905±405
254-S	29857±8837 a)	2377±461 b)

Biological comparison of antitumor activity was performed on the basis of the antitumor activity of patients plasma using antitumor index (ATI) which was defined as the area under the percent colony suppression versus time curve obtained by bioassay and calculated by means of trapezoidal rule. ATI/SCLC and ATI/NSCLC revealed ATIs when NCI-H-69 and PC-9 were used as target cells of bioassay, respectively. AUCs were determined from the computer generated fit by the trapezoidal rule.
a) Significantly higher than ATI/SCLC of cisplatin ($p < 0.05$)
b) Significantly higher than ATI/NSCLC of carboplatin ($p < 0.05$)

The ATIs revealed no statistical difference in the ATI/NSCLCs for cisplatin vs. carboplatin and for cisplatin vs. 254-S. However, 254-S had a significantly higher ATI/NSCLC value than did carboplatin. The ATI/SCLCs for carboplatin and 254-S were significantly higher than that of cisplatin. The ATIs have no correlation with AUCs of free platinum (Table III.).

The correlation between the ATIs and the clinical response for cisplatin and carboplatin for SCLC and NSCLC were plotted. Significantly high correlation between two factors were indicated.

From these retrospective analysis, the clinical efficacy of 254-S against SCLC and NSCLC was prospectively predicted using this relationship. The response rate for 254-S against SCLC and NSCLC were predicted to be 40%-65% and 14%-16%, respectively and Dr. Ariyoshi, Aichi Cancer Center , reported clinical result of 254-S revealing 44% for SCLC and 19% for NSCLC, respectively [7]. This approach based on the sensitivity of cancer cell line may be one of the useful method for understanding clinical effect of platinum compounds.

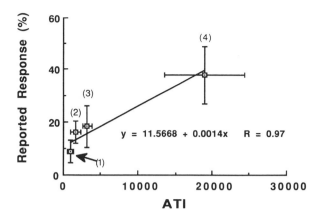

Fig. 2. The correlation between ATI calculated in Table 3 by the result of bioassay and reported clinical response rates of cisplatin and carboplatin against SCLC and NSCLC which were reviewed in Table 4. (1); carboplatin against NSCLC, (2); cisplatin against NSCLC, (3); cisplatin against SCLC, (4); carboplatin against SCLC. Each point represents mean response rate and its 95% confidence interval and mean ±SD of ATI. The response rates of 254-S against SCLC and NSCLC are predicted as 57-67% and 16-23%, respectively by the formula of [Reported Response (%)]=11.5668 + 0.0014 x [ATI].

Prediction of thrombocytopenia for 254-S by creatinine clearance (Ccr.):

Dr. Egorin, University of Maryland Cancer Center, reported interesting approach to predict thrombocytopenia for carboplatin. His rationales were as follows; (1) pretreatment Ccr. correlates with Total body clearance, (2) AUCs negatively correlates with Ccr. and (3) AUCs also correlates platelet reduction and finally he predicted platelet reduction by Ccr [8]. As I mentioned previously, both carboplatin and 254-S have similar pharmacological characteristics.

We reported the equation between nadir platelet count (NPC) and Ccr. by retrospective analysis in 38 "Training Set" patients [9];

$$[NPC] = 2{,}783.4 \times [Ccr.] - 64{,}264.7$$

We retrospectively and prospectively analysed the relationship between pretreatment Ccr. and platelet nadir counts in the "Training Set" and "Test Set" patients.

To evaluate prospectively the equation in the "Test Set" patient and to refine it. Thirty four patients who entered phase II study of 254-S for NSCLC were prospectively analysed. Significant correlation was observed between observed NPC and predicted NPC which was calculated by the equation (R = 0.51) (Fig. 3).

Table IV. Characteristics of Patients

Characteristics	Training set	Test set
Number of patients	38	34
Evaluable courses	38	34
Age		
60>	17	12
60-70	12	13
70<	9	9
Sex		
Male	23	19
Female	15	15
Performance status		
0	1	0
1	18	32
2	11	1
3	8	0
Tumor type		
Lung	33	34
Adenocarcinoma	23	27
Adenosquamous	2	0
Squamous cell	5	5
Large cell	2	2
Undifferentiated	1	0
Colon	3	0
Uterus	2	0
Prior therapy		
None	19	20
Chemotherapy	19	8
Chemotherapy with CDDP	14	6

To refine the equation, we reanalysed the patient characteristics which may influence platelet reduction by multivariate analysis in all of the 72 patients in the "Training Set" and "Test Set". Only Ccr. has been identified as the prognostic variable for platelet reduction by multivariate analysis.

We, then, compared three models including simple linear least regression mode, Hill's equation and E max. model to analyze the relationship between Ccr. and platelet nadir counts and simple linear model describes most successfully this relationship although no significant difference was observed in these three model.

The revised equation is:

[Nadir platelet count] = 2,201.7 x [Ccr.] -17695

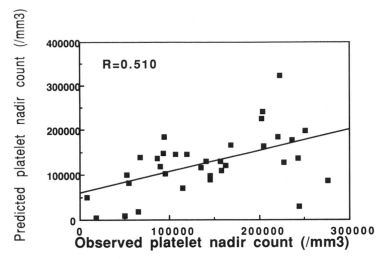

Fig. 3. *The relationship between observed platelet nadir count and predicted platelet nadir count in 34 Test Set patients.*

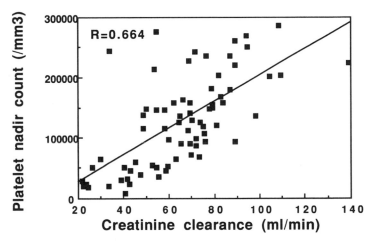

Fig 4. *The relationship between creatinine clearance and platelet nadir count in all of 72 patients.*

This work suggests that empirical approach will be useful to predict platelet nadir count in such drug as 254-S which has similar pharmacokinetic and pharmacodynamic profile as carboplatin. The works of Oncological Pharmacology remain to be extensively explored in Japan.

This series of works had been conducted in Department of Medical Oncology and Pharmacology Division, National Cancer Center of Japan between 1988 and 1990.

Acknowledgements.This work was supported in part by a Grant-in Aid for Cancer Research and for the Comprehensive 10-Year Strategy for Cancer Control from the Ministry of Health and Welfare and grants from the Foundation for the Promotion of Cancer Research.

The author thanks Dr. Shinkai, Dr. Eguchi,Dr. Tamura and Dr. Ohe for their assistance in obtaining clinical samples and advises. The author wish to thank Harumi Taniguchi for her secretary help.

References

1. Terasaki T, Kameya T, Nakajima T, Tsumuraya M, Shimosato Y, Kato K, Ichinose H, Nagatsu T (1984) Interconversion of biological characteristics of small cell lung cancer depending on culture conditions. Gann 75: 1089

2. Carney D N, Gazdar A F, Bepler G, Guccion J G, Marangos P J., Moody T W, Zweig M H, Minna J D (1985) Establishment and identification of small cell lung cancer cell lines having classic and variant features. Cancer Res 45: 2913

3. Hayata Y, Tsuji K (1975) Lung cancer: In: Culture of human cancer cells (written in Japanese). Asakurashoten, Tokyo, p 131

4. Salmon S E (1984) Human tumor colony assay and chemosensitivity testing. Cancer Treat Rep 68: 117

5. Takahashi K, Seki T, Nishikawa K, Minamide S, Iwabuchi M, Ono M, Nagamine S, Horinishi H (1985) Antitumor activity and toxicity of serum protein-bound platinum formed from cisplatin. Jpn J Cancer Res (Gann) 76: 68

6. Yamaoka K, Tanigawara Y, Nakagawa T, Uno T (1980) Pharmacokinetic analysis program (MULTI) for microcompiuter. J Pharm Dyn 4: 879

7. Ariyoshi Y, Fujii M, Kurita Y, Ohshima S, Tamura M, Inoue S, Nishiwaki Y, Kimura I, Niitani H. (1989) Phase II clinical study of (glycolato-0,0') diammine platinum (II) (254-S), a new platinum complex, for primary lung cancer. Proc Am Soc Clin Oncol 8: 927

8. Egorin M J, Van Echo D A, Tippin S J, Olman E A , Whitacre M Y , Thompson B W, Aisner J (1984) Pharmacokinetics and dosage reduction of cis-diammine(1,1-cyclobutanedecarboxylato)platinum in patients with impaired renal function. Cancer Res 44: 5432

9. Sasaki Y, Fukuda M, Morita M, Shinkai T, Eguchi K, Tamura T, Ohe Y, Yamada K, Kojima A, Nakagawa K, Saijo N. (1990) Prediction by creatinine clearance of thrombocytopenia and recommended dose in patients receiving (glycolato-0,0')-diammine platinum (II) (NSC 375101D). Jpn J Cancer Res 81: 196

Pharmacokinetically guided dose escalation in phase I trials—current status and future prospects

David R. Newell

Cancer Research Unit, University of Newcastle upon Tyne Medical School, Newcastle, UK

INTRODUCTION - THE FUNCTION OF THE PHASE I TRIAL

Despite notable successes in the chemotherapy of childhood malignancies (1,2), the impact of cytotoxic drugs in the treatment of common adult solid tumours has been more limited (3). As a response to the need for more effective systemic therapies, extensive drug discovery and development programmes are ongoing in both academia and the pharmaceutical industry. These programmes continue to produce compounds for clinical evaluation and with the recent advances in our understanding of the molecular basis of cancer, and the novel targets for drug development thereby exposed, the rate of drug discovery will hopefully increase.

Historically, the role of the Phase I trial in drug development has been to identify a safe dose and schedule such that the activity of the drug against a range of tumour types can be determined in Phase II studies (4,5). Since established anticancer drugs only show reproducible activity at or near the maximum tolerated dose (MTD), it is assumed that Phase II studies should be carried out at doses close to the MTD. Hence the end points of a Phase I trial include defining the MTD and describing in both qualitative and quantitative terms the toxicities encountered. To avoid life threatening toxicity, Phase I studies employ dose escalation from an initial non-toxic starting dose until the MTD is reached. The starting dose is chosen on the basis of preclinical toxicity studies and the National Cancer Institute (NCI, USA), Cancer Research Campaign (CRC, UK), and European Organisation for Research and Treatment on Cancer (EORTC, Europe) all use 1/10th of the dose lethal to 10% of mice (1/10th LD10) as a guide to the starting dose. Toxicity is also studied in a second species although experience with a very large number of agents has shown that, with one exception (fludarabine), 1/10th the LD10 is a safe starting dose (data reviewed in 6). Indeed, in a number of studies the lack of toxicity seen in the second species has led to Phase I entry doses of greater than 1/10th the mouse LD10. For example, in the cases of merbarone, deoxyspergualin and hexamethylene bisacetamide acute lethality following bolus adminstration in mice was not seen in dogs given continuous iv infusions, the proposed clinical schedule. Hence Phase I starting doses were calculated on the basis of data from dogs with considerable savings in the number of patients and dose escalation steps required

249

to reach the MTD (data reviewed by Collins *et al.*, 7).

Traditionally empirical dose escalation schemes have been used to calculate dose increments in Phase I trials, for example an arithmetic scheme or the modified Fibonacci number series. However, a number of groups have pointed out the negative impact that these empirical dose escalation methods can have on drug development (7-11). The central problem is that whilst 1/10th the mouse LD10 is almost invariably a safe starting dose, the MTD may be anywhere between 1x and 700x this value (for NCI data see Collins *et al.*, 7,8; for UK CRC data see below). If the MTD of a drug is close to the starting dose there is a serious risk of life threatening toxicity due to rapid initial dose escalation, conversely, if the MTD is far greater than the starting dose the trial will take a long time, require a large number of patients and use more hospital resources. In addition, the fact that most agents are only active at or near the MTD means that, for the majority of patients treated with drugs whose MTD is far greater than the Phase I starting dose, there is little chance of therapeutic benefit. Since most patients will not receive even potentially therapeutic doses, serious ethical problems arise because, in reality, patients only agree to therapy with Phase I drugs because they hope that they may benefit.

In an attempt to improve dose escalation, Collins and colleagues proposed, in 1986 (8), that preclinical pharmacokinetic data should be used to guide dose escalation in Phase I trials. The central hypothesis in this approach is that discrepancies between toxic doses in patients and mice can be explained in part by differences in the pharmacokinetics of the drug in the two species and that by compensating for the pharmacokinetic differences more efficient dose escalation can be undertaken. Before considering these proposals in detail the recent Phase I experience of the Phase I/II Committee of the UK CRC will be reviewed with particular emphasis on the number of escalation steps and patients required to reach an MTD for each compound.

PHASE I CLINICAL STUDIES CONDUCTED UNDER THE AUSPICES OF THE UK CRC PHASE I/II CLINICAL TRIALS COMMITTEE

The major body for coordinating new drug trials with antitumour agents in the UK is the CRC Phase I/II Trials Committee. Table I summarizes the results from a number of the studies performed under the auspices of this committee. The major conclusion to be drawn from the data in Table I concerns the size of the trials and the length of time taken to complete them. Most of the studies have used empirical dose escalation with the result that up to 20 steps have been required to achieve an MTD. Indeed, for those compounds undergoing evaluation for the first time, only in the case of methylene dimethane sulphonate (MDMS) was an MTD reached in less than 10 steps. In the case of amphethinile, a large (5

TABLE I: RECENT PHASE I STUDIES CONDUCTED UNDER THE
            AUSPICES OF THE CRC PHASE I/II CLINICAL TRAILS
            COMMITTEE

Drug	Schedule	Number of Patients	Escalation Steps	Ref.
MDMS	iv bolus x1	39	8	12
LM985	0.1-1h inf.	26	13	13
FAA	1-6h inf.	54	15	14
Amphethinile[1]	iv bolus x1	15	5	15
Trimelamol	0.1-1h inf.	49	12	16
	iv inf. dx3	33	5	16
MZPES	1-24h inf.	68	20	17
LY195448[2]	2x 10min inf. weekly x3	9	3	18
Didox	30min inf.	34	13	19
	36h inf.	12	3	20
DUP941[1]	iv bolus x1	44	10	21
	weekly x3	41	10	22
Temozolomide	iv/po x1	49	15	23
CB10-277	5-20min inf.	36	12	24
	24h inf.	22	4	24

Notes
1.   Studies performed with pharmacokinetic input. For DUP941 see below.
2.   Trial discontinued before reaching an MTD.

fold) initial dose escalation was made on the basis of pharmacokinetic results and this greatly reduced the duration of the study. Thus the UK CRC results mirror the recent US NCI experience (7); lengthy Phase I studies remain a significant problem. An additional point to be noted from Table I is the high incidence of schedule alteration during the Phase I trial. Thus for flavone acetic acid (FAA), trimelamol, didox and CB10-277 the trials were all extended to include a more prolonged adminstration schedule. The reasons for this alteration vary, however, it argues strongly for careful schedule dependency studies in preclinical efficacy studies and then use of the most effective schedule for preclinical toxicological evaluation. A move towards compound orientated toxicity testing is already under way (25) and is to be welcomed.

Not included in Table I are a number of anti-endocrine agents which have also undergone clinical trial under the aegis of the CRC Phase I/II Clinical Trials committee.

These compounds are particularly interesting as they are analogous to the new agents which are being developed to interact with tumour growth factor receptors and second messenger pathways. Hence lessons learnt with anti-endocrine drugs may expedite the clinical evaluation of such new agents. In the case of anti-endocrine agents there is often a quantitative pharmacodynamic parameter which can be measured and this greatly assists dose escalation as well as the identification of the most effective route and schedule of adminstration. For example, in the study of the novel anti-oestrogen zindoxifene, Stein and colleagues used elevations in the levels of sex hormone binding globulin to conclude that biologically active levels of drug were being achieved (26). In studies with the aromatase inhibitor 4-hydroxyandrostenedione (4-OHA), suppression of plasma oestradiol was used, again to show that the required pharmacodynamic effect was being achieved. Using oestradiol measurements, as well as conventional pharmacokinetic studies of the levels of 4-OHA, Dowsett et al. (27) were able to study the effect of dose, route and schedule in only 55 patients. This study involved an evaluation of two routes of adminstration, 4 dose levels and 4 schedules. A similar approach has been applied to the evaluation of another aromatase inhibitor, pyridoglutethimide (28). Taken together, these studies with anti-endocrine agents illustrate the value of including pharmacokinetic *and* pharmacodynamic studies in Phase I trials.

PROPOSALS FOR PHARMACOKINETICALLY GUIDED DOSE ESCALATION (PGDE) IN PHASE I TRIALS

As discussed above, the central hypothesis in PGDE is that the discrepancy between the LD10 in mice and the MTD in patients may be due in part to pharmacokinetic differences. To test this hypothesis Collins et al., in their original paper (8), calculated the MTD/LD10 ratio for a number of cytotoxic drugs and also the ratio of the area under the plasma drug concentration *versus* time curves (AUCs) in the two species at these doses. If the AUC ratio is closer to unity than the dose ratio it implies that the difference in toxic doses is partially or totally due to pharmacokinetic differences. The most compelling example given by Collins et al. was doxorubicin where almost identical plasma concentration *versus* time profiles were observed following 18mg/m² in mice, the LD10, and in patients at 90mg/m², the MTD. A similar, though less striking, correlation between AUC values was found for a number of drugs and these authors have recently updated their experiences (7). These data and those from other retrospective analyses are given in Table II.

From the data in Table II it is clear that for the platinum complexes, alkylating agents, DNA binding drugs, trimelamol and indicine-N-oxide the discrepancy, where it exists, between the LD10 and the MTD can largely be explained by pharmacokinetics, ie. different

COMPARISON OF DOSES AND AREAS UNDER PLASMA CONCENTRATION V. TIMES CURVES (AUCs) IN MICE (LD10 DOSE) AND PATIENTS (MTD)[1]

Drug	MTD/LD10 Dose ratio	MTD/LD10 AUC ratio
Alkylating agents/ platinum complexes		
Carboplatin[2]	1.1	1.0
Cisplatin[2]	2.2	1.3
JM40[2]	4.0	1.3
Diaziquone	1.0	1.0
Teroxirone	4.3	0.8
Thio-TEPA	0.4	1.0
Antimetabolites		
5-Azacytidine	6.0	1.1
Dihydroazacytidine	1.2	0.3
Fludarabine	0.1	0.1
PALA	2.8	3.3
Pentostatin/DCF	0.7	1.1
Tiazofurin	0.7	0.9
DNA binding drugs		
Amsacrine	0.8	1.3
Doxorubicin	5.0	0.8
Miscellaneous		
Indicine-N-oxide	0.9	0.6
Trimelamol[3]	4.8	1.3

Notes

1. Data are from Collins *et al.* (7) except:
2. Van Hennik *et al.* (29)
3. Judson *et al.* (16)

doses are required in mice and patients to achieve to same AUC. The inherent sensitivity of the dose-limiting normal tissue in these cases is not species dependent. In contrast, for antimetabolites, the relationship between AUC values is no better than the already poor relationship for dose. The inability of pharmacokinetic differences to explain the dose discrepancy for antimetabolites is not, however, surprising. Antimetabolites usually require intracellular metabolic activation, their toxicity is primarily time dependent once a given threshold concentration has been reached and cytotoxicity can often be reversed by extracellular nucleosides and/or bases, the levels of which are highly species dependent. A better guide for antimetabolite dose escalation is the intracellular level of the active metabolite or, where appropriate, inhibition of the target enzyme.

Having identified pharmacokinetic variation as a major reason for inter species differences in cytotoxic drug tolerance, Collins *et al.* went on to propose the use of preclinical pharmacokinetic data to guide dose escalation in Phase I trials (8). Briefly, it was proposed that the LD10 and the AUC at the LD10 dose in mice should be determined and then the Phase I trial started at 1/10th the LD10 dose. Measurement of the AUC in patients at the starting dose would then allow estimation of how close the starting dose was to the probable MTD. If the Phase I starting dose AUC was <40% of the mouse LD10 AUC, doses could be escalated rapidly, for example, at least doubled. Once 40% of the LD10 AUC was achieved it was proposed that a modified Fibonacci scheme should be used until the MTD was reached. The Pharmacology and Molecular Mechanisms (PAMM) Group of the EORTC produced similar, though more detailed, guidelines for PGDE (9). In particular, the need for a sensitive assay to detect drugs at 1/10th LD10 doses was stressed as was the need to study the linearity of the pharmacokinetics, the impact of drug metabolism on toxicity and the role of protein binding. In addition, the EORTC PAMM Group emphasized the need to match the preclinical and clinical studies in terms of route of administration, schedule and vehicle. Finally, the importance of coordinating the preclinical pharmacokinetic and toxicity studies was noted so as to avoid possible pharmacogenetic or chronobiological variation. Following the proposals of Collins *et al.* and the EORTC PAMM Group a number of studies have attempted to apply PGDE. These studies, which have served to highlight some of the problems anticipated by the EORTC PAMM Group, will now be considered.

PROSPECTIVE EVALUATION OF PGDE

Four studies on 3 compounds have now been reported in detail (21,30-32). The drugs are all DNA binding agents thought to act primarily through DNA topoisomerase II inhibition. Two of the compounds, piroxantrone and DUP941, are anthrapyrazoles developed in the search for a compound with equal or superior activity to doxorubicin, but without significant cardiotoxicity. The third agent, 4'-iodo-4'-deoxydoxorubicin (I-DOX), is an anthracycline with both reduced cardiotoxicity in experimental models and activity in multidrug resistant cells lines. It is interesting that all four agents are DNA binding drugs in that doxorubicin, the archetypal DNA binder, was amongst the agents with the largest dose ratio discrepancy in retrospective studies. This discrepancy could be entirely explained when the AUC was taken into account (Table II). Thus these new DNA binding drugs were good candidates for PGDE.

The preclinical and clinical data for I-DOX, DUP941 and piroxantrone are summarized in Table III with the numbers of dose escalations steps that would have been used in a Fibonacci scheme also being given. Thus for both piroxantrone and I-DOX there was a saving of 1 step by using PGDE whilst in the case of DUP941 fewer steps would have been needed had a modified Fibonacci scheme been used. However, in all of the studies problems were encountered which complicated the application of the PGDE approach and as such the modest success achieved should not be dismissed. In the case of piroxantrone assay problems precluded the satisfactory analysis of plasma levels at the initial starting

TABLE III: PRECLINICAL AND CLINICAL PHARMACOKINETIC AND
               TOXICITY DATA FOR COMPOUNDS USED IN PROSPECTIVE
               PGDE STUDIES

Compound	I-DOX(30)	DUP941(21)	Piroxantrone[2] (31,32)
Mouse LD10 mg/m^2	18	60	75
Human MTD mg/m^2	80	55	150-160
AUC at mouse LD10 (μM.h)	6.2[1]	4.6	5.1
AUC at human MTD (μM.h)	4.4 ± 1.4[1]	4.9	3.3-8.3
MTD/LD10 Dose ratio	4.4	0.9	2.1
MTD/LD10 AUC ratio	0.7	1.1	1.0
Escalation steps used	9	9	7,7
Escalation steps needed using Fibonacci scheme	10	6	8

Notes
1.   The AUC data for I-DOX is the sum of the parent drug and the 4'-iodo-4'-
      deoxydoxorubicin-13-ol AUC values.
2.   The data for piroxantrone are the range of results from the two studies.

doses. With I-DOX there were substantial differences between mice and patients in the metabolism of I-DOX to the corresponding 13-OH compound (I-DOXOL) and this only become apparent during the clinical trial. Thus it was necessary to suspend PGDE whilst the preclinical toxicity and pharmacokinetics of I-DOXOL were defined. However, once this was done Gianni and co-workers successfully added in the metabolite contribution and completed the study with PGDE. Finally, with DUP941, inter patient variability at the initial doses precluded the application of PGDE although it was subsequently found that the variability did not have a major impact on toxicity. Assay insensitivity, inter species differences in metabolism and inter patient variability had all been anticipated as potential problems with PGDE (9) and future PGDE studies should address these aspects more carefully. Perhaps the most interesting point to arise from the studies with these three compounds is that the MTD/LD10 AUC ratio was as close or closer to unity that the dose ratio (Table III) and this again lends weight to the central PGDE hypothesis. Overall, the PGDE hypothesis has withstood the first test and the priority now is to expand the range of compounds prospectively evaluated.

FUTURE STUDIES WITH PGDE

As originally envisaged, PGDE was a method of expediting Phase I clinical trials in order to save resources as well as hasten the evaluation of new therapies. However, it is already clear that *pharmacologically* guided dose escalation has far more to offer that simply more rapid or safer dose escalation. The first major area were improvements can be envisaged is in the application of molecular pharmacodynamics to Phase I studies. As discussed previously, the value of pharmacodynamic investigations in Phase I trials is already clear from studies with anti-endocrine drugs. Modern analytical methodology makes such studies feasible for most drug classes.

The second major development that may be anticipated with PGDE is the use of adaptive control of drug adminstration to allow PGDE where it is AUC that is escalated rather than dose. For example, an AUC escalation study with carboplatin has already been reported (33). In the future the combined application of pharmacokinetic, pharmacodynamic and adaptive control dosing methods should allow safer *and* more rational Phase I drug evaluation.

REFERENCES

1. Craft AW and Pearson ADJ (1989) Cancer Surveys 8:605
2. Stiller CA and Bunch KJ (1990) Br J Cancer 62:806
3. Frei E III (1985) Cancer Res 45:6523
4. EORTC New Drug Development Committee (1985) Eur J Cancer Clin Oncol 21:1005
5. Von Hoff DD, Kuhn J & Clark GM (1984) In: Buyse ME, Staquet MJ & Sylvester RJ, (eds) Cancer Clinical Trials. Methods and Practice. Oxford University Press, Oxford, pp210-220

6. Grieshaber CK and Marsoni S (1986) Cancer Treat Rep 70:65

7. Collins JM, Grieshaber CK, Chabner BA (1990) JNCI 82:1321

8. Collins JM, Zaharko DS, Dedrick RL, *et al.* (1986) Cancer Treat Rep 70:73

9. EORTC PAM Group (1987) Eur J Cancer Clin Oncol 23:1083

10. Newell DR (1990) Br J Cancer 61:189

11. Edler L (1990) Onkologie 13:90

12. Smith DB, Fox BW, Thatcher N *et al.* (1987) Cancer Treat Rep 71:817

13. Kerr DJ, Kaye SB, Graham J *et al.* (1986) Cancer Res 46:3142

14. Kerr DJ, Kaye SB, Cassidy J *et al.* (1987) Cancer Res 47:6776

15. Smith DB, Ewen C, Mackintosh J *et al.* (1988) Br J Cancer 57:623

16. Judson IR, Calvert AH, Rutty CJ *et al.* (1989) Cancer Res 49:5475

17. Stuart NSA, Crawford SM, Blackledge GRP *et al.* (1989) Cancer Chemother Pharmacol 23:308

18. Cassidy J, Lewis C, Adams L *et al.* (1989) Cancer Chemother Pharmacol 24:233

19. Veale D, Carmichael J, Cantwell BMJ (1988) Br J Cancer 58:70

20. Carmichael J, Cantwell BMJ, Mannix KA *et al.* (1990) Br J Cancer 61:447

21. Foster BJ, Newell DR, Graham MA *et al.* (In Press) Europ J Cancer

22. Allan SG, Cummings J, Evans S *et al.* (1991) Cancer Chemother Pharmacol 28:55

23. Newlands ES, Blackledge GRP, Slack J *et al.* (1990) In: Giraldi T, Connors TA, Cartei G (eds) Triazenes. Plenum Press, New York, pp185-193

24. Newell DR, Foster BJ, Carmichael J *et al.* (1990) In: Giraldi T, Connors TA, Cartei G (eds) Triazenes. Plenum Press, New York, pp119-131

25. Greishaber CK (1991) In: Powis G, Hacker MP (eds) The toxicity of anticancer drugs. Pergammon Press, New York, pp10-27

26. Stein RC, Dowsett M, Cunningham DC *et al.* (1990) Br J Cancer 61:451

27. Dowsett M, Goss PE, Powles TJ *et al.* (1987) Cancer Res 47:1957

28. Dowsett M (1990) J Steroid Biochem Mol Biol 37:1037

29. van Hennik MB, van der Vijgh WJF, Klein I *et al.* (1987) Cancer Res 47:6297

30. Gianni L, Vigano L, Antonella S *et al.* (1990) JNCI 82:469

31. Ames MM, Loprinzi CL, Collins JM *et al.* (1990) Cancer Res 50:3905

32. Hantel A, Donehower RC, Rowinsky EK *et al.* (1990) Cancer Res 50:3284

33. Calvert AH, Newell DR, Gumbrell LA *et al.* (1989) J Clin Oncol 7:1748

Discussion

Professor William M. Hryniuk (Ontario Cancer Treatment and Research Foundation, Hamilton Regional Cancer Centre, Hamilton, Ontario, Canada): Dr Jodrell, in the carboplatin data, the AUC was shown. It was not clear to me whether that was the summation or the average of a number of cycles of treatment.

Dr Jodrell: The AUC that was shown was that for the first course of therapy, so it was not clouded by data on total dose. We did not have data for the total AUC administered. Obviously the AUC at course 1 can easily be related to the toxicity which was also measured during that course, but I agree that there is some question about whether it is fair to relate that to response. I think if you look at it on an intention-to-treat basis, then it is valid to do so.

Professor Hryniuk: What was the interval between courses?

Dr Jodrell: Most patients were receiving 400 mg/m^2 on a 4-weekly schedule, and they were all single-agent studies—there were no combination data included in the analysis.

Professor Hryniuk: If you wanted to convert that to AUC/m^2 per week you would divide that by 4, if you just wanted to correlate that with AUC using carboplatin on a q3 week schedule.

Dr Jodrell: I did not have time to show all the data comparing the likelihood of response and toxicity to dose as opposed to AUC. We were unable to demonstrate sigmoidal relationships, particularly for toxicity, because the patients who received the lower doses were those with impaired renal function, and therefore they had high AUCs and high toxicity. Therefore the incidence of toxicity at the lower doses was greater than the incidence of toxicity at 400 mg/m^2.

Professor Hryniuk: The inflection dose intensity or the inflection AUC was between 4–6 and 6–7 mg/mL per min. What would that correspond to in an average adult for carboplatin, recognizing the intraindividual variation?

Dr Jodrell: The AUC of 7 approximates to 400 mg/m^2 in an average patient, but due to the spread of glomerular filtration rate that you see in a population, a single dose of 400 mg/m^2 can relate to an AUC ranging from about 3 to 12.

Professor Hryniuk: That would be 400 mg/m^2 every 4 weeks. If the ratio of carboplatin to cisplatin is 4:1 or similar, it would be about 100 mg of platinum every 4 weeks, which is about 25 mg of platinum/square meter per week as the inflection dose intensity counterpart for carboplatin. I am just trying to identify the point at which you stop giving platinum or carboplatin when you reach that inflection point.

Dr Jodrell: I think it is difficult to go from the one drug to another, but I take that point.

Dr Masanori Shimoyama (National Cancer Center Hospital, Tokyo, Japan): Dr Jodrell, we know that the optimal drug dose is usually less in Japanese than in US or European people. Do you have any data on differences in dosages between races?

Dr Jodrell: No, I do not.

Professor Kiyoji Kimura (National Nagoya Hospital, Nagoya, Japan): Dr Jodrell, as you have said, concerning the effects and side effects of a drug it is important to observe blood components, such as decreases in white blood cells, red blood cells, and platelets. I think it is much more necessary to know how much of the drug reaches the target end-organ and to what extent this influences its effect.

Dr Jodrell: I agree that we are measuring plasma concentration and it is not the target end-organ. I think in most cases it is very difficult to measure the effect at the end-organ, although obviously we are attempting to do this in studies with antimetabolites such as thymidylate synthase inhibitors and also with adduct formation using platinum drugs. It is important that plasma samples are easily obtainable and therefore if we can develop such relations with something that is easily measurable, it is going to be very useful in the clinic rather than having to try to take tumor biopsies for each individual patient.

Professor Kimura: What we really want to know is how much of the drug administered reaches the target tissue. We need to work in cooperation with surgeons. I think that the effective dose can only be decided when drugs are given for fixed periods, followed by operation to measure cancerous tissue drug concentrations.

Dr Jodrell: Yes, I think that is true.

Professor Hryniuk: It would depend then on the organ as to how much variation there would be between individuals. Now you are looking primarily at myelotoxicity and the bone marrow, which is a very vascular organ. Because there is so little variation between individuals there might not be much variation in vascularity as a second factor determining scatter, or rather more importantly in the blood levels, as you have shown. Perhaps for the liver or kidney it might be quite a different relationship with much more scatter, as Professor Kimura has suggested.

Dr Jodrell: We have attempted to look at toxicities such as mucositis, but as you mentioned, there is a lot of scatter in such data. Dr Sasaki, the studies that we did with carboplatin suggested that the platelet nadir was also related to the pretreatment platelet count and that maybe percentage change in platelets could be better related to the AUC. Have you looked at that for 254-S?

Dr Sasaki: Yes, we calculated the relationship between creatinine clearance and the percentage of white blood cell count reduction. Higher correlation was observed between creatinine clearance and nadir platelet count in this series, however.

Dr Newell: Were the data you presented on correlation with creatinine clearance from calculated or measured creatinine clearance?

Dr Sasaki: It was measured. We used the average of 2 measurements from each patient.

Dr Newell: That is important. Did you have a chance to compare the renal clearance of your compound with creatinine clearance in those patients?

Dr Sasaki: Not yet.

Professor Hryniuk: The in vitro system that you used to show us the results of the non-small cell lung cancer line sensitivity suggests to me that you might be able to detect differences in sensitivity between stage of disease and correlate the stage of the disease as the source of the material. For example, after resection for stage I or stage II disease you might see different chemosensitivity than for stage III or IV non-small cell lung cancer. Do you have sufficient material to make that kind of correlation?

Dr Sasaki: No. We used only lung cancer cell lines. However, we previously checked using clonogenic assays to determine the sensitivity of various kinds of anticancer agents in freshly isolated materials, but we could not identify any tendency according to the staging of the patient.

Dr Shigeru Tsukagoshi (Cancer Chemotherapy Center, Cancer Institute, Tokyo, Japan): Dr Newell, that is a very interesting explanation for PGDE. It is undoubtedly a useful means for assessing dose escalation. In our experience, however, some drugs are very sensitive to dog or monkey, but not necessarily to mouse. Also, you mentioned the interspecies variation of drug metabolism. Is it possible to apply your escalation to any drugs sensitive to other animal species?

Dr Newell: Yes, I think that in theory there is no reason why, once you have defined a target AUC in whatever happens to be the most sensitive species in toxicological studies, one cannot then target toward that AUC. Dr J.M. Collins, Food and Drug Administration, Rockville, MD, USA, has been doing work recently or has been helping to coordinate work where, due to the difficulties of giving the prolonged infusions necessary to obtain activity in mice, the researchers have been relying heavily on dog data. That seems to be an adequate way of doing it. If you do know what the most sensitive species is, then there is no reason why you cannot use data from that species instead.

Dr Sasaki: Unfortunately we have no experience of PGDE in Japan. We must check the hypothesis of Dr Collins during the early steps of this strategy. I personally feel that the Italian study is very informative on this hypothesis. Do you agree? What kind of endpoint is important for continuation of this strategy, or for stopping and converting to traditional methods?

Dr Newell: I do not believe that there is a simple answer to that. I think the single most important thing that PGDE has done for phase I studies is to put more science into them. So the answer to your question is, it will depend on the compound concerned. I think where we still fail is in the molecular pharmacodynamics area. With the absence of that, PGDE is going to be really quite limited. It seems good for platinum complexes, and probably for simple DNA binders as well. Beyond that I think it will have limitations, but providing pharmacodynamic data are obtained, I think it is going to be valuable. Of course, the days when we selected compounds randomly for phase I studies are thankfully beginning to pass now. Rational drug development is now established. If a compound is developed for a particular target, then I think we must try to determine whether that target is being hit as soon as we possibly can.

Professor Hryniuk: Dr Newell, the LD_{10} for a mouse for cyclophosphamide depends on how the drug is administered and at what intervals of time. You can kill 10% of the mice with one injection, or you can give 2 lower doses and wait a week, or give 3 lower doses and wait 2 or 3 weeks. There is a whole matrix of LD_{10}s. It was not clear to me from your presentation what the relation is between LD_{10} and the scheduling that was given to the patients which allows you to make this conversion.

Dr Newell: In terms of the schema that I showed for the EORTC PAM group, where our first question is does metabolism affect the activity, with a drug like cyclophosphamide you would immediately stop at that stage, and measuring patient drug levels would not be useful. You would have to develop assays for the active metabolites, which is very difficult for the oxazaphosphorenes. In terms of the more general issue though, there is still a problem with exploiting preclinical information. Studies with TOPO isomerase I inhibitors are ongoing at the moment, where we know from in vitro studies they are phenomenally more cytotoxic with prolonged exposure and yet there are phase I studies underway of relatively short duration. The preclinical and clinical schedules must be matched closely before this conversion is made. Second, the preclinical work should be done to define the most efficacious schedule, ie, the schedule with the best therapeutic index before phase II studies are started. I do not think that phase II studies are where you should find that out.

Professor Hryniuk: Were the LD_{10} data that you showed for mice one-shot LD_{10}?

Dr Newell: The LD_{10} data that I presented for the prospective studies were obtained using an identical schedule to the one that was subsequently used clinically, which in those cases was all single-shot data.

Dr Ryuzo Ohno (The Branch Hospital, Nagoya University School of Medicine,

Nagoya, Japan): Did you do the CI941 studies according to the EORTC schedule?

Dr Newell: No, that study was done as a prospective evaluation of PGDE. At the first dose level we treated 3 patients, one of whom had an AUC that was 50% of our target AUC. We felt that if we doubled the dose and had the same variability, we would run into serious problems with vastly overshooting and hence putting patients at risk of life-threatening toxicity. Retrospectively, that would not have been the case, but prospectively that is the dilemma we were faced with. So in answer to the question, did we follow the schedule, for the first step, yes, but then we immediately concluded that there was too much variability.

Professor Franco M. Muggia (Kenneth Norris Cancer Center, University of Southern California, Los Angeles, California, USA): I noted that the one drug that took the most steps was a lipophilic antifolate not familiar to me. I would wonder whether you could comment further on it, based on your PGDE?

Dr Newell: I think that the way forward with antifolates, and in general with antimetabolites, is to identify the loci of drug action within the tumor cell, determine whether peripheral white cells are useful to model that loci, and then carry out dose escalation on the basis of that. There have been studies recently where this has in fact been done, but that particular antifolate was not one of them, that was a prodrug for a lipophilic antifolate. It carried a positive charge on a nitrogen and, not surprisingly, it was neurotoxic. We learn as we go.

Dr Jodrell: We have done some studies again with data from the study on the anthrapyrazole CI941, showing that it is possible to develop a population pharmacokinetic model on quite a small set of patients, 12 or 14. Obviously this is a preliminary pharmacokinetic model. It is also possible to use the data accrued in the limited sampling sets to update that population model at a later stage. There are various computer programs, among which the most well known is NONMEM (Nonlinear Mixed Effect Modeling), which are able to generate population pharmacokinetic models using a limited number of samples from each patient, sometimes as few as 1 or 2. At the University of Maryland we used an approach known as the iterative 2-stage approach, developed by Dr Alan Forrest, Department of Developmental Therapeutics, University of Maryland Cancer Center, Baltimore, MD, USA, and again that is very useful for updating population pharmacokinetic models, using 2 or 3 samples from each patient. That does use a bayesian algorithm.

Professor Hryniuk: Dr Sasaki, your ATI calculation was extremely interesting. I did not understand how you converted from an in vitro model to a percentage response in vivo as CR plus PR.

Dr Sasaki: We used the data of both CR and PR percentages of patients reported in the literature.

Professor Hryniuk: How do you make the conversion?

Dr Sasaki: We analyze the correlation between ATIs of carboplatin and cisplatin for small cell lung cancer and non-small cell lung cancer and thus the response rate is reported.

Administration methods of anticancer drugs

A pharmacokinetic hypothesis for the clinical efficacy of etoposide in small cell lung cancer (SCLC) and the activity of a prolonged schedule of etoposide in patients with SCLC

Peter I. Clark

Mersey Regional Centre for Radiotherapy and Oncology, Clatterbridge Hospital, Wirral, Merseyside, UK

INTRODUCTION

Etoposide is a semi-synthetic derivative of podophyllotoxin, an anti-cancer drug that has been in use for over a thousand years. In 900-950 A.D., an early medieval English book [1], the Leech Book of Bald, records the treatment of cancer with the roots of wild chervil which contain deoxypodophyllotoxin. For several hundred years, North American Indians used an extract of the plant Podophyllum Peltatin as a cancer remedy [2]. In Solzhenitysyn's Cancer Ward [3], the hero who suffered from metastatic seminoma improved with treatment with the mandrake root of Issyk Kul', a podophyllotoxin-containing extract.

Etoposide has been the most successful of the podophyllotoxin derivatives and currently has first-line use in the management of small cell lung cancer, Hodgkin's and non-Hodgkin's lymphomas, acute leukaemia and testicular cancer. The phase-specificity of its cytotoxic action and its schedule-dependent efficacy in vitro have meant that the clinical pharmacology of etoposide was always likely to be of great potential significance.

It is only recently that pharmacodynamic studies have begun to direct the testing of potentially more efficacious etoposide treatment schedules and it is such investigations that will be discussed below.

Etoposide is a phase-specfic drug, acting in the late S or early G2 phases of the cell cycle (4). In vitro studies have clearly demonstrated that the duration of exposure of cells to etoposide dictates the degree of cytotoxicity (4). For the same degree of cell kill in small cell lung cancer lines, one hundred times the dose of etoposide was required in a 1-hour exposure than in a 24-hour incubation (5).

FIRST SCHEDULING STUDY - 24-HOUR REGIMEN VERSUS 5-DAY SCHEDULE

Clinical confirmation of the schedule-dependency of etoposide has only relatively recently been made (6). 39 patients with previously untreated extensive small cell lung cancer were randomised to receive one of two schedules of the same total dose of single-agent etoposide. One arm received a 24-hour continuous infusion of 500 mg/m² and the second arm were treated with 5 consecutive daily 2-hour infusions each of 100 mg/m². Both schedules were repeated every 3 weeks for a maximum of 6 cycles. The results are shown in Table 1. The response rate in the 5-day arm was 90%, dramatically superior to the 10% achieved in the 24-hour regimen. The bone marrow toxicity as assessed on day 10 of the first treatment cycle was similar in both treatment arms, thereby further demonstrating the greater therapeutic index of the longer schedule of etoposide administration.

An important part of this study was also to examine the pharmacokinetics of etoposide in these patients in order to examine the drug pharmacodynamics. The great majority of patients consented to have serial blood samples taken on several of the treatment days.

The mean pharmacokinetic profiles of the two schedules are shown in Figure 1 and the relevant data in Table 1. The pharmacokinetic parameters examined were the area under the concentration versus

Table 1   Results of 24-hour versus 5-day etoposide study

	24-hour arm		5-day arm
Number of patients	20		19
Response rate (%)	10	*	90
Median remission duration (months)	-		5.2
Median nadir neutrophils x 10^9/l	2.5		2.5
Median drug AUC (ug/ml.hr)	483		472
Median peak plasma level (ug/ml)	17.5		15.0
Median duration >10 ug/ml (hours)	24	*	12
Median duration >5 ug/ml (hours)	32		34
Median duration >1 ug/ml (hours)	49	*	97
Number of etoposide peaks	1		5

Mean plasma etoposide over 1 and 5 days

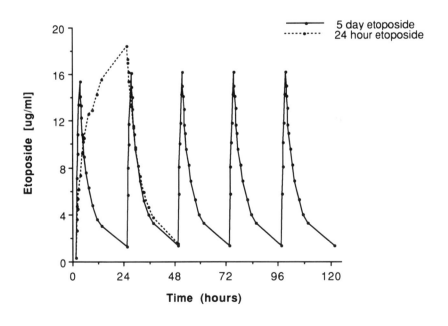

Figure 1

time curve (AUC) and the total duration per schedule for which the plasma concentration of etoposide exceeded 1, 5 and 10 ug/ml.

The two modes of etoposide administration had almost identical AUCs and very similar durations of plasma concentrations of etoposide exceeding 5 ug/ml per cycle of therapy. However, the two schedules differed in two important aspects. The 5-day arm offered 5 discrete, daily pulses, whereas the 24-hour infusion resulted in a broad, sustained exposure. The duration of plasma concentrations exceeding 1 ug/ml per course of treatment in the 5-day arm was twice that in the 24-hour regimen. There are thus two possible pharmacodynamic explanations for the greater efficacy of the 5-day schedule in this study: the presence of 5 separate daily exposures to etoposide or the greater duration of low plasma concentrations of etoposide (>1 ug/ml).

SECOND SCHEDULING STUDY - 5 DAY VERSUS 8-DAY REGIMEN

A second scheduling study was therefore conducted to try and differentiate between these two pharmacokinetic features but without changing the total dose of etoposide in both treatment arms. A pilot study demonstrated that an 8-day schedule of etoposide would provide a similar duration of plasma concentrations of etoposide exceeding 1 ug/ml as a 5-day regimen, but would of course offer an extra 3 pulsed exposures. 59 patients with previously untreated extensive small cell lung cancer were therefore randomised to receive etoposide 500 mg/m² per course, either as 5 consecutive daily 2-hour infusions each of 100 mg/m² or 8 daily consecutive 75-min infusions each of 62.5 mg/m². Both schedules were repeated every 3 weeks for a maximum of 6 cycles.

A similar pharmacokinetic analysis was performed as in the

previous study. The pharmacokinetic profiles are shown in Figure 2 and the patient and pharmacokinetic data in Table 2. As had been predicted, the 8-day schedule provided a very similar total duration of plasma concentrations of etoposide above 1 ug/ml per cycle of therapy as the 5-day arm. The response rates of about 75% and median durations of remission of 5-6 months were also very similar, although the small numbers in this study cannot rule out a modest (but not clinically meaningful) difference.

Thus, the 8-day schedule achieved 3 more pulsed exposures than the 5-day arm (representing an increase of 60%), reduced durations of plasma concentrations of etoposide at higher concentrations (5 and 10 ug/ml) but a similar duration of plasma concentration above 1 ug/ml per course of treatment. These data therefore suggest that the cytotoxicity of etoposide, at least in small cell lung cancer, is

Table 2   Results of 5-day versus 8-day etoposide study

	5-day arm		8-day arm
Number of patients	31		28
Response rate (%)	71		79
Median remission duration (months)	5.4		6.1
Median nadir neutrophils x 10^9/l	0.8	*	1.7
Median drug AUC (ug/ml.hr)	496		453
Median peak plasma level (ug/ml)	15.5		12.4
Median duration >10 ug/ml (hours)	11	*	4
Median duration >5 ug/ml (hours)	33	*	26
Median duration >1 ug/ml (hours)	98		106
Number of etoposide peaks	5		8

(* $p < 0.05$)

271

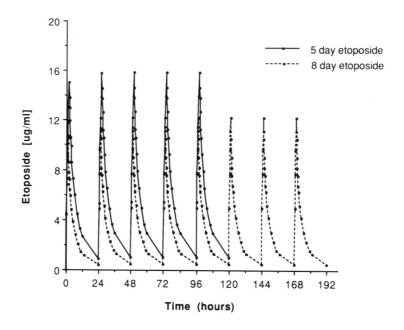

Mean plasma etoposide over 5 and 8 days

Figure 2

related to the maintenance of low plasma concentrations of drug, for example 1 ug/ml (7). This hypothesis is thus in direct agreement with the in vitro evidence for the schedule-dependency of etoposide.

Before further discussing the scheduling of etoposide, one further pharmacodynamic observation can be made. In the above 5-day versus 8-day study, the nadir neutrophil counts were examined. The median nadir neutrophil count in the 5-day regimen was $0.8 \times 10^9/l$, significantly less than $1.7 \times 10^9/l$ in the 8-day schedule (p=0.03). In terms of pharmacokinetics therefore, it would seem possible that bone marrow toxicity may be partly related to the duration of higher plasma concentrations of etoposide (e.g. >5 and 10 ug/ml) since these were the only pharmacokinetic parameters which were greater in the 5-day study compared with the 8-day schedule.

The bone marrow toxicity in the first study was equal (see Table 1), as was the duration of plasma etoposide concentrations exceeding 5 ug/ml. (The 5-day patients in the second study suffered lower blood counts than the 5-day patients in the first study, probably because as a whole they were less fit patients.) It would therefore seem possible that bone marrow toxicity may be partly related to the duration of etoposide blood levels exceeding 5 ug/ml. This observation raises the possibility of being able to partly differentiate anti-tumour efficacy in small cell lung cancer (duration >1 ug/ml) from that of bone marrow toxicity (duration >5 ug/ml) by manipulating the schedule of etoposide administration.

The results of these two scheduling studies raise several questions. The first asks whether low doses of etoposide are effective in small cell lung cancer and the second whether much longer exposure to low doses of etoposide determines the degree of response. The final question is the most fundamental of all and relates to the optimal schedule of etoposide.

It is possible that the optimal schedule of etoposide administration may vary from tumour to tumour or even from person to person, depending on the variable proportion of cycling cells open to attack by the phase-specific action of etoposide. At present, there are answers to the first question and anecdotal hints to the second.

A STUDY OF PROLONGED ORAL ETOPOSIDE ADMINISTRATION

The first question asked whether low doses of etoposide are effective in small cell lung cancer. A phase II study has been conducted examining the efficacy of a prolonged schedule of single-agent oral etoposide in 60 patients previously untreated with small cell lung cancer. Patients were eligible if they had extensive disease or if they had limited disease and either a WHO performance score of 3 or were >70 years old and had a WHO performance score of 2 or more. Patients were not staged routinely and only had investigations performed on symptomatic grounds. It is likely therefore that many of the patients staged as having limited disease did in fact have extensive disease.

42 patients were classed as having extensive disease and 18 as limited. The median age was 62 years (range 42-78, 18 patients >70 years) and the median WHO performance score was 2. The schedule for 35 patients was a 14-day regimen of oral etoposide 50 mg twice daily, repeated 3-weekly. 25 patients were either >70 years old or had a WHO performance score of 3 and these patients received a 10-day schedule of oral etoposide 50 mg twice daily, again repeated every 3 weeks. Patients received a maximum of 6 cycles. Pharmacokinetic studies were also performed to examine the bioavailability of a 50 mg dose of oral etoposide by comparing it with a short intravenous infusion of 50 mg of etoposide.

All patients are eligible for analysis. 42 patients had extensive disease and 18 had limited disease. 18 patients were older than 70 years and the median WHO performance score was 2, reflecting the generally poor fitness of the patients treated. The response rate was 70%, nearly all of the responses being partial and the median time to response was 14 days. The median duration of remission was 5.5 months and that of survival was 8.0 months.

Alopecia was found in all but 1 patient. Most patients did not suffer nausea and vomiting but if it occurred, it was mild and easily controlled with simple anti-emetics. In most patients, the blood count nadir was on day 22, the day on which the next course was initiated. Details of marrow suppression are shown in Table 3.

Although the median white cell and neutrophil nadir counts are not low, some patients suffered very considerable falls in their counts

Table 3   Day 15 and day 22 blood counts during 1st course

	Median White Cells	Median Neutrophils
Day 15	4.5 x 10⁹/l (range 1.0-13.5)	2.8 x 10⁹/l (range 0.6-11.3)
Day 22	4.0 x 10⁹/l (range 1.3-7.3)	2.1 x 10⁹/l (range 0.3-4.5)

(see the ranges quoted in Table 3), mainly those with very extensive disease amd poor WHO performance status.

The pharmacokinetic studies have shown that the bioavailability of a 50 mg dose of oral etoposide is about 60% and exhibits considerable within and between patient variability (8). The pharmacokinetic profile of this schedule is shown in Figure 3.

The mean peak plasma concentration of etoposide following a 50 mg dose was 2.3 ug/ml, as contrasted with a value of 15.0 ug/ml, the mean peak plasma concentration achieved with a 2-hour infusion of etoposide 100 mg/^{2} (the 5-day schedule). A 24-hour profile of these two schedules is shown in Figure 4.

It is therefore clear that a prolonged schedule of small individual doses of etoposide is very active in small cell lung cancer and supports the hypothesis that the schedule-dependency of etoposide, at least in part, is related to the prolonged maintenance of low plasma concentrations of drug. Anti-tumour activity was achieved in most patients at the cost of modest bone marrow toxicity considering the generally poor fitness of the patients treated.

Mean plasma etoposide after oral   dosing (50 mg bd)

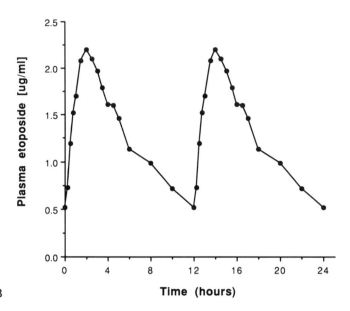

Figure 3

Mean plasma etoposide after oral   and IV administration

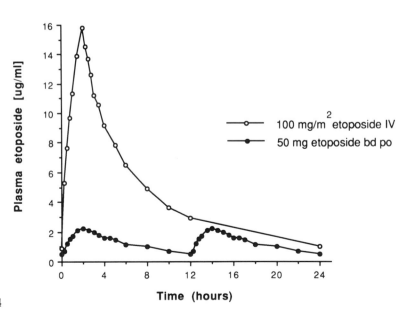

Figure 4

276

Etoposide has now been proven to be schedule-dependent in man and the case for using more prolonged schedules in the treatment of cancer is undoubted. With reference to the three questions posed above, the first has been answered and low doses are clearly very active in small cell lung cancer. The second question as to whether greater durations of low individual doses of etoposide are more active has yet to be formally determined. The remission durations achieved in the prolonged oral etoposide study were similar to those recorded in the 5- and 8-day schedules. It may be that exposure to etoposide need only last about 5 days or the use of remission as the model for efficacy in small cell lung cancer in such scheduling studies is limited.

That this may be so is illustrated by reports of patients with germ cell tumours who failed standard chemotherapy containing etoposide given over 3-5 days and yet who subsequently responded to prolonged schedules of low doses of etoposide (Kaye S B, personal communication).

The final question related to the optimal schedule of etoposide administration and is clearly yet unanswered. Pharmacodynamic studies have pointed in the direction of more prolonged schedules but much work needs to be done. Etoposide has been in use for many years and while the search continues for new drugs, it is ironic that we still do not know the best way to administer an anti-cancer drug that is increasingly used every day.

References

1. Cockayne T O.
    Leech Book of Bald. In: Leechdon, Wartcurings and Starcraft of Early England, vol III.
    London: Holland Press, 1961: p313

2. Lombard L H.
    Medicinal plants of our Maine Indians.
    In: The Maine Writer's Research Club (Eds)
    Maine Indinas in history and legends.
    Portland: Severn-Wylie-Jennett, 1952: 96-102

3. Solzhenitsyn A.
    Cancer Ward
    New York: farrar, Straus and Giroux, Inc 1969

4. Clark P I and Slevin M L.
    The clinical pharmacology of etoposide and teniposide.
    Clin Pharmacokinet 1987; 12: 223-252

5. Roed H, Vindelov L L, Christensen I J, et al.
    The effect of the two epipodophyllotoxin derivatives etoposide
    (VP-16) and teniposide (VM-26) on cell lines established from
    patients with small cell carcinoma of the lung.
    Cancer Chemother Pharmacol 1987; 19: 16-20

6. Slevin M L, Clark P I, Joel S P, et al.
    A randomised trial to evaluate the effect of schedule on the
    activity of etoposide in small cell lung cancer.
    J Clin Oncol 1989; 7: 1333-1340

7. Clark P I, Slevin M L and Joel S P.
    A pharmacokinetic hypothesis for the clinical efficacy of
    etoposide in small cell lung cancer.
    Proc Amer Soc Clin Oncol 1989; 8: 66 (abstract)

8. Joel S P, Dolega-Ossowski E, Jones K, et al.
    The bioavailability of oral etoposide during prolonged
    administration and development of a limited sampling strategy
    for the estimation of AUC after an oral dose
    Proc Amer Assoc Cancer Research 1991; 32: 178 (abstract)

Combination of cisplatin and carboplatin in vitro and in clinical practice

Kunihiko Kobayashi, Akinobu Yoshimura, Mitsunori Hino, Akihiko Gemma, Kouzou Yoshimori, Masahiko Shibuya, Toshiro Takemoto, Kenji Hayashihara, Mie Matsuzaka, Satsuki Wasai, Hisanobu Niitani

Nippon Medical School, Tokyo, Japan

INTRODUCTION

Cisplatin (CDDP) and its derivative Carboplatin (CBDCA) are four valence platinum compounds with the same carrier ligands and different leaving ligands. For both drugs to have their cytotoxicity, leaving ligands must be dissociated by hydroxylation (Fig.1). It was reported that, though the rate to dissociate leaving ligands of CDDP was rapid whereas it of CBDCA was slow, CDDP and CBDCA finally changed to the same active substance, diamminedihydroxy cisplatin (1). Thus the action of both drugs is thought to be mainly the same DNA alkylation. This fact seems to indicate that, if diamminedihydroxy cisplatin is increased by the combination of CDDP and CBDCA, the antineoplastic activity could possibly be enhanced.

Based on these facts, in vitro experiment was first carried out to investigate the advantage of combining CDDP and CBDCA, and then a clinical study combining both drugs was put in practice.

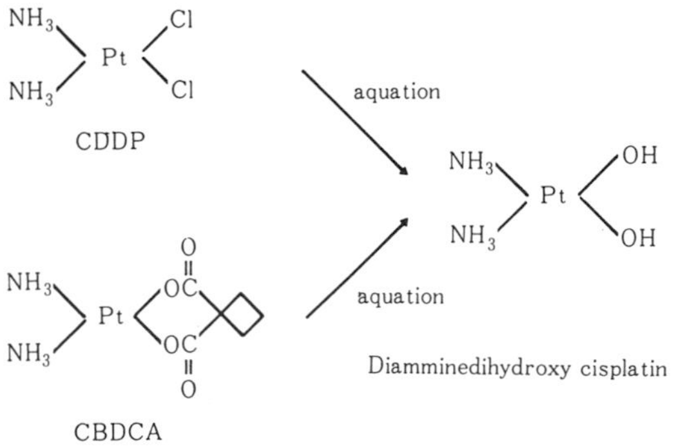

Fig. 1 Structures of CDDP, CBDCA, and Their Active Form

MATERIAL AND METHODS

In vitro

Estimation of AUC dependent drug or time dependent one. To estimate it, HTCA
(HUman Tumor Clonogenic Assay), in which PC-9 cells derived from a lung adenocarcinoma patient were exposed to each of CDDP and CBDCA for several times of 1,
2, 4, 8, and 24 hours, was performed. The IC50 value of each drug, the concentration reducing the survival fraction to 50% of the control, was determined
from dose-response curve for each exposure period, and whether each drug was AUC
(Area Under Curve) dependent drug or not was investigated by log-log relationship
between IC50 and its exposure time devised by Ozawa et al (2). Drugs showing a
straight line with a slope of -1 in the log-log relationship are defined as AUC
dependent drugs.

AUC of free platinum in Exposure Medium. To determine of AUC of free platinum
(free Pt; non-protein bound platinum) from CDDP and CBDCA in Exposure Medium,
which consisted of McCoy's 5A + 10% fetal bovine serum, the concentration of free
Pt was measured at each period of incubation times (0, 1 hour for CDDP and 0, 3
hours for CBDCA) by atomic absorption spectrophotometry, and concentration times
the time of free platinum, that was AUC of free Pt in Exposure medium, was
calculated by trapezoidal rule.

Combination effect of CDDP and CBDCA. To investigate the combination effect of
CDDP and CBDCA, HTCA which had exposure times of 1 hour for CDDP and 3 hours for
CBDCA was performed using PC-9 cells and PC-14 (human lung adenocarcinoma cell
line) cells, and it was investigated by median effect analysis devised by Chou
and Talaley (3). Combination Index (CI) was calculated by the formulas.

$$CI = \frac{(D)_1}{(D_x)_1} + \frac{(D)_2}{(D_x)_2} + \frac{\alpha (D)_1 (D)_2}{(D_x)_1 (D_x)_2}$$

where $(D_x)_1$ is the dose of Drug 1 required to produce x% effect alone. $(D)_1$
is the dose of that drug required to produce the same x% effect in combination
with $(D)_2$. Similarly, $(D_x)_2$ is the dose of Drug 2 required to produce x% effect
alone, and $(D)_2$ is the dose required to produce the same effect in combination.
If the drugs mutually exclusive, then α is 0; if mutually nonexclusive, then α
is 1. An additive effect is shown when Combination Index is 1, a synergistic
effect is shown when it's less than 1, and when greater than 1, an antagonistic
effect is shown.

In clinical practice

Patient selection. Patients with histologically or cytologically proven
advanced non-small lung cancer (NSCLC) were entered in this phase I study.
Eligibility criteria included the following: measurable or evaluable disease, a
performance status of ECOG 0-3, and age of 80 years old or less. All patients,

who were given informed consent, had adequate bone marrow (WBC count ≥4,000/ul, platelet count ≥10,000/ul), normal liver function, and normal renal function (creatinin clearance ≥60ml/min).

Drug administration. Briefly, CBDCA and CDDP were administered as sequential infusions on day 1. After pre-hydration of 1,500ml, CBDCA was given in 250ml of physiological saline by i.v. drip infusion over 30 minutes, and CDDP was sequentially administered by i.v. drip infusion over 1 hour. Then mannitol of 60g, post-hydration of 1,500ml, furosemide of 20mg, and antiemetics were administered. Courses were repeated every 4 weeks.

The starting doses of CBDCA and CDDP were 300mg/m² and 80mg/m², respectively. Dose of each agent was escalated to be 350/80mg/m² or 300/100mg/m² of CBDCA/CDDP.

Evaluation of toxicity and tumor response. The patients were evaluated for toxicity and tumor response according to the criteria of Japan Society for Cancer Therapy, which was modified from WHO criteria.

RESULTS

In vitro

Estimation of AUC dependent drug or time dependent one. Fig. 2 shows the log-log relationships between various exposure times and IC50. The log-log

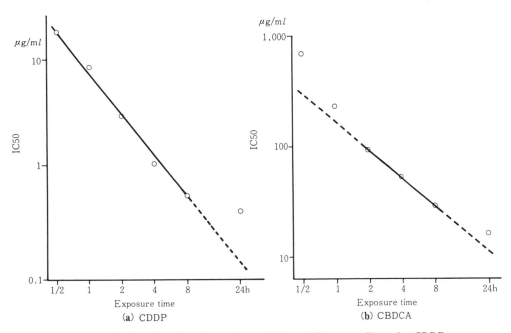

Fig. 2 Log-log Relationships between IC50 and Exposure Time for CDDP and CBDCA by HTCA Using PC-9 cells

relationships of CDDP was shown as a straight line with a slope of -1 up to 8 hours of exposure time, and this indicated that CDDP was an AUC dependent drug. From two hours of exposure time CBDCA had a straight line of -1, and this indicated that CBDCA had AUC dependency, but that it had time dependency up to 2

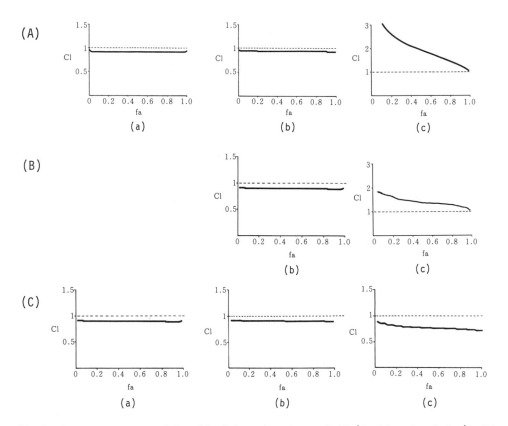

Fig.3   Computer-generated Graphical Presentations of CI (Combination Index) with respect to fraction affected (fa) for the inhibition of colony formation by HTCA.
(A),(B) CI with respect to fa for the inhibition of colony formation of (A) PC-9 or (B) PC-14 cells by "CBDCA+CDDP exposure" at molar ratios of (a) CBDCA/CDDP≑1, (b) 2, and (c) 6.
(C) CI with respect to fa for the inhibition of PC-9 colony formation by (a) "CDDP→CBDCA sequential exposure", (b) "CBDCA+CDDP exposure", and (c) "CBDCA→CDDP sequential exposure" at a molar ratio of about 4 (CBDCA/CDDP).
CI <1, =1, and >1 represent synergistic, additive, and antagonistic effect, respectively.

hours of exposure time.

AUC of free platinum in Exposure Medium. From the concentrations of free Pt (data not shown) in Exposure Medium, AUC of free platinum were calculated by trapezoidal rule. When the molar ratios of CBDCA to CDDP in Exposure Medium were raised from 1, 2, 4, to 6, the AUC ratios of free Pt increased from 3, 7, 14, to 20, accordingly.

Combination effet of CDDP and CBDCA. Fig. 3 represents the computer-generated graphycal presentations of combination index with the respect to fraction affected (fa) for the inhibition of PC-9 or PC-14 colony formation when CDDP and CBDCA were combined under various conditions.

From Fig.3(A), 3(B), and 3(C)(b), in both PC-9 and PC-14 cells, the combination effect of CBDCA and CDDP by "CBDCA + CDDP exposure", which was carried out by exposing tumor cells to CBDCA alone for 2 hours and, without washing it, CBDCA and CDDP in combination for 1 hour, indicated to be almost additive at the molar ratios up to about 4 of CBDCA to CDDP, but it was antagonistic at a molar ratio of about 6. From the above results almost additive effect was shown at the AUC of free Pt ratio up to 14 of CBDCA to CDDP, but antagonistic effect was indicated at that of 20.

From Fig.3(C), Combination Index of "CBDCA → CDDP sequential exposure", which was the schedule of exposing PC-9 cells to CBDCA for 3 hours and, after washing

TABLE 1

PATIENTS CHARACTERISTICS

| | CDDP(mg/sqm) / CBDCA(mg/sqm) | | |
	80/300	80/350	100/300
No. of patients	8	6	3
Sex (M/F)	5/3	4/2	2/1
Median age in year (range)	59	60	61
	(43-76)	(45-77)	(39/68)
Performance status (0-1/2-3)	6/2	5/1	1/2
Clinical stage (III_B/IV/recurrence)	2/2/4	1/4/1	1/1/1
Histologic type (Ad/Sq/Ad-Sq)*	5/3/0	3/2/1	3/0/0
Prior therapy (none/chemo/chemo+RT)**	4/3/1	5/1/0	2/1/0

* Ad; Adenocarcinoma, Sq; Squamous cell carcinoma, Ad-Sq; Adeno-squamous cell carcinoma

** chemo; chemotherapy only, chemo + RT; chemotherapy plus radiotherapy

it, CDDP for 1 hour, at the molar ratio of about 4 of CBDCA to CDDP, that is an AUC of free Pt rate of 14 was from 0.74 to 0.86, and it indicated a slightly synergistic effect.

In clinical practice

Table 1 shows the patient characteristics. Seventeen patients were entered in this study. Table 2 represents side effects. Three of 6 patients receiving CBDCA of 350mg/m2 and CDDP of 80mg/m2 had grade 3 or 4 of leukopenia according to the Japan Society for Cancer Therapy. In all of the 3 patients treated with

TABLE 2(A)

LEUKOPENIA DURING FIRST CYCLE OF THE COMBINATION CHEMOTHERAPY OF CDDP AND CBDCA

	CDDP(mg/sqm) / CBDCA(mg/sqm)		
	80/300	80/350	100/300
Median wbc count nadir (range)	2,600	2,100	700
(/μl)	(1,500-4,400)	(300-3,500)	(300-1,400)
No. of patients			
with leukopenia of grade 3-4*	3/8	3/6	3/3*
	(37.5%)	(50.0%)	(100%)

* Three patients were given G-CSF because of severe leukopenia.

TABLE 2(B)

THROMBOCYTOPENIA DURING FIRST CYCLE OF THE COMBINATION CHEMOTHERAPY OF CDDP AND CBDCA

	CDDP(mg/sqm) / CBDCA(mg/sqm)		
	80/300	80/350	100/300
Median platelet count nadir (range)	72	80	16
$(x10^3/\mu l)$	(40-131)	(20-98)	(8-17)
No. of patients			
with thrombocytopenia of grade 3-4*	2/8	2/6	3/3
	(25.0%)	(33.3%)	(100%)

* Gradings of leukopenia and thrombocytopenia are assessed according to the criteria of the Japan Society for Cancer Therapy, which is modified from WHO criteria.

TABLE 3

TUMOR RESPONSE OF THE COMBINATION CHEMOTHERAPY OF CDOP AND CBDCA BY EACH DOSAGE

CDDP(mg/sqm) /CBDCA(mg/sqm)	No. of patients	PR	MR	NC	PD	Response rate
80/300	8	3	1	4	0	3/ 8 (37.5%)
80/350	6	1	0	5	0	1/ 6 (16.7%)
100/300	3	0	0	3	0	0/ 3 (0 %)
	17	4	1	12	0	4/17 (28.6%)

The patients are evaluated for response according to the criteria of the Japan Society for Cancer Therapy, which is modified from WHO criteria.

CBDCA of $300mg/m^2$ and CDDP of $100mg/m^2$, severe thrombocytopenia and leukopenia were observed beyond our expectation. It was thought that both of the combinations of these doses were maximum tolerated doses, and that thrombocytopenia and leukopenia were dose limiting factors of this combination. CBDCA and CDDP were safely given in combination at the doses of $300mg/m^2$ and $80mg/m^2$, respectively.

Tumor response according to the doses of CBDCA and CDDP was shown in Table 3. In 8 patients treated with CBDCA of $300mg/m^2$ and CDDP of $80mg/m^2$, which was the optimal doses of this combination, 3 patients achieved partial response, and response rate was 37.5%. Overall response rate was 28.6%.

DISCUSSION

Recently the concept of AUC dependent drug whose cytotoxicity was determined only by the product of concentration times the time was clarified (2). So it is thought that the experiment to investigate the combination effect of two AUC dependent drugs should be done based on AUC of the drugs.

As CDDP and CBDCA were found to be fundamentally AUC dependent drugs from Fig. 2, it seems to be indicate that, if the AUC of diamminedihydroxy cisplatin from CDDP and CBDCA is increased by the combination of both drugs, the antineoplastic activity could possibly be enhanced.

From Fig. 3 almost additive effect was shown at AUC of free platinum (free Pt) rate up to 14 of CBDCA to CDDP, and especially in "CBDCA → CDDP sequential exposure" at an AUC of free Pt rate of 14 of CBDCA to CDDP, the Combination Index was from 0.74 to 0.86, and it indicated a slightly synergistic effect. But antagonistic effect was indicated at that of 20.

As it was reported that, when 80mg/m^2 of CDDP or 450mg/m^2 of CBDCA was given by i.v. drip infusion in clinical practice, the AUC of free platinum for CDDP and CBDCA were 3.47ug/m^2 × h and 57.4ug/m^2 × h, respectively (4). If 80mg/m^2 of CDDP and 450mg/m^2 of CBDCA in combination should be given, AUC of free platinum for CBDCA would be 17 times higher than that for CDDP. It would be needed to increase the dose of CDDP or to reduce that of CBDCA.

So based on the results of these experiments, we are caring out phase I study of the CBDCA → CDDP sequential combination by the doses from 300 to 350mg/m^2 of CBDCA and from 80 to 100mg/m^2 of CDDP for non-small cell lung cancer patients (5).

From this phase I study it was thought that the combinations by the doses of 350/80mg/m^2 and 300/100mg/m^2 of CBDCA/CDDP were maximum tolerated doses, and that thrombocytopenia and leukopenia were dose limiting factors of this combination. The recommended doses for phase 2 study were 300mg/m^2 of CBDCA and 80mg/m of CDDP.

It was reported the response rate of the combination by the doses of 350/50 mg/m^2 of CBDCA/CDDP, which was thought to be the antagonistic ratio of AUC of free platinum from this experiment, was not good for NSCLC patients (6). But in our study the response by the doses of 300/80mg/m^2 of CBDCA/CDDP was 37.5%, and higher than in the above study. As the doses of 300/80mg/m^2 of CBDCA/CDDP in clinical practice thought to have the AUC ratio of less than 14, the combination was seemed to get more than additive effect.

We are going to increase the number of cases in phase II study. And if results similar to those in this study, further comparison studies with other regimens should be warranted.

REFERENCES

1. Knox, R.J., Friedros, F., Lydall, D.A., Roberts, J.J. (1986) Cancer Res., 46 : 1972

2. Ozawa, S., Sugiyama, Y., Mitsuhashi, Y., Kobayashi, T., Inaba, M. (1988) Cancer Chemother Pharmacol 21 : 185

3. Chou, T.C., Talalay, P. (1981) Eur. J. Biochem. 115 : 207

4. Sasaki, Y., Tamura, T., Eguchi, K., Shinkai, T., Fujiwara, Y., Fukuda, M., Ohe, Y., Bungo, M., Horichi, N., Niimi, S., Minato, K., Nakagawa, K., Saijo, N. (1989) Cancer Chemother Pharmacol 23 : 243

5. Kreisman H., Goutsou M., Modeas C., Graziano S.L., Costanza M.E., Green M.R. (1990) Eur J Cancer 26(10) : 1057

Individualized administration of anticancer drugs

Mary V. Relling, John H. Rodman, William R. Crom, Ching-Hon Pui,
William E. Evans

St. Jude Children's Research Hospital, University of Tennessee, Memphis, Tennessee, USA

INTRODUCTION

Variability in the pharmacokinetics of and thus the systemic exposure to some anticancer drugs has been shown to translate into variability in drug response (Evans & Relling 1989; Evans 1988; Ratain et al 1990; Powis 1985; Dodwell et al 1990; and elsewhere in these proceedings). Systemic exposure in individual patients can be measured as area-under-the-plasma-concentration-versus-time-curve or AUC, steady-state plasma or other tissue concentrations, period of time above a certain threshold plasma concentration, etc. In all cases where a significant relationship has been established, *higher* systemic exposure to antineoplastics has been associated with greater anticancer response. Unfortunately, higher systemic exposure is often also associated with greater toxicity. Recently, significant pharmacodynamic relationships between antineoplastic drug exposure and response have been identified for several drugs. Unlike prognostic factors such as race, sex, age, etc., which are unalterable, systemic exposure is a prognostic variable that may be *modified* if one prospectively monitors anticancer drug pharmacokinetics and adaptively controls each individual patient's blood or plasma concentrations of drugs by altering the dosage of antineoplastic. However, the value of adjusting dosages to achieve targeted blood concentrations of specific drugs and for specific diseases should preferably be established in prospective trials. Establishing the utility of therapeutic drug monitoring of antineoplastics is particularly challenging in the setting of *combination chemotherapy* as employed in most Phase III trials.

Herein, we briefly review examples of pharmacodynamic relationships which have been elucidated, and some of the practical aspects of adaptive control of anticancer drug doses in patients.

287

PHARMACODYNAMIC RELATIONSHIPS

Obviously, the setting with the fewest confounding variables is best suited to identifying potentially important pharmacodynamic relationships. Pharmacokinetic information from Phase I trials helps to define toxicity/exposure relationships. The disadvantage of completely characterizing pharmacodynamic relationships at the level of Phase I studies is that many Phase I agents turn out to lack significant clinical utility. Therefore, resources will sometimes be expended on inactive drugs. However, even for inactive drugs, it may be helpful to know that inactivity was demonstrated despite the presence of active drug concentrations known to be tumoricidal in pre-clinical systems.

Pharmacokinetics may be incorporated into Phase I-II trials in one of two ways. The first is the traditional strategy, wherein the doses of the new drug are determined using a dose-escalation procedure is conducted according to the Fibonacci or some other scheme (Collins et al 1986). Collection of pharmacokinetic data for each patient may allow the retrospective identification of relationships linking toxicity with systemic exposure, as has been reported for drugs such as carboplatin, menogaril, amsacrine, teniposide (VM26), etc. (Hall et al 1983; Egorin et al 1984, 1987; Rodman et al 1987; Pratt et al 1991; Kerr et al 1990; Bailey et al 1991). The second strategy is to determine dosages not by an escalation of dose *per se*, but by escalation of systemic exposure level (also been termed *pharmacologically guided dose escalation*) (EORTC 1987; Collins et al 1990; Evans et al 1991a). This concept is the topic of other participants in this congress. Examples of drugs for which prospective studies have been conducted using this strategy include teniposide, piroxantrone, and iododeoxydoxorubicin (Rodman et al 1989; Gianni et al 1990; Hantel et al 1990).

In a Phase I-II trial of escalating doses of teniposide, 28 children with relapsed solid tumors and leukemia were treated with 300 to 750 mg/m^2 as a 72 hour continuous infusion (Rodman et al 1987). Both tumor response and toxicity were found to be correlated with teniposide Cp_{ss} (steady-state plasma concentration), while there was no significant relationship between clinical response and dose. All ten patients with Cp_{ss} > 12 mg/l exhibited a clinical response versus only 5 of 13 patients with Cp_{ss} < 12 mg/l. Moreover, significant inter-patient variability (4-6 fold) in clearance resulted in overlap of systemic exposure at various dosage levels, making the determination of a recommended Phase III dosage difficult.

288

Pharmacodynamic relationships demonstrating a correlation between exposure and either toxicity or efficacy have been identified retrospectively in many Phase III studies, often in conjunction with multi-agent chemotherapy. Examples include 6-mercaptopurine (Lennard et al 1983, 1989), 5-fluorouracil (Au et al 1982, Santini et al 1989), teniposide (Petros et al 1991), and many others (reviewed in Ratain et al 1990; Powis 1985; Dodwell et al 1990; Evans et al 1988, 1989, 1991a). In one front-line Phase III trial (St. Jude Total X) for childhood acute lymphocytic leukemia (ALL), a major component of maintenance therapy was 15 courses of high-dose MTX (1 g/m^2 over 24 hours) over the course of 2 years. It was shown that relapse-free survival was improved in a group of 49 children whose median MTX Cp_{ss} exceeded 16 μM, compared to a group of 59 children whose median Cp_{ss} was < 16 μM (Evans et al 1986). Moreover, children with higher MTX Cp_{ss} had a significantly better continuous complete remission rate at 4 years (74%) than a historic control group (50%) who received similar therapy but no HD-MTX (p = .004) (Abromowitch et al 1988). Interestingly, with a median follow-up of 7.3 years, MTX clearance is no longer statistically significant as a predictor of disease-free survival in the very low-risk subgroup of 82 children, while it has maintained its prognostic significance in worse-risk patients (Evans et al 1990). Because the impact of any prognostic factor is highly dependent on the overall efficacy of the treatment administered, it is not surprising that MTX systemic exposure retained significance in only a subgroup of high-risk cases.

PROSPECTIVE TRIAL

Given the above retrospective studies suggesting a pharmacodynamic relationship for teniposide and methotrexate, we have designed a prospective study to adaptively control systemic exposure to these agents in children. Our current Phase III randomized trial (Total XII) for childhood ALL test the efficacy and toxicity of targeted systemic exposure (TSE) versus conventional (CONV) dosing methods (Evans et al 1991b). After a six-drug induction regimen (Rivera et al 1991), backbone therapy consisting of weekly MTX (40 mg/m^2) and daily oral 6-mercaptopurine (75 mg/m^2/day) is given for 2 years. Backbone therapy is interrupted by five pulses of MTX (CONV dose = 1.5 g/m^2) alternated every 6 weeks with five pulses of teniposide (200 mg/m^2) and Ara-C (cytarabine) (300 mg/m^2) given every 6 weeks for the first year of therapy. The dose of

MTX was chosen so that the average MTX Cp_{ss} would exceed the 16 μM plasma concentration which has been associated with favorable outcome in our previous study (Evans et al 1986). The doses of teniposide and Ara-C were chosen so that a patient with average clearance of both agents would have an exposure expected to have an acceptable degree of toxicity. Moreover, the target AUC for teniposide was that associated with a higher probability of oncolytic response (Rodman et al 1987).

The major goal in the TSE arm is to avoid low systemic exposure (lowest 50th percentile) in children with high clearance of these agents, and to avoid unusually high exposure (top 10th percentile) in those with unusually low clearance. The expected range of clearance estimates was predicated on several prior studies of MTX, teniposide, and Ara-C disposition in children (Sinkule et al 1983, 1984; Rodman et al 1987). In this way, it is hoped to avoid both sub-therapeutic and unusually toxic systemic exposure to the major anticancer drugs. Toxicities and long-term efficacy in the TSE versus the CONV arms will be compared. The overall strategies for dosage adjustments for teniposide and MTX are depicted in the following figure.

MTX is given as a 200 mg/m^2 intravenous (IV) loading dose over 1 hour and followed with 1300 mg/m^2 over the next 23 hours. Appropriate hydration, alkalinization with sodium bicarbonate, and leucovorin rescue are given. Blood samples are obtained from all children pre-dose and at 1, 6, and 23 hours from the start of infusion.

In the 50% of children who are randomized to the TSE arm, plasma from the 1 and 6 hour blood samples is immediately assayed for MTX using a fluorescence polarization immunoassay (TDx, Abbot Laboratories, Chicago, USA). Estimates of clearance and predicted Cp_{ss} are made using a Bayesian algorithm and a two-compartment model with pediatric population prior estimates of the appropriate model parameters (volume of the central compartment, elimination rate constant, and intercompartmental rate constants), using a modification of the ADAPT software (USC, Los Angeles, USA).

Estimates of clearance and Cp_{ss} are used in children on the TSE arm to determine the infusion rate necessary to achieve a predicted AUC within the target range, which is 640 to 900 μM•hr. If the predicted AUC is within these bounds, no dosage adjustment is made, and the CONV dosing rate is continued. Children with very low clearance estimates (about 10% of the population), such that their predicted AUC is >

290

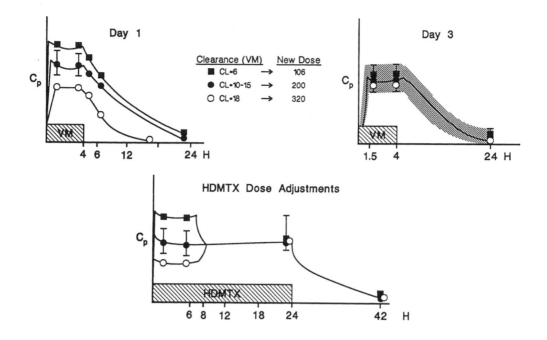

Figure legend: Illustration of dosage individualization between doses for teniposide (VM, upper panel) and during MTX infusions (lower panel) in patients with either high or low clearance. Examples of clearances (ml/min/m²) and dose (mg/m²) are depicted for teniposide.

900, have an infusion rate reduction (8 hours into the infusion) to achieve the target AUC of 800 μM. However, the rate can not be reduced to such an extent that the predicted Cp_{ss} would be < 20 μM. Children with clearance estimates lower than the population median, such that their predicted AUC is < 640 μM•hrs, have an infusion rate increase (8 hours into the infusion) to achieve the target AUC of 800 μM.

The final clearance and actual AUC and Cp_{ss} obtained in each patient is estimated again using the 1, 6, and 23 hour MTX plasma concentrations and the Bayesian algorithm described above. This clearance estimate is then used to determine whether the patient will achieve an AUC in the target range if they are administered the conventional dose of 1500 mg/m². If their clearance is estimated as either too high (> 86 ml/min/m²) or too low (< 61 ml/min/m²), then a new dose is chosen to tailor the patient's AUC to achieve the target AUC of 800 μM. The MTX is always administered as a 200 mg/m² loading dose over 1 hour with the remainder given over 23 hours. The same process of measuring MTX plasma concentrations, estimating clearance, and adaptively controlling infusion rates is repeated with each course of high-dose MTX.

Pulses of teniposide and Ara-C have been administered as concurrent 4 hour IV infusions on Day 1 and Day 3, every 12 weeks. The CONV dose (and starting dose in the TSE patients) of teniposide is 200 mg/m², with 45% of the dose (90 mg/m²) given over 1 hour, and the remainder given over the following 3 hours. The conventional dose of Ara-C is 300 mg/m², given as a 30 mg/m² loading dose IV push, with the remainder given as an IV infusion over the next 4 hours. Blood samples are obtained in all children with both Day 1 and Day 3 doses at 1 and 3 hours (both during the infusions), 8 hours, and approximately 20 hours from the start of the infusions. In patients randomized to the TSE arm, plasma from the Day 1 dose is assayed by separate HPLC assays for Ara-C and teniposide (Sinkule et al 1984, 1983). Clearance is estimated as described above; a one-compartment model using the 1 and 3 hour concentrations is used for Ara-C and a two-compartment model with all 4 concentrations is used to obtain teniposide clearance estimates. For teniposide, the AUC target range is 400-500 μM•hr, with the target AUC being 450 μM. For Ara-C, the AUC target range is 25-57 μM•hr, with the target AUC being 42 μM•hr. Again, if the patient has clearance estimates such that the CONV dose would be predicted to have an AUC within the target range, no dosage alteration is made for the Day 3 doses. In patients with clearance estimates such that their predicted AUC is either too high or too low, the appropriate dosage adjustments are made for the Day 3 doses to attempt to achieve the target AUCs for both teniposide and Ara-C.

Plasma concentrations of teniposide (all 8 plasma samples) and Ara-C (all 4 intra-infusion plasma samples) are then used to obtain a total-course estimate of clearance of both drugs. These overall clearance estimates are then used to determine the starting doses for the next pulse of teniposide and Ara-C. As for MTX, if the clearance estimates are too high (> 49.3 l/hr/m² for Ara-C or > 12.7 ml/min/m² for teniposide) or too low (< 21.6 l/hr/m² for Ara-C or < 10.2 ml/min/m² for teniposide), the conventional doses are altered starting with the Day 1 dose of the subsequent pulse. Again, the process of measuring teniposide and Ara-C plasma concentrations and estimating clearance is repeated with every dose of every course, so that doses are continuously adaptively controlled in the TSE patients.

For all children (CONV and TSE), if a child has two consecutive pulses that are followed by unacceptable toxicity, the dose is decreased by 25% from the toxic dose for all subsequent courses.

This procedure has proven to be quite feasible. We have now performed these dosage adjustments in over 320 courses of MTX and over 600 doses of teniposide/Ara-C. Adverse effects have been similar in the TSE and CONV arms, despite the fact that the average doses of MTX, teniposide, and Ara-C are 1.4 times higher in the TSE arm for all 3 drugs. This equivalent tolerance between the two arms probably results from our ability to avoid unnecessarily high exposure in the children on the TSE arm who have clearances in the lowest 10th percentile. Whether the long-term outcome will differ between the two arms will not be known for several more years.

In summary, we have found that it is feasible to adaptively control patients' exposure to multiple anticancer drugs in a Phase III trial using limited sampling and a Bayesian algorithm to estimate clearances. We have found that it is possible to avoid both very high and low systemic exposure in patients by this control strategy. Whether there are any long term-differences in overall toxicity or efficacy has yet to be determined.

ACKNOWLEDGEMENTS

Supported by Cancer Center CORE grant CA21765, by a Center of Excellence grant from the State of Tennessee, and American Lebanese Syrian Associated Charities.

REFERENCES

Abromowitch M, Ochs J, Pui C-H, Kalwinsky D, Rivera GK, Fairclough D, Look AT, Hustu O, Murphy SB, Evans WE, Dahl GV, Bowman WP. High-dose methotrexate improves clinical outcome in children with acute lymphoblastic Leukemia: St. Jude Total Therapy Study X. Med Pediatr Oncol 16:297-303, 1988.

Au JLS, Rustum YM, Ledesma EJ, Mittelman A, Creaven PJ. Clinical pharmacological studies of concurrent infusion of 5-fluorouracil and thymidine in treatment of colorectal carcinomas. Cancer Res 42:2930-2937, 1982.

Bailey H, Tutsch KD, Arzoomanian RZ, Tombes MB, Alberti D, Bruggink J. Phase I clinical trial of fazarabine as a twenty-four hour continuous infusion. Cancer Res 51:1105-8, 1991.

Collins JM, Zaharko DS, Dedrick Rl et al. Potential roles for preclinical pharmacology in Phase I clinical trials. Can Treat Rep 70:73-80, 1986.

Collins JM, Grieshaber CK, Chabner BA. Pharmacologically guided Phase I clinical trials based upon preclinical drug development. J Natl Cancer Inst 82:1321-1326, 1990.

Dodwell DJ, Gurney H, Thatcher N. Dose intensity in cancer chemotherapy. Br J Cancer 61:789-94, 1990.

Egorin MJ, Conley BA, Forrest A, et al. Phase I study and pharmacokinetics of menogaril (NSC 269148) in patients with hepatic dysfunction. Cancer Res 47:6104-6110, 1987.

Egorin MJ, Van Echo SJ, Tipping EA et al. Pharmacokinetics and dosage reduction of carboplatin in patients with impaired renal function. Cancer Res. 44:5432-5438, 1984.

EORTC Pharmacokinetic and Metabolism Group: Pharmacokinetically guided dose escalation in Phase I clinical trials. Commentary and proposed guidelines. Eur.J.Cancer Clin Oncol. 23:1083-1087, 1987

Evans WE, Relling MV. Clinical pharmacodynamics of antineoplastics agents in humans. Clin Pharmacokinet 16: 327-336, 1989.

Evans WE, Rodman JR, Relling MV, Crom WR, Rivera GK, Crist WM, Pui C-H. Individualized dosages of chemotherapy as a strategy to improve response for acute lymphocytic leukemia. Semin Hematology 1991b;28:(suppl 4) 15-21.
Evans WE, Rodman JH, Relling MV, Crom WR, Rivera DK, Pratt CB, Crist WM. The concept of maximum tolerated systemic exposure (MTSE) and its application to Phase I-II studies of anticancer drugs. Med Pediatr Oncol 1991a;19:153-9.

Evans WE, Crom WR, Abromowitch M, Dodge R, Look T, Bowman P, George SL, Clinical pharmacodynamics of high-dose methotrexate in acute lymphocytic leukemia: Identification of a concentration-effect relationship. N Engl J Med 314:471-477, 1986.

Evans WE, Pui C-H, Schell MJ. MTX clearance more important for intermediate-risk ALL (Letter). J Clin Oncol 8:1115-1116, 1990.

Evans WE. Clinical pharmacodynamics of anticancer drugs: A basis for extending the concept of dose-intensity. Blut 56:241-248, 1988.

Evans WE, Relling MV, Rodman JH, Crom WR. Anticancer therapy as a pediatric pharmacodynamic paradigm. Dev Pharmacol Ther 13:85-95, 1989.

Gianni L, Vigano L, Surbone A, Ballinari D, Casali P, Tarella C, Collins JM, Bonadonna G. Pharmacology and clinical toxicity of 4'-iodo-4'-deoxydoxorubicin: an example of successful application of pharmacokinetics to dose escalation in Phase I trials. J Natl Cancer Inst 82:469-477, 1990.

Hall SW, Friedman J, Legha SS, Benjamin RS, Gutterman JU, Loo TL. Human Pharmacokinetics of a new acridine derivative, 4'-(9-acridinylamino) methanesulfon-m-anisidide (NSC 249992). Cancer Res 43:3422-3426, 1983.

Hantel A, Donehower RC, Rowinsky EK, Vance E, Clarke BV, McGuire WP, Ettinger DS, Noe DA, Grochow LB. Phase I study of pharmacodynamics of piroxantrone, a new anthrapyrazole. Cancer Res 50:3284-88, 1990.

Kerr DJ, Slack JA, Secrett P, Stevens MFG, Blackledge GRP, Bradley C, Kaye SB. Relationship between the pharmacokinetics and toxicity of mitozolomide. Cancer Chemother Pharmacol 25:352-354, 1990.

Lennard L, Rees CA, Lilleyman JS, et al. Childhood leukemia: A relationship between intracellular 6-mercaptopurine metabolism and neutropenia. Br J Clin Pharmacol 1983; 16:359-63.

Lennard L, and Lilleyman JS. Variable mercaptopurine metabolism and treatment outcome in childhood lymphoblastic leukemia. J Clin Oncol 1989; 7:1816-23.

Petros WP, Rodman JH, Mirro J, Evans WE. Pharmacokinetics of continuous infusion amsacrine and teniposide for the treatment of relapsed childhood acute nonlymphocytic leukemia. Can Chemo Pharmacol 27:397-400, 1991.

Pratt CB, Relling MV, Meyer WH, Douglass EC, Kellie SJ, Avery L. Phase I study of flavone acetic acid (NSC 347512, LM975) in patients with pediatric malignant solid tumors. Am J Clin Oncol (in press)

Powis G. Anticancer drug pharmacodynamics. Cancer Chemo Pharmacol 14:177-183, 1985.

Ratain MJ, Schilsky RL, Conley BA, Egorin MJ. Pharmacodynamics in cancer therapy. J Clin Oncol 8:1739-53, 1990.

Rivera GK, Raimondi SC, Hancock ML, Behm FG, Pui C-H, Abromowitch M, Mirro J, Ochs J, Look AT, Murphy SB, Dahl GV, Kalwinsky DK, Evans WE, Kun L, Simone JV, Crist WM. Reinforcement of early therapy with teniposide-cytarabine and high-dose methotrexate followed by rotational combination chemotherapy in childhood acute lymphocytic leukemia. Lancet 1991; 337:61-66.

Rodman JH, Abromowich M, Sinkule JA et al. Clinical Pharmacodynamics os Continuous Infusion Teniposide: Systemic Exposure as a Determinant of Response in a Phase I trial. J Clin Oncol. 7: 1007-1014, 1987.

Rodman JH, Sunderland M, Furman WA, Rivera G. Prospective evaluation of patient specific teniposide dosage regimens for pediatric cancer patients. Clin Pharmacol Ther 45:240, 1989.

Santini J, Milano G, Thyss A, Rennee N, Viens P, Ayela P, Schneider M, Demard F. 5-FU therapeutic monitoring with dose adjustment leads to an improved therapeutic index in head and neck cancer. Br J Cancer 59:287-290, 1989.

Sinkule JA, Stewart CF, Crom WR et al. Teniposide (VM-26) disposition in children with leukemia. Cancer Research 44:1235-1237, 1984.

Sinkule J, Evans WE. High performance liquid chromatography (HPLC) assay of cytosine arabinoside. J Chrom 274:87-93, 1983.

Sinkule JA, Evans WE. High-performance liquid chromatographic analysis of the semi-synthetic epipodophyllotoxins, teniposide (VM26) and etoposide (VP16) using electrochemical detection. J Pharm Sci 73:164-168, 1984.

Disussion

Dr Hiroshi Fujita (School of Dental Medicine, Tsurumi University, Yokohama, Japan): I am very interested in cancer drug pharmacology. You showed that the bioavailability of oral etoposide at a dose of 50 mg is about 60%. This is very good bioavailability, but according to some papers etoposide at doses over 300 mg orally is not absorbed as well.

Dr Clark: That is right.

Dr Fujita: Why do you think this phenomenon occurs?

Dr Clark: I am not sure. Studies that as yet are unpublished show that etoposide is absorbed in the upper small bowel and etoposide is not that stable in gastric juice, although it is much more stable in gastric juice than it is in duodenal juice. Etoposide comes out of solution very quickly in duodenal juice. In vitro studies that I have been involved in have shown that this loss of stability is very concentration dependent. I suspect that the variable bioavailability relates to stability in the duodenum, but clearly, with the advent of etoposide phosphate, we may not need to worry about that too much.

Dr Hideo Saka (Nagoya University, Nagoya, Japan): Now many clinical investigations utilizing the chronic oral or low-dose use of etoposide are ongoing worldwide, including ours. What do you think about the future role of low-dose administration of etoposide in combination chemotherapy in small cell lung cancer or other solid tumors?

Dr Clark: I have not used this schedule of administration of etoposide in combination with anything. So I cannot say, because my interest is in the scheduling of etoposide. From discussions I have had, such a schedule does not appear to be bone marrow toxic in the great majority of patients, although in some it clearly is. Once you begin to add other drugs, I am told that the bone marrow toxicity, especially over a 21-day schedule, is highly significant. I think that with a drug with variable absorption, we first need to get reproducible absorption from day to day. Then we must work out what the best schedule is, whether it is smaller doses 3 times a day, whether the duration is 1, 2, or 3 weeks; there is clearly a lot of work to be done. However, I think that what it offers small cell lung cancer patients, certainly in our institution in Liverpool at the moment, is reasonable palliation at the expense of very modest toxicity. Combining it with less marrow-toxic drugs, such as cisplatin, would be the obvious thing to do in small cell lung cancer.

Dr Martin E. Blackstein (Mount Sinai Hospital, Toronto, Ontario, Canada): The ways of administering etoposide are becoming more complex. A paper presented at the 1990 ASCO meeting on the use of platinum and etoposide in small cell lung cancer appeared to show that the sequence of the administration of cisplatin and etoposide played a role. The response rates were much higher and the duration of response was much higher if the cisplatin was given first, followed by the etoposide. Is there any possible reason for these sorts of interactions?

Dr Clark: Not that I am aware of.

Professor Hryniuk: Are you planning to do any pump infusion studies to search for where that magic level is?

Dr Clark: That is very interesting, because even 3 years ago, pump technology was not sufficiently advanced to be able to give long-term infusions of etoposide. Patients were given infusions of etoposide, but using relatively small-volume syringes. The big problem with etoposide is precipitation in the Hickman catheter line. Now that there are much better pumps that can be used to administer etoposide, with less solution, and 100 mL or 250 mL bags per day can be infused, Professor Hryniuk is correct in believing that that is the most constant way of seeking out the therapeutic level.

Professor Hryniuk: What, if any, effect does the known chronobiologic disposition of the drug have to do with your scheduling or your observations?

Dr Clark: I have no knowledge about that with regard to efficacy. I can tell you that measurements of pharmacokinetics have shown there is no difference between night-time and daytime etoposide pharmacokinetics.

Professor H. Rodney Withers (UCLA Medical Center, Los Angeles, California, USA): As one of the few radiation oncologists here, I would like to make 2 points. One is that a cycle-active drug, particularly one that kills cells in S phase, can be a very useful adjunct in radiotherapy because the cell cycle phase that is so resistant to radiation is S phase. Combining an S phase-specific drug with radiation makes biological sense. Second, with careful beam direction, you can minimize the bone marrow damage so that radiation therapy can be an agent that need not be very bone marrow toxic. In your considerations of multidrug treatments, radiation is a very useful addition.

Dr Clark: As someone once said, radiation is one of the more active single agents, but I think at my institution, etoposide and radiotherapy are now combined. They have had to be very careful because several of the patients have had very severe esophagitis.

Professor Withers: Yes, that was also the problem with hydroxyurea.

Professor Franco M. Muggia (Kenneth Norris Cancer Center, UCLA, Los Angeles, California, USA): Dr Kobayashi, I was very interested in the rationale for your study. What was the sequence of carboplatin and cisplatin? Was there an interval between them when you administered them?

298

Dr Kobayashi: We did not test the interval between them. We think carboplatin/cisplatin sequential exposure is a good method, but the combination does not have a time lag.

Dr Muggia: Did you give them together?

Dr Hisanobu Niitani (Nippon Medical School, Tokyo, Japan): I am the collaborator in this study, so I can tell you that we have no interval; cisplatin is given immediately after the infusion of carboplatin.

Dr Nagahiro Saijo (National Cancer Center, Tokyo, Japan): I am interested in the in vitro pharmacokinetics of cisplatin and carboplatin. The intracellular concentration of platinum increases dose dependently and concentration dependently. Does the intracellular concentration of platinum increase if you combine carboplatin and cisplatin? Second, are the DNA interstrand cross-links induced by platinum increased by the combination of cisplatin and carboplatin?

Dr Kobayashi: I have no data on this.

Dr David R. Newell (University of Newcastle upon Tyne Medical School, Newcastle upon Tyne, UK): Do you have any pharmacokinetic data? I would imagine that unless the glomerular filtration rate was very close for all your patients, administering a fixed dose of carboplatin would give a wide range of AUC values.

Dr Kobayashi: We measured free platinum in clinical use, but carboplatin has a large AUC of free platinum, whereas cisplatin has a little. Thus measuring free platinum by atomic absorption spectrophotometry cannot detect the AUC ratios of cisplatin to carboplatin in clinical practice. We must measure this by HPLC in vitro and in clinical practice.

Dr Atsuya Karato (National Cancer Center, Tokyo, Japan): In your phase I studies did you observe any neurotoxicity or renal toxicity? Did you evaluate rate toxicities?

Dr Kobayashi: Other toxicities, such as renal, neurogenic, and others, are very mild.

Dr Ryuzo Ohno (The Branch Hospital, Nagoya University School of Medicine, Nagoya, Japan): I think your TSE strategy is a good way to administer chemotherapy, but have you ever examined why there is so much variety in the clearance of methotrexate or teniposide?

Dr Relling: Yes. A major focus of our research is aimed at characterizing variability in hepatic metabolism and renal excretion of anticancer drugs. Those are some of the interesting points we have learned from this trial so far—things that you might not pay much attention to. For instance, we found a really dramatic, over 2-fold higher teniposide clearance in children who were treated with anticonvulsants concurrently.

There was no overlap between the clearances of the 2 groups. That is not totally surprising, and phenobarbitone and phenytoin would be expected to increase the clearance of almost any drug that is hepatically metabolized. Even a single dose of pentobarbital, however, which is sometimes given to our pediatric patients before bone marrow procedures or lumbar punctures which are done the day before they receive their pulses, result in enhanced clearance of teniposide. So whenever possible, we are trying to find clinical indicators of how we could try to predict clearance in patients better so that we do not have to measure it every single time. There is a great deal of variability that we have not been able to explain by the methods we have employed so far.

Dr Ohno: You are calculating an administration dose on a per square meter basis. Nowadays the younger Japanese generation is becoming bigger and I believe that when we compare the toxicity of chemotherapeutic drugs to young, very tall children with an older, smaller Japanese generation, the younger generation do not experience as much toxicity when we administer on the per square meter basis. I am not sure whether we are really doing the right thing in administering drugs on the per square meter basis. Have you ever looked at this?

Dr Relling: Are you proposing using a per kilogram basis instead?

Dr Ohno: Not exactly, but you have so many patients. Do you take data from patients of the same height and weight and compare the clearance, and still have such variation?

Dr Relling: Yes, there is always an excellent correlation between either body surface area or weight and unnormalized clearance. There is an R^2 of over 0.9. In children, although it may not be true in adults, body size is an important determinant or covariant of clearance. All of the values that I showed are normalized. We always tend to see more of a correlation in clearance among the pediatric age-group versus age when it is normalized per body weight than per body surface area. I think it is for that reason that dosing per body surface area has perhaps become so standard for adjusting doses.

Professor Hryniuk: Are you concerned at all that the interindividual variation in handling of 6MP and methotrexate may produce events the frequency of which will obscure the reduction in events that you are going to manage with this very sophisticated and I must say very necessary experimental approach?

Dr Relling: Yes, I am very concerned. We are measuring red blood cell 6TGN concentrations as the active metabolite of 6MP, and methotrexate polyglutamates at least 6 times per patient over a 2-year period. We are seeing, especially for the 6TGNs, more variability than has been reported by Dr Lynne Lennard, University Department of Therapeutics, Royal Hallamshire Hospital, Sheffield, UK, in her study of children with acute lymphocytic leukemia. 6TGN exposure could be one of the most important determinants of acute toxicity of the chemotherapy. So yes, I am worried that that is going to obscure the picture.

Professor Hryniuk: On the other hand, you are measuring, so you will know in the end.

Dr Relling: Yes, we will know what it is, but in retrospect it might have been nice to go ahead and adjust 6-mercaptopurine.

Dr Clark: What is the concordance between the patients in whom you have to raise or lower the methotrexate? For how many patients will you change the methotrexate and for how many the teniposide?

Dr Relling: It is totally unrelated. Within the same course, we may have to decrease the cytarabine and double the teniposide.

Dr Yutaka Ariyoshi (Aichi Cancer Center, Nagoya, Japan): Do you measure every time to adjust the variables?

Dr Relling: Yes, we do. It is going to be important to look at how we do this. If we took into account all those things that we suspect affect clearance: for example, if we estimated creatinine clearance for methotrexate, and assessed for low serum albumins and/or high bilirubins for teniposide, and assessed all possible drug interactions, how much intrapatient variability could we account for? We believe that some variability in clearance would remain which we cannot a priori predict. There are definitely cases where we see a 2-fold change in clearance within the same patient from course to course with no clinically evident variable that is changing, but we cannot explain it.

SPECIAL LECTURE

Importance of pharmacokinetics for developing new therapies

Franco Muggia, Kenneth Chan, Anil Tulpule, Anastassios Retzios

University of Southern California School of Medicine and School of Pharmacy, Kenneth Norris Jr Comprehensive Cancer Center, Los Angeles, California, USA

INTRODUCTION

Examples of pharmacokinetics guiding the development of newly introduced anticancer drugs have become commonplace, and are also illustrated by others in this symposium. We shall cite several additional examples whereby optimal treatment strategies are being developed based on a pharmacokinetic rationale or new pharmacological findings. Pharmacokinetic information can be used to develop new methods for clinical dosing (i.e., adaptively controlled), to introduce new schedules of administration (i.e., continuous infusion, circadian-based), to guide towards resolving clinical issues such as the role of dose-intensity, and to establish the rationale for locoregional therapy with drugs. In this overview, we shall describe the impact of pharmacokinetics on such important developments in clinical oncology.

THERAPY WITH ESTABLISHED DRUGS

Fluoropyrimidines

These drugs, originally introduced by Heidelberger in the 1950s are now playing a major role in the treatment of gastrointestinal cancer, and have again become the subject of much laboratory and clinical research as will be briefly summarized.

Biochemical modulation with leucovorin. This subject has been extensively reviewed in several monographs, and the improved clinical performance of 5-fluorouracil (FU) + leucovorin (LV) regimens has been generally accepted. LV has been demonstrated to work through biochemical effects as a precursor of 5,10-methylene tetrahydrofolate on stabilizing the ternary complex of thymidylate synthase, 5-fluorodeoxyuridylate and this folate cofactor. However, much debate continues on the optimal dose and schedules of both the effector (FU) and modulator (LV) drugs, and on whether the dose-intensity of FU can be generally enhanced and yield similarly improved results.

Other biochemical modulation. The use of several other 'modulators' such as hydroxyurea, PALA, and alpha-interferon have been proposed in conjunction with fluoropyrimidines; however, how their actions are mediated is less certain. For example, alpha-interferon may affect the pharmacokinetics of FU (J. Grem, Educational Session, Phase I working group, March, 1991), and the improved effects may therefore merely reflect dose-intensification. Modulation with LV plus other drugs affecting DNA and RNA synthetic pathways is under active investigation.

Continuous infusion schedules. Leichman and coworkers[1], and Lokich and coworkers[2] have employed protracted (>5 day) infusion schedules with the rationale that one may deliver greater amounts of FU than by intermittent doses. The toxicity pattern of FU is rather drastically altered by protracted infusions, with hand-foot syndromes becoming most prominent while lower gastrointestinal toxicities and hematologic toxicities become very infrequent. Although initially, the protracted infusion schedule was not totally driven by a pharmacokinetic rationale, the clinical outcome and pharmacology is highly consistent with pharmacokinetic principles. The short half life and the readily saturable hepatic catabolism favors the use of protracted infusion. Additionally, the protracted infusion may increase the CxT value of the active anabolites which supports the greater efficacy of this regimen. Biochemical modulation with LV in these protracted infusion schedules have been tested by these workers, and the amount of LV to modulate safely a dose of 200 mg/m2/day is much lower (i.e., 20 mg/m2/week) than for briefer schedules. This is consistent with experimental observations from the laboratory of Moran.[3]

Circadian schedules. Diasio and coworkers[4] convincingly demonstrated a circadian rhythm for the catabolism of FU by dihydropyrimidine dehydrogenase. French investigators[5] have devised circadian dose schedules for FU in combination with a platinum analog and reported improved tolerance and striking clinical results. Similarly, American investigators reported activity of 5-fluoro-2'-deoxyuridine (FUdR) against renal cell carcinoma using circadian-based dosing. Questions concerning circadian schedules include the relevance of animal models, the role of normal tissue kinetics, and the applicability to circumstances of differing analogues and modulator drugs. For example, if the buccal mucosa has the highest S-phase during late morning hours; would dosing of LV best be accomplished in late evening? Both laboratory and clinical studies are required to answer these questions.

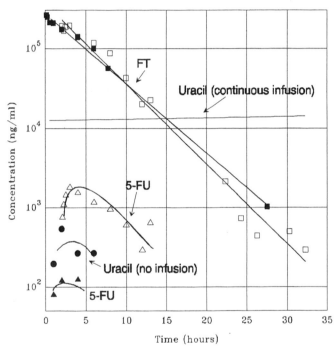

Figure 1: Plasma FT, uracil, and 5-FU levels in the rat. Open symbols denote concentrations under continuous infusion of uracil; closed symbols denote concentrations without uracil infusion.

Pharmacologically-based analogues. UFT (Taiho) has recently undergone clinical testing in the United States, with the purpose of providing an oral form of fluoropyrimidine, an alternative to continuous infusion schedules of FU. The 4:1 ratio of uracil to prodrug FT presumably allows optimal inhibition of FU catabolism and prolongs its CxT. Our preliminary results on an animal model on FT dosing with and without constant infusion of uracil supports this contention (Figure 1). Our initial experience indicates better tolerance with a divided (every 8 h) dose schedule not exceeding 400 mg/m2 daily and some correlation of hematologic toxicity with FU levels[6,7]. Some individual variation in FU AUCs is observed, as has been noted for FU itself. Further testing of UFT with LV as a biochemical modulator appears attractive. Trials employing UFT + LV will be of interest and will address three major variables: 1) dose of UFT, 2) dose of LV, and 3) duration of therapy (length of cycle). The relationship of dose, schedule, and AUC to the toxicities observed promise to provide important information on the development of fluoropyrimidines in general.

Epipodophyllotoxins.

Etoposide's role in cancer treatment is expanding as a result of greater understanding of its mechanisms of action, and of its interaction with other drugs, coupled with the achievement of improved clinical outcome from safe dose-intensification[8] and new chronic dosing schedules[9]. Similarly expanded applications are taking place with teniposide[10], and the pharmacologic differences between the two analogues may provide additional clues as to the selectivity of these compounds.

Mechanism of action and interaction with other drugs. Study of the effects of etoposide on topoisomerase II-directed DNA cleavage has stimulated hypotheses concerning drug resistance and drug synergy[11]. These must be taken into account when considering the pharmacologically-based exploration of dose intensity and dose scheduling.

Dose-intensity. Ratain and coworkers[8] have utilized pharmacologic information to devise an individually safe 72-hour dose of etoposide. In their initial study they demonstrated that the extent of dose-limiting leukopenia achieved is a function of the pretreatment white cell count, the serum albumin, the performance status, and the bone marrow function as assessed from prior transfusion needs. They have subsequently shown in a randomized study of fixed versus individualized dosing, that the latter allowed a 22% dose increase with a safe decrease in white cell count while the variability of the nadir count was lessened. Evans and coworkers[10] have utilized an analogous adaptive controlled dosing with teniposide in children with acute leukemia. In an initial study they had demonstrated that doses of teniposide ranging from 100 to 250 mg/m2/day for 3 days gave progressively higher concentration of steady state, but the individual variability was substantial. When they analyzed their data in terms of toxic events and responses there was no clear relationship to dose given, but a steep relationship appeared with AUCs. A trial is ongoing at St Jude Children's Hospital randomizing conventional versus Bayesian dose-adjusted regimens of teniposide plus cytarabine. Based on measurements on day 1, in the non-fixed arm, doses are adjusted on day 3 and on a subsequent cycle. From this experience, the evolution of drug regimens than seek to define the maximum tolerated systemic exposure, beyond what appears to be the maximum tolerated dose (MTD) is likely. Such evolution is desirable when the response clearly relates to AUC.

Chronic scheduling. Preclinical studies have suggested a remarkable schedule dependence of teniposide and etoposide activity in L1210 leukemia[12]. Only recently have protracted schedules of etoposide received attention[9], and some of the results achieved suggest that antitumor activity may bear a relationship to days above a certain threshold concentration (1 mcg/ml) whereas dose-limiting leukopenia relates to AUC. Clark and Slevin[13] in this volume and in prior reports provide evidence for a gain in therapeutic index from chronic dosing schedules of etoposide in small cell lung cancer. Schedules that have been explored include the 5 and 8 day infusion schedules, and oral administration of daily and twice daily etoposide for 14 days, and daily drug for 21 days. A number of drug combination studies have been launched following on the antitumor activity noted with etoposide alone in these schedules.

THERAPY WITH INVESTIGATIONAL DRUGS
New platinum analogues

Cisplatin and carboplatin are both in widespread use in cancer treatment. The clinical development of carboplatin lived up to the promise of a 'gentler' platinum while demonstrating equivalent antitumor activity, at least against ovarian cancer. It relative absence of non-hematologic toxicity has allowed greater focus on dose-intensity issues. Because of carboplatin's dose-limiting thrombocytopenia, however, cisplatin may prove to be the preferred component[14] in some combinations regimens. The more predictable pharmacologic behaviour of carboplatin than cisplatin has provided correlations between AUCs and toxicity as well as response. Identification of platinum-DNA adducts in cells may provide a pharmacodynamic expression of drug action.

Rationale for new analogues. The second and third generation platinum analogues were introduced in an effort to decrease the non-hematologic toxicities of cisplatin. More recently, Harrap and colleagues[15] have continued extensive structure-activity relationships to define drugs

307

with a different spectrum of toxicity, that are not cross-resistant with cisplatin or carboplatin, and that are orally active. In preclinical studies, some of these analogues have a striking improvement in therapeutic index. At present, several derivatives by other groups have undergone clinical testing and have given indications of a shift in dose-limiting toxicities towards leukopenia. In addition, the prospects of overcoming cisplatin resistance will be tested as clinical trials with ormaplatin (tetraplatin) proceed beyond Phase I. This water soluble Pt(IV) analogue presumably delivers an intracellular platinum species that is converted to the active Pt(II) species *in vivo*. As our knowledge of the mechanisms involved in acquired and intrinsic resistance to cisplatin expands, the clinical applications of these compounds may be further enhanced. In addition, the identification of platinum-induced DNA damage recognition proteins may have a great impact in future drug development.

Dose-intensity issues. Egorin and colleagues[16] have reviewed data on response and toxicity of patients with ovarian cancer enrolled in carboplatin trials. Since carboplatin's AUC is primarily related to its renal clearance, by knowing a patient's GFR one could calculate the AUC of carboplatin that was achieved. In turn, it was possible to correlate outcome with AUCs. The degree of thrombocytopenia increased linearly with the AUC whereas response in patients with ovarian cancer increased only to an AUC of 7 or 8 mcg.h/ml, up to a plateau varying from 25 to over 50% in accordance with patient characteristics. For example, an untreated patient with good performance status would have a higher probability of a response 'maxima' than a previously treated patient, with poorer performance status. These concepts will aid in the development of future platinum analogues.

Pharmacodynamics of platinum-DNA adducts. Immunocytochemical and chemical methods permit the identification of platinum-DNA adducts in tissues following treatment with cisplatin and carboplatin. We have been involved in collaborative studies to identify patterns of such adduct formation in leukocytes and in buccal cells following treatment with carboplatin on day 1 and cisplatin on day 3. These investigations have suggested a relationship of signal intensity by immunocytochemistry with the calculated AUC of carboplatin, and of quantitation of platinum-DNA adducts 24 h after carboplatin with probability of response. In addition, we have established a contribution to these adducts by cisplatin at 50, 75, and 100 mg/m2. Cisplatin contributed an average of 5 times the amount of adducts compared to carboplatin on a weight equivalence basis, but the range was quite wide indicating that a number of factors modify adduct formation following cisplatin, as for example, serum albumin[17,18]. Although drugs such as ormaplatin may lead to a different array of inter- and intrastrand platinum-DNA adducts, similar studies as these may shed light on the selectivity of these new compounds.

Camptothecin analogues

Although sodium camptothecin was introduced into clinical study by the National Cancer Institute in 1969, and preliminary investigations on its unique mechanism of action were done shortly after, new clinical studies with this family of drugs are very recent. Recent developments have followed the recognition of the role of topoisomerase I in mediating cytotoxicity, the striking efficacy of camptothecin analogues against colon cancer in nude mice [11].

Mechanism of action. Horwitz and colleagues[19] first identified the need for the closed lactone form for activity. Such observation possibly explained some of the disappointing results with the sodium salt, and also the cystitis resulting from excretion of the drug in an active form in acidic urine. Studies of the effects of topoisomerases on DNA eventually identified camptothecin as a topoisomerase I-directed drug, and further studies worked out structural requirements for interaction with this enzyme. Additional studies promise to identify mechanisms of drug resistance, and exploitable relationships between topoisomerase I and II-directed drugs.

Analogue development. Clinical studies have been initiated with CPT-11, a camptothecin analogue, in Japan, and now in the United States, and topotecan in the United States and Europe.

308

Pharmacologic studies with topotecan have focused on the fate of the lactone form versus the inactive carboxylate upon administration. Since CPT-11 is a prodrug of the active topoisomerase I-directed drug[20], pharmacokinetic assessments must take into consideration the fate of both the parent compound and its active metabolite. Introduction of other analogues such as 9-amino camptothecin is based on activity against human colon cancer xenografts; an activity that is also striking with the parent compound[11]. Clinical activity has been noted in a number of these trials presented at the 1991 American Society of Clinical Oncology meetings.

Scheduling. Prominent hematologic and gastrointestinal toxicities, as well as antitumor effects may be schedule dependent and be related to a threshold concentration. In the original studies of sodium camptothecin, high intermittent doses appeared more advantageous than daily x 5 schedules[21]; and Gottlieb[22] was able to escalate the dose severalfold to individual tolerance on an every two week basis. However, with administration of the active forms of the drug, it is possible that prolonged infusion above a certain threshold might be cytotoxic to tumors containing high levels of topoisomerase I while not leading to dose-limiting toxicities. If so, as in the case of etoposide, a protracted schedule of administration might prove advantageous. Modelling to minimize marrow and other target tissue damage, while maximizing tumor destruction may prove helpful and must be tested[23].

LOCOREGIONAL THERAPY
Rationale for intraperitoneal therapy

Depth of penetration of drugs administered via the intraperitoneal (IP) route, and the relationship of the tumor to the peritoneal surfaces are the factors that determine the 'therapeutic advantage' for the IP route over systemic administration of drugs. The depth of penetration is a function of the IP concentration that is achieved, and other inadequately studied factors. Since most studies have used surgical endpoints to assess response, the value of IP drug administration remains largely anecdotal[24]. Clinical trials are ongoing that will test what benefit, if any, results from IP cisplatin in patients with optimally resected ovarian cancer. We have performed sequential trials of IP carboplatin alone, and in combination with etoposide. We are now testing carboplatin with deep hyperthermia to overcome drug resistance and to facilitate uptake of platinum compounds[25]. In gastrointestinal cancer, the only comparative trial employed IP versus IV FU, and no difference was noted in survival, even though an effect was noted on peritoneal recurrence rates[26]. We have been developing the rationale for IP FUdR and modulators for both gastrointestinal and ovarian cancers, and more recently for IP suramin. The issues involved in the evaluation of such therapies are applicable to those of other locoregionally directed drugs.

IP fluoropyrimidines and modulation. FUdR has yielded a 2 to 3 log advantage in IP over plasma AUCs[27]. Its enhanced potency and greater modulatory capacity with LV relative to FU, make it an attractive drug via this route. Study #8835 by the Southwest Oncology Group in ovarian cancer, confirms the tolerance of the 3 g x 3 day schedule of FUdR. In addition, this cooperative group trial has provided information on the prognostic value of pretreatment CA-125 while also raising questions as to the optimal endpoints by which to assess efficacy in such studies[28]. Presently, definition of response remains elusive, but more rigorous definitions of time to failure as surrogate endpoints to survival has emerged: a rise in CA-125 is an indicator of 'undeterminate' progression (after therapy), while both extra- and intraperitoneal recurrences are evidence for progression during or after treatment.

Modulation with 6(R,S)-leucovorin and FUdR at the dose given above has been tested in 15 patients, with no apparent increase in toxicity[29]. Current studies are exploring 6(S)-leucovorin, and also combinations of LV with FUdR and cisplatin IP in ovarian cancers. Serial pharmacokinetic studies have provided indications of changes in peritoneal clearance for both FUdR and LV in some patients (Figure 2). This suggests that the peritoneum may be altered during treatment resulting in

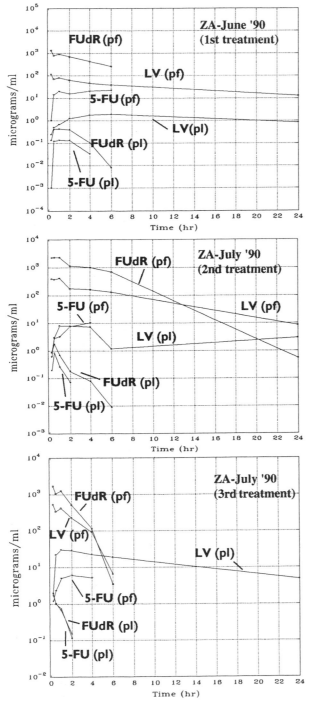

Figure 2: Pharmacokinetic profiles of FUdR, leucovorin and 5-FU following repeated FUdR/leucovorin IP treatment. The FUdR dose remained constant at 3 g but leucovorin dose was increased from 160 mg for the first treatment to 320 mg for the second and 640 mg for the third treatment.

altered pharmacology. The circumstances leading to such an occurrence must be defined while continuing to explore the role of IP therapy in ovarian and in gastric cancer.

IP carboplatin. Cisplatin has been shown to have significant pharmacologic advantages when given IP to patients with ovarian cancer and minimal residual disease. This pharmacologic advantage can be predicted by the IP pharmacokinetic model of Dedrick et al[30]. With the subjectively better tolerated analogue, carboplatin, its IP administration has also given rise to some encouraging clinical results, although conclusive evidence of superiority over systemic treatment is lacking. With Dr. Michael Sapozink (Radiation Oncology) we have been studying the pharmacokinetic behavior of IP carboplatin when given alone, and when combined with hyperthermia. Interest in hyperthermia combined with platinum compounds is derived from the enhanced penetrance of both cisplatin and carboplatin into experimental tumors that may be shown when temperatures of 40' and 42'C are achieved[25]. Representative pharmacokinetic profiles are shown in Figure 3. These preliminary pharmacologic data indicated a more rapid initial disappearance from the peritoneal fluid suggesting either its rapid

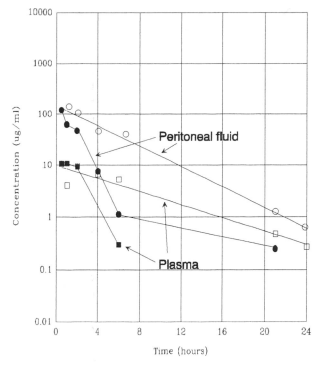

Figure 3: Plasma and peritoneal levels of ultrafiltrable platinum following IP carboplatin treatment with and without hyperthermia. Open symbols denote levels without hyperthermia, closed symbols indicate levels with hyperthermia.

distribution or degradation. The subsequent elimination, however, was less affected. Additional study is needed to verify the suggestion that treatment with hyperthermia (radiofrequency heating to 42'C for 30 min) alters carboplatin pharmacokinetics. Enhanced IP carboplatin clearance relative to other studies in the literature may also reflect altered pharmacokinetics from preceding exposure to IP drugs.

ACKNOWLEDGEMENTS

This work was supported in part by R01-CA50412-01A1 and by Cancer Center Core Grants from the National Cancer Institute, NIH, USPHS and by an unrestricted institutional grant from the Bristol Myers Squibb Foundation.

REFERENCES

1. Leichman CG, Leichman L, Spears CG, Rosen P, Muggia FM, Jeffers S, Waugh W (1989) A dose-ranging study of leucovorin plus low-dose continuous infusion 5-fluorouracil in gastrointestinal cancers. Cancer Chemother Pharmacol 26:57-61.

2. Lokich J, Anderson N, Bern M, Coco F, Zipoli T, Moore C, Gonsalves L (1991) Dual modulation of 5-fluorouracil using leucovorin and hydroxyurea. Cancer 68:744-746

3. Moran RG, Scanlon KL (1991) Schedule dependent enhancement of cytotoxicity of fluoropyrimidines to human carcinoma cells in the presence of folinic acid. Cancer Res 51:4618-4623.

4. Harris BE, Song R, Soong S-J, Diasio RB (1990) Relationship between dihydropyrimidine dehydrogenase activity and 5-fluorouracil levels with evidence of circadian variation of enzyme activity and plasma drug levels in cancer patients receiving 5-fluorouracil by protracted continuous infusion. Cancer Res 50:197-201.

5.   Levi F, Misset JL, Brienza S, Adam R, Kunstlinger F, Metzger G, Le Couturier S, Gastiaburu J, Bismuth H (1991) Circadian-rhythm modulated venous chemotherapy against metastatic colorectal cancer: efficcacy of pump delivered 5-fluorouracil, folinic acid and oxaliplatin. Proc ASCO 10:155

6.   Spicer D, Muggia F, Tulpule A, Chan K, Leichman G, Spears P, Jeffers S (1991) Phase I circadian dosing of daily oral uracil (U) plus 1-(tetrahydro-2-furanyl)-5-fluorouracil (FT) with leucovorin (LV). Proc ASCO 10:118 (Abstract # 342)

7.   Tulpule A, Chan K, Muggia FM, Spears CP, Spicer D, Jeffers S (1991) Uracil (U) + Ftorafur (FT): pharmacokinetic profile of an orally active 5-fluorouracil (FU) prodrug. Clin Res 29:374A

8.   Ratain MJ, Mick R, Schilsky RL, Vogelzng NJ, Berezin F (1991) Pharmacologically based dosing of etoposide: a means of safely increasing dose intensity. J Clin Oncol 9:1480-1486

9.   Greco FA, Johnson DH, Hainsworth JD (1991) Chronic oral etoposide Cancer 67:303-309

10.   Evans WE, Rodman JH, Petros WP, Madden T, Crom WR, Relling MV, Rivera GK, Kalwinsky DK, Crist WM (1990) Individualized doses of chemotherapy for children with acute lymphocytic leukemia (ALL). Proc ASCO 9:69

11.   Potmesil M, Kohn KW (Eds, 1991) DNA topoisomerases in cancer. Oxford University Press, New York, pp.331

        Rozencweig M, Von Hoff HH, Henney JE, Muggia FM (1977) VM-26 and VP 16-213: a ⅄parative analysis. Cancer 40:34-342.

13.   Clark PI, Slevin ML (1987) The clinical pharmacology of etoposide and teniposide. Clin Pharmacokinet 12:223-252.

14.   Muggia FM (1989) Overview of carboplatin: replacing, complementing and extending the therapeutic horizons of cisplatin. Sem Oncol 16(suppl 5):7-13.

.15.   Abstracts of the Sixth International Symposium on Platinum and Other Metal Coordination Compounds in Cancer Chemotherapy (1991) Cancer Center, University of California, San Diego, January 23-26.

16.   Egorin MJ, Van Echo DA, Tipping SJ, et al (1984) Pharmacokinetics and dose reduction of cis-diammine (1,1-cyclobutanedicarboxylato) platinum in patients with impaired renal function. Cancer Res 44:5432-5438.

17.   Parker RJ, Gill I, Tarone R, Vionnet JA, Grunberg S, Muggia FM, Reed E (1991) Platinum-DNA damage in leukocyte DNA of patients receiving carboplatin and cisplatin chemotherapy, measured by atomic absorption spectrometry. Carcinogenesis 12:1253-1258

18.   Gill I, Muggia FM, Terheggen PMAB et al (1991). Dose-escalation study of carboplatin (day 1) and cisplatin (day 3): tolerance and relation to leukocyte and buccal cell platinum-DNA adducts. Ann Oncol 2:115-121.

19.   Horwitz MS, Horwitz SB (1971) Intracellular degradation of HeLa and adenovirus type 2 DNA induced by camptothecin. Biochem Biophys Res Commun 45z;723.

20.   Kawato Y, Aonuma M, Hirota Y, Kuga H, Sato K (1991). Intracellular roles of SN-38, a metabolite of the camptothecin derivative CPT-11, in the antitumor effect of CPT-11. Cancer Res 51:4187-4191.

21.   Muggia FM, Creaven PJ, Hansen HH, Cohen MH, Selawry OS (1972). Phase I clinical trial of weekly and daily treatment with camptothecin (NSC-100880): correlation with preclinical studies. Cancer Chemotherap Rep 56:95-101.

22.   Gottlieb JA, Luce JK (1972). Treatment of malignant melanoma with camptothecin (NSC-100880). Cancer Chhemotherap Rep 56:103-105.

23.   Agur Z (1986) The effect of drug schedule on responsiveness to chemotherapy. Ann NY Acad Sci 504:274

24.   Muggia FM, Alberts DS (1991) Intraperitoneal therapy in ovarian cancer: time's not up. J Clin Oncol 9:1510.

25.   Los G, Sminia P, Wondergem J, et al (1991) Optimization of intraperitoneal chemotherapy with regional hyperthermia. Eur J Cancer 27:706-713.

26.   Sugarbaker PH, Gianola FJ, Speyer JC, et al (1985) Prospective randomized trial of intravenous versus intraperitoneal 5-fluorouracil in patients with advanced primary colon or rectal cancer. Surgery 98:414-421.

27.   Muggia FM, Chan KK, Russell C (1991) Phase I and pharmacologic study of intraperitoneal 5-fluoro-2'-deoxyuridine. Cancer Chemother Pharmacol 28:241-250.

28.   Truesdel C, Muggia FM, Alberts DS, Liu PY, O'Sullivan J, Wallace D (1991) CA-125: a predictor of outcome from intraperitoneal therapy in Southwest Oncology Group study 8835. Proc ASCO 10:195

29.   Muggia FM, Chan K, Tulpule A, Jeffers S, Retzios A (1991) Intraperitoneal floxuridine and (d-l) leucovorin: rationale and results of pharmacologic studies. Clin Res 39:375A.

30.   Los G, McVie JG (1990) Experimental and clinical status of intraperitoneal chemotherapy. Eur J Cancer 26:755-762.

Discussion

Dr Kunihiko Kobayashi (Nippon Medical School, Tokyo, Japan): My in vitro data indicate that, when cisplatin and carboplatin are given in combination, a better effect is achieved with higher cisplatin doses. We planned our phase I study based on this. Did you use several doses in your study and what type of response, ie, antitumor effect, did you obtain with those doses?

Professor Muggia: The question relates to the responses seen in our phase I trial. We actually have observed responses with most of the dose levels studied, but of course this was a very heterogeneous population of patients with a variety of tumors. We have 7 responses scattered throughout many of the dose levels. So I do not think we can conclude anything about the preference for any one dose combination over the other.

Dr Kobayashi: What type of dosage schedule do you have in mind? Which drug do you give first, cisplatin or carboplatin, and at what intervals?

Professor Muggia: We gave the carboplatin on the 1st day and then, because we were particularly interested in studying the adduct formation and the different contributions of the 2 platinums, cisplatin was administered 2 days later. So it is day 1, day 3 treatment. I do not know that it pertains necessarily to your experimental conditions, but I was interested to learn that you had optimal dosing in terms of synergy.

CLOSING REMARKS

Closing remarks

Makoto Ogawa*

Japanese Foundation for Cancer Research, Tokyo, Japan
Current address: Aichi Cancer Center, Nagoya, Japan

This symposium began with a keynote address by Dr Robert C. Bast, Jr, who reviewed several important issues, including abnormalities of autocrine growth related to oncogenes and suppressor genes in relation to the biological characteristics of ovarian and breast cancer. He also discussed strategies by which this knowledge could be utilized in the treatment of both types of tumor.

Session 1 covered the biology of tumor progression and regulation, a rapidly expanding research area. Oncologists now recognize that cancer is related to abnormalities of genes. Of these, the RB and p53 genes were reviewed during this session. Dr Wen-Hwa Lee reported that inactivation of the RB gene is observed not only in retinoblastoma, but also in many other cancers including osteosarcoma, small cell lung cancer, bladder cancer, and prostatic cancer. Dr David P. Lane and Dr Takashi Takahashi reported their results on mutation of the p53 gene, which is frequently found in cases of gastric, lung, colon, and other malignant tumors. After examination of polyclonal and monoclonal antibodies against the p53 gene protein, about 60% of human cancers demonstrated a high level of this protein. The presence of this mutant protein may therefore represent a prognostic factor. Dr Lee also suggested that new antitumor agents that can destroy the protein might be developed as a new group of drugs.

Dr Riccardo Dalla-Favera reported on the role of c-*myc* oncogene activation in B cell malignancies and suggested that specific interactions may exist between c-*myc* and P53.

Variations between protein C kinase including products of c-*erb*B-2, *fyn*, and *lyn* and tumorigenesis were presented by Dr Tadashi Yamamoto, who suggested that c-*erb*B-2 gene products are involved in the loss of signal transduction.

The second subject in session 1 was drug resistance. Dr Helen S.L. Chan demonstrated that P glycoprotein expression at diagnosis has a profound impact on treatment outcome, including response rate, relapse-free survival, and survival in pediatric tumors. Dr Michihiko Kawano presented his results on synthetic isoprenoid and dihydropyridine; both reversed drug resistance. He also presented data on the MDR gene promoters.

The topic of the final session on the first day was dose intensity. Professor William M. Hryniuk demonstrated that dose intensity correlated well with treatment outcome in a retrospective analysis of single-agent efficacy or combination chemotherapy against breast, lung, ovarian, and other tumors. Results so far from prospective, randomized studies to test dose intensity have been controversial. Dr Martin E. Blackstein reported that dose escalation of epirubicin in non-small cell lung cancer appears useful

317

in the treatment of this disease. Dr Masaaki Kawahara studied dose intensity employing a weekly regimen with G-CSF (figrastim) support in small cell and non-small cell lung cancer. Response rates obtained were higher in the G-CSF arm, but survival gain appears to be minimal. Although dose intensity is still under investigation, the introduction of G-CSF to treatment regimens could be incorporated in future study designs to test these hypotheses.

Session 3 on the second day began with a presentation by Dr H. Rodney Withers on the optimal delivery of radiotherapy and optimal duration of chemotherapy in adjuvant and neoadjuvant settings. He suggested that dose intensity is important in both radiotherapy and chemotherapy. The subsequent session covered neoadjuvant chemotherapy for lung cancer. Although concurrent use of chemotherapy and radiotherapy yields high response rates, toxicity is also increased. Ways of reducing toxicity are thus necessary. Dr Karin V. Mattson reported the results of an interesting combination of interferons and cytotoxic drugs in lung cancer based upon preclinical evidence. Nearly all studies on the efficacy of adjuvant chemotherapy after curative operation for non-small cell lung cancer have shown negative results, and therefore the efficacy of neoadjuvant chemotherapy is being investigated currently. Dr Nael Martini presented promising results from a pilot study employing neoadjuvant chemotherapy with 2–3 cycles of MVP. Dr Nobuyuki Hara suggested that chemoradiotherapy before operation may improve both response rate and survival duration. However, both speakers stressed that prospective, randomized trials are necessary to confirm these results.

In session 5, clinical trials based on pharmacology were presented. Three speakers, Drs Duncan I. Jodrell, Yasutsuna Sasaki, and David R. Newell, discussed the role of pharmacokinetics and pharmacodynamics extensively. It appears that molecular pharmacology techniques, such as utilizing DNA adducts, will be employed in this field in the near future.

Studies relating to the optimal dose and schedule in phase II trials were reported in the second part of the session. Dr Peter I. Clark demonstrated that the daily, chronic, oral administration of etoposide is effective in treating small cell lung cancer. He explained that this effect is due to prolonged maintenance of plasma levels of the minimal effective dose of etoposide.

Dr Franco M. Muggia summarized his results obtained in biochemical modulation, including leucovorin plus 5FU, and UFT, intraperitoneal use of FUDR plus leucovorin, intraperitoneal carboplatin plus cisplatin, and current protocols using intraperitoneal carboplatin plus hyperthermia, and stressed the pharmacokinetic advantage of intraperitoneal platinum compounds.

On behalf of the Organizing Committee, I would like to thank all the speakers for excellent presentations, and all those who participated in this symposium. I would also like to thank Bristol-Myers Squibb for their continued generous support of this symposium.

AUTHOR INDEX

Author index